Endovascular Therapies

Current Evidence

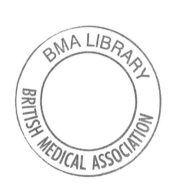

Edited by

Michael G Wyatt &

Anthony F Watkinson

tfm Publishing Limited
Castle Hill Barns
Harley
Shrewsbury
SY5 6LX
UK

Tel: +44 (0)1952 510061
Fax: +44 (0)1952 510192
E-mail: nikki@tfmpublishing.com
Web site: www.tfmpublishing.com

Design: Nikki Bramhill, tfm publishing Ltd.
Typesetting: Nikki Bramhill, tfm publishing Ltd.
Cover image: Courtesy of Robert Morgan

First Edition   © June 2006

ISBN 1 903378 46 X

Printed by Gutenberg Press Ltd., Gudja Road, Tarxien, PLA 19, Malta.

Tel: +356 21897037; Fax: +356 21800069.

Contents

PART V: VENOUS DISEASE

PART VI: MISCELLANEOUS

Contributors

Mo Adiseshiah MA MS FRCS FRCP Consultant Vascular & Endovascular Surgeon, University College Hospital, London, UK

Sherif Awad MB MRCS Senior House Officer in Surgery, Leicester Royal Infirmary, Leicester, UK

Jonathan D Beard ChM MEd FRCS Consultant Vascular Surgeon, Sheffield Vascular Institute, The Northern General Hospital, Sheffield, UK

Viktor Berczi MD PhD Endovascular Fellow, Sheffield Vascular Institute, The Northern General Hospital, Sheffield, UK

Raj Bhat MS FRCS FRCR Specialist Registrar in Radiology, Ninewells Hospital, Dundee, UK

Colin Bicknell MD MRCS Specialist Registrar, North West Thames, St. Mary's Hospital, London, UK

Andrew W Bradbury BSc MD MBA FRCS (Ed) Professor of Vascular Surgery, Birmingham University Department of Vascular Surgery, Heart of England NHS Foundation Trust, Birmingham, UK

John Brennan MD FRCS Consultant Vascular Surgeon, Royal Liverpool University Hospital, Liverpool, UK

Marcus Brooks MA MD FRCS (Gen Surg) Specialist Registrar, St. George's Vascular Institute, St. George's Hospital, London, UK

Sam Chakraverty MA MRCP FRCR Consultant Radiologist, Ninewells Hospital, Dundee, UK

Nick Chalmers FRCR Consultant Vascular Radiologist, Manchester Royal Infirmary, Manchester, UK

Nick Cheshire MD FRCS Professor of Vascular Surgery, St. Mary's Hospital, London, UK

Siew Chng MD Clinical Surgical Fellow, Leicester Royal Infirmary, Leicester, UK

Trevor J Cleveland FRCS FRCR Consultant Vascular Radiologist, Sheffield Vascular Institute, The Northern General Hospital, Sheffield, UK

Philip Coleridge Smith DM FRCS Reader in Surgery, UCL Medical School, London, UK

Robert K Fisher MD FRCS Endovascular Fellow, Northern Vascular Centre, Freeman Hospital, Newcastle upon Tyne, UK

Peter Gaines FRCP FRCR Consultant Vascular Radiologist, Sheffield Vascular Institute, The Northern General Hospital, Sheffield, UK

Ivancarmine Gambardella MD BVS Clinical Fellow in Vascular Surgery, Royal Liverpool University Hospital, Liverpool, UK

Ian Gillespie MB ChB DMRD FRCSE FRCR Consultant Vascular Radiologist, Edinburgh Royal Infirmary, Edinburgh, Scotland

Geoffrey Gilling-Smith MS FRCS Consultant Vascular Surgeon, Royal Liverpool University Hospital, Liverpool, UK

Michael J Gough ChM FRCS Consultant Vascular Surgeon, The General Infirmary at Leeds, Leeds, UK

Derek A Gould MB ChB FRCP FRCR Consultant Interventional Radiologist, Royal Liverpool University Hospital, Liverpool, UK

Mo Hamady MB ChB FRCR Consultant, Interventional Radiology, St. Mary's Hospital, London, UK

Ralph W Jackson MB BS MRCP FRCR Consultant Vascular and Interventional Radiologist, Northern Vascular Centre, Freeman Hospital, Newcastle upon Tyne, UK

Keith G Jones MS FRCS Consultant Vascular Surgeon, King's College Hospital, London, UK

David Kessel MA MRCP FRCR Consultant Vascular Radiologist, Leeds Teaching Hospitals NHS Trust, St. James's University Hospital, Leeds, UK

Bernard Lee FRCS Consultant Vascular Surgeon, Belfast City Hospital, Belfast, Ireland

Tim Lees MB ChB FRCS MD Consultant Vascular Surgeon, Northern Vascular Centre, Freeman Hospital, Newcastle upon Tyne, UK

William Loan FRCR Consultant Radiologist, Belfast City Hospital, Belfast, Ireland

Ian Loftus BSc MB ChB FRCS MD Consultant Vascular Surgeon, St. George's Vascular Institute, St. George's Hospital, London, UK

Sumaira Macdonald MB ChB (Comm.) MRCP FRCR PhD Consultant Vascular Radiologist & Honorary Clinical Senior Lecturer, Freeman Hospital, Newcastle upon Tyne, UK

James E McCaslin MB BS MRCS (Eng) Vascular Research Fellow, Queen Elizabeth Hospital, Gateshead, UK

Richard G McWilliams FRCS FRCR Consultant Interventional Radiologist, Royal Liverpool University Hospital, Liverpool, UK

Robert Morgan MRCP FRCR Consultant Radiologist, St. George's Vascular Institute, St. George's Hospital, London, UK

Graham Munneke MRCP FRCR Clinical Fellow, Interventional Radiology, St. George's Vascular Institute, St. George's Hospital, London, UK

Micheal Murphy FRCSI FRCR Consultant Interventional Radiologist, Royal Liverpool University Hospital, Liverpool, UK

A Ross Naylor MD FRCS Professor of Vascular Surgery, Leicester Royal Infirmary, Leicester, UK

Tony Nicholson MSc FRCR Consultant Vascular Radiologist, Leeds Teaching Hospitals NHS Trust, The General Infirmary at Leeds, Leeds, UK

Andrew Platts FRCS FRCR Consultant Radiologist, Royal Free Hospital, London, UK

Janet T Powell MD PhD FRCPath Professor, Section of Vascular Surgery, Imperial College at Charing Cross, London, UK

John Rose FRCP FRCR Consultant Interventional Radiologist, Northern Vascular Centre, Freeman Hospital, Newcastle upon Tyne, UK

Chee V Soong MD FRCS Consultant Vascular Surgeon, Belfast City Hospital, Belfast, Ireland

Sriram Subramonia MB BS MS FRCS Specialist Registrar, General Surgery, Grantham and District Hospital, Grantham, UK

David Thompson FRCR Specialist Registrar in Radiology, Manchester Royal Infirmary, Manchester, UK

Matt Thompson MD FRCS Professor of Vascular Surgery, St. George's Vascular Institute, St. George's Hospital, London, UK

Anthony F Watkinson, BSc MSc (Oxon) FRCS FRCR Honorary Professor of Radiology, The Peninsula Medical School and Consultant Radiologist, The Royal Devon and Exeter Hospital, Exeter, UK

Nick Woodward MRCP FRCR Specialist Registrar, Radiology, Royal Free Hospital, London, UK

Michael G Wyatt, MSc MD FRCS Consultant Vascular Surgeon, Northern Vascular Centre, Freeman Hospital, Newcastle upon Tyne, UK

Foreword

Since its inception towards the end of the last millennium, minimally invasive therapy has undergone a revolution in the number of techniques, which has been fuelled by the enthusiasm of interventionists and their patients. These techniques are now practised by a wide range of physicians and the range of procedures encompasses almost the whole sphere of medicine.

Endovascular techniques are undergoing constant evolution and refinement. The indications for treatment are subject to regular evaluation, as a result of new device designs and publications reporting the outcomes of these relatively new minimally invasive procedures. Consequently, from these developments it is very useful to review the status of endovascular procedures on a regular basis. This tome is a successor to the book *Endovascular Intervention: Current Controversies*, which was published in 2004. This new book aims to provide information on developments in this field since that time.

Among the subjects under discussion in this book are chapters on the implications of the results of the EVAR and DREAM trials, which evaluated endovascular aneurysm repair, new developments in abdominal aneurysm repair such as fenestrated stents, the current designs of thoracic endografts including their advantages and drawbacks, and the new hybrid treatments for patients with thoraco-abdominal aortic aneurysms.

This book will be of interest to anybody who is involved in the treatment of patients by endovascular procedures. These will include interventional radiologists, vascular surgeons, cardiologists, angiologists, trainee interventionists, radiographic technologists, and nurses.

We would like to congratulate the authors of the chapters and the Editors, Mike Wyatt and Tony Watkinson, who have worked hard to produce a textbook in a timely manner which is up-to-date and reflects the current state of the art of endovascular therapy. Finally, we would like to thank Nikki Bramhill of tfm Publishing Limited who has been of great help in facilitating the publication of this book in a relatively short time.

Robert Morgan and Matt Thompson
St. George's Hospital, London, June 2006

Chapter 1

Aortic stent grafts: current availability and applicability

John Brennan MD FRCS, Consultant Vascular Surgeon

Ivancarmine Gambardella MD BVS, Clinical Fellow in Vascular Surgery

Royal Liverpool University Hospital, Liverpool, UK

Introduction

Endovascular aneurysm repair (EVAR) is now firmly established as a valid treatment option for the management of infrarenal abdominal aortic aneurysms (AAA). While some sceptics remain to be convinced, increasing numbers of specialists involved in the management of AAA recognise this fact. Perhaps of even more significance is the fact that well informed patients will wish to consider EVAR as a potential management option when discussing intervention for their aneurysm. The end result of this is that there will inevitably be a considerable increase in the number of EVAR procedures being performed in the UK over the next few years. In the short term, the majority of these procedures will continue to be performed in centres which have built up a large experience over the last decade or so, but it is inevitable that new centres will develop the knowledge and skills to start their own programmes in order to cope with the increasing demand. With this in mind it is timely to consider the level to which aortic stent grafting has evolved in terms of determining patient suitability for EVAR, and then considering the options in terms of currently available stent grafts.

This chapter will be restricted to endovascular repair of infrarenal AAA in the elective setting.

Indication for intervention

In current UK practice, the indications for intervention in AAA remain unchanged and are the same whether one is considering conventional open repair or EVAR. For the overwhelming majority, with an asymptomatic aneurysm, intervention is considered when maximal aneurysm diameter reaches 5.5cm. It is our practice to routinely assess all patients whose aneurysm is deemed to warrant intervention, to determine their potential suitability for EVAR. If an endovascular approach is feasible, this then forms part of the discussion with the patient over potential treatment options.

The decision to intervene must also take into account an assessment of the patients' fitness, and again this remains true for both options. The potential for reducing operative risk by early intervention with open repair in aneurysms smaller than 5.5cm failed to show any advantage [1] and in the UK, practice will continue to advocate surveillance for small aneurysms, even with EVAR being more widely available.

The other principal grounds for considering intervention are an aneurysm which becomes symptomatic and one which demonstrates rapid expansion over a short period, usually >1cm in six months.

One relatively strong indication for EVAR over open repair is the synchronous presentation of a large AAA and a potentially curable malignancy. Exclusion of the aneurysm with a stent graft means that the malignancy can be tackled on its merits with minimal delay due to the much shorter postoperative recovery associated with EVAR.

Anatomical suitability for EVAR

When EVAR was first introduced, the anatomical selection criteria were fairly conservative, with publications indicating that only 20% of cases were considered suitable. With increasing experience, the proportion of cases deemed suitable has increased considerably, due to an inevitable relaxing of the original criteria along with rapid development of stent graft technology [2, 3]. In the early days, aortic morphology was assessed with a combination of axial CT scanning and conventional aortography, but this approach has now been superceded by multislice CT analysed at a workstation [4]. It is eminently feasible that, with appropriate training, any clinician with an interest in EVAR can rapidly become proficient at image analysis on a workstation in order to determine whether a given case is suitable for an endovascular approach.

For practical purposes, the overwhelming majority of elective EVAR procedures involve delivery of a bifurcated device, and for this reason, the key areas to assess at the workstation are the infrarenal aortic neck and the common iliac arteries, since these are the principal sealing zones (Figures 1 and 2). Other factors, while of lesser overall importance, need to be considered in conjunction with this initial analysis before making a final decision regarding suitability.

The infrarenal aortic neck

An adequate infrarenal neck remains the single most important factor for both initial successful deployment and long-term durability. The ideal neck should be a straight tube, at least 15mm long, and no more than 30mm in diameter (Figure 1). It is generally recommended that the diameter of the aortic segment of a stent graft should be oversized by 20% in relation to the neck into which it is being deployed. The largest devices routinely available have an aortic body

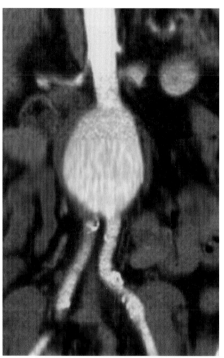

Figure 1. CT angiogram demonstrating the features of an ideal case for EVAR: a long straight neck and long straight common iliac arteries.

Planning measurements

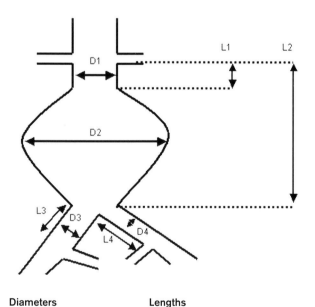

Diameters	Lengths
D1: proximal neck	L1: proximal neck
D2: maximum	L2: lowermost renal to
D3, 4: iliac	aortic bifurcation
	L3, 4: common iliac

Figure 2. The principal measurements necessary.

Adverse anatomical features

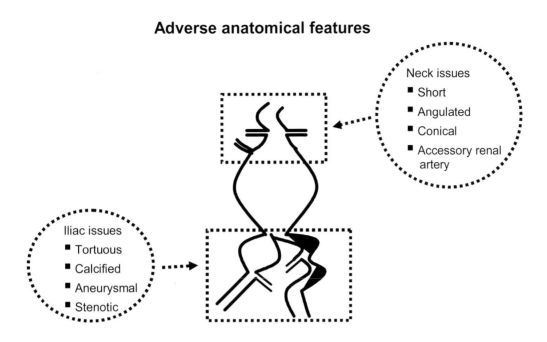

Figure 3. The principal adverse anatomical features encountered when assessing suitability for EVAR.

diameter of 36mm, which means that one is compromising the degree of oversize if the neck diameter is >30mm. It remains one of life's little anomalies that when performing open repair most surgeons use a tube graft ranging from 16 to 20mm without noticing anything unusual and yet the infrarenal neck diameter on CT usually measures 24 to 30mm.

In addition, the neck should be free from intraluminal thrombus, minimally calcified and not angulated in relation to the aneurysm. Not surprisingly, the 'perfect' aortic neck is seen relatively infrequently, and one must accept a compromise in one or more of these criteria in most cases. The degree to which one can deviate from the ideal configuration is largely a function of the experience of the team involved. In a large percentage of cases, the neck is not a straight tube, but is conical to a varying degree, whereby the diameter just below the lowermost renal artery is smaller than the diameter just before the start of the aneurysm. There are no hard and fast rules about how much of a diameter difference over what length is acceptable, but it is logical that a relatively small diameter change (e.g. <5mm) over a reasonably long

neck (e.g. 20mm) is more acceptable than a larger change in a neck of borderline length.

If one elects to use a neck of barely adequate length, then there is clearly a need to ensure that deployment is as accurate as possible, so that all the available neck is used to form the sealing zone, without encroaching on the renal arteries. This situation is encountered relatively frequently and prompted the development of devices with an uncovered proximal stent which crosses the renal artery origins, allowing a longer segment of fixation. It is still necessary in these cases to ensure that the fabric-covered second stent of the device is deployed as accurately as possible, since it is this segment which provides the all important proximal seal.

Adverse neck anatomy

As alluded to above, there are a number of different factors which lead to one concluding that the infrarenal neck will not produce an adequate sealing zone (Figure 3). Probably the most frequent reason for turning a case down is the presence of a short, wide neck, usually associated with a degree of conicality, before it becomes truly aneurysmal. In some cases, it is fairly evident that there is no effective neck and it is quite easy to turn the case down. It is more common, however, to see a neck that is of borderline length and/or diameter and it is useful to review these cases in a multidisciplinary setting in order to gain a consensus view [5].

Mural thrombus lining the neck is of concern on a number of fronts [6]. The first is that the thrombus may be disrupted during delivery and deployment of the device, resulting in atheromatous embolisation, especially to the kidneys. The second is that, while the device may produce a seal with no obvious endoleak, a thick layer of thrombus may still allow pressure to be transmitted to the aneurysm sac (e.g. endotension), and the possibility of continued expansion [7]. Finally, a layer of thrombus may impair the degree of fixation, leaving the graft at risk of migration and possible development of a late proximal endoleak.

Angulation of the aortic neck is a relative contraindication and is actually difficult to quantify, as there is no standardisation as to the baseline from which the angle is measured (e.g. is it relative to the true vertical, or to the line of the aneurysm? What if the aneurysm is angulated as well? etc.). It is easier to appreciate severe angulation by direct observation of the images without necessarily trying to measure any angles as such. If the neck seems to be deviating by more than 45 degrees to the flow channel, then this is going to create difficulties in both device delivery and deployment [8].

Calcification of the neck is only a relative contraindication. An effective proximal seal requires some degree of conformability of the aorta, and this is clearly reduced as the degree of calcification increases. It is more common to observe a ring of calcification at the junction between neck and aneurysm. If this is completely circumferential, it may prevent full expansion of the stent graft with subsequent failure to secure an adequate seal in the neck above this.

It is not uncommon to see multiple renal arteries, and occasionally there is a lower pole artery fairly low down in an otherwise suitable neck. It is preferable to cover such a vessel rather than compromise the seal in this situation. Whilst there is obvious concern about some loss of functional renal mass, it is very unlikely to result in clinically significant renal impairment in someone with pre-existing normal renal function. It goes without saying that this must be fully discussed with the patient [9].

Distal sealing zone

The simplest configuration for an aortic stent graft would be a tube which sealed in the distal aorta, mimicking the standard tube graft repair used during open surgery. There is virtually never a sufficient length of relatively normal aorta in which to land such a device, since the aneurysmal process generally extends to the aortic bifurcation. It is for this reason that EVAR for AAA necessitates deployment of a bifurcated system.

The distal sealing zone is, therefore, the common iliac artery which in ideal circumstances would be a long straight tube, preferably at least 3cm long and no wider than 16mm (Figure 1). It is common practice to oversize the iliac limbs by 2mm in order to effect a seal.

In addition, a general principle is that the iliac limbs should occupy as much of the common iliac segment as possible, thus ensuring a long sealing zone, without encroaching on the internal iliac origins. There is much more flexibility over the absolute criteria than with the proximal neck, and again experience is an important factor, but it is unusual to turn down a case on the basis of unfavourable iliac anatomy alone.

Adverse iliac anatomy (Figure 3)

The commonest adverse feature encountered in the iliac segments is ectasia which can range from a wide artery, i.e. >16mm, to a frank aneurysm. Provided the artery is a relatively straight tube, the problem of simple ectasia can be overcome by using an appropriately oversized iliac limb [10,11]. A definite iliac aneurysm is more challenging as they usually almost always extend to the iliac bifurcation, and there is no distal sealing zone in the common iliac. The solution in this case is to embolise the internal iliac artery, usually as a separate elective procedure, and extend the limb into the external iliac artery. It is generally felt that provided at least one internal iliac remains patent then there are good prospects for cross pelvic collateralisation. Whilst this runs the theoretical risk of colonic ischaemia, it is surprisingly well tolerated, although the patient should be warned about buttock claudication [12].

If bilateral iliac aneurysms are present it is probably not advisable to embolise both internal iliacs and this is for some an indication for open repair. One option is to consider surgical transposition of at least one of the internals to create a landing zone in the external whilst maintaining internal iliac patency. A fairly recent development is iliac branched graft technology in which a smaller bifurcated system is deployed within the iliac aneurysm and internal iliac patency maintained via a covered stent. This inevitably increases the complexity of the procedure but is an illustration of the ingenious way in which such technical problems can be overcome.

Tortuosity of the iliac segments is frequently encountered, and if severe can present major problems in device delivery. It is usually possible, however, to overcome surprisingly marked tortuosity with stiff wires such as the Lunderquvist (Cook). Tortuosity is much more of a problem when associated with calcification, and the two must be assessed in tandem. Even if the iliacs appear relatively uncalcified it is quite common to see a ring of calcification at the aortic bifurcation, something frequently encountered during open repair, and this can cause difficulties when trying to negotiate large diameter delivery systems into the aorta.

Occlusive disease of the iliac segments is clearly a potential obstacle to device delivery, but is actually encountered relatively infrequently. A short segment stenosis may require predilation, and can sometimes be overcome with the tapered nosecone of the delivery system. Diffuse disease of the external iliac can very occasionally warrant retroperitoneal exposure of the iliac bifurcation and suturing of a conduit to the common iliac through which the system is then introduced.

Collateral branches

Patent vessels from the aneurysm itself, i.e. lumbar arteries and the inferior mesenteric artery (IMA), are conventionally oversewn during open surgery. As they are not dealt with directly during EVAR, however, they form a potential channel for continued blood flow into the aneurysm sac, known as a Type 2 endoleak. It was quite reasonably assumed that any perfusion of the sac following EVAR left the aneurysm at risk of continued expansion and possibly late rupture. This in turn led to a lot of attention focusing on the problem of Type 2 endoleaks, with numerous reports relating to their detection and management. There is now, however, an increasingly general consensus that Type 2 endoleaks pose very little threat in reality and, in the majority of instances, they can be observed as part of the follow-up programme. Thus, while assessment of lumbar and IMA patency used to be regarded as an integral part of the pre-operative assessment, this is no longer the case [13, 14].

Currently available devices

Having determined suitability for an endovascular approach it is then necessary to select an appropriate device to exclude the aneurysm. The initial descriptions of EVAR involved devices which were constructed in relatively crude fashion by sewing together available stents and arterial grafts and inserting them into a large delivery system. This process often took place in theatre as part of the procedure. Rather unsurprisingly, these early procedures were complicated by numerous technical failures, but never to such an extent that the concept itself was deemed unworkable. Rather, these pioneering efforts resulted in a number of basic principles being identified as important for a successful outcome, which have been incorporated in devices in current use [15].

Basic stent graft construction

The devices used in current practice are now all commercially manufactured using materials of

Table 1. The currently available devices, including a comparison of their key features.

Device	Material	Configuration	Deployment	Fixation	Aortic graft diameters	Iliac graft diameters	Suprarenal stent
				Endograft characteristics			
Zenith (Cook)	Polyester	Modular	Self-expanding	Compression-fit and barbs	22-36	8-24	Yes
Talent (Medtronic)	Polyester	Modular	Self-expanding	Compression-fit	24-34	8-24	Yes
Excluder (Gore)	ePTFE	Modular	Self-expanding	Compression-fit and anchors	23/26/28.5	12--14.5	No
Anaconda (Terumo)	Twillweave	Modular	Self-expanding	Compression-fit and hooks	19.5-34	9-18	No
Powerlink (Edwards Lifesciences)	ePTFE	Unipiece	Self-expanding	Compression-fit	25/28	16	Optional

appropriately high standard (Table 1). They each consist of a metal framework (usually steel or nitinol), of varying design, which supports a fabric graft (either Dacron or PTFE). There are various technical differences between devices which are important to understand when actually using the system (e.g. whether the stents are inside or outside the fabric), but they are essentially fairly similar. All of the systems currently available in the UK use self-expanding stents.

Device design and manufacture is in large part a compromise between developing a sufficiently robust stent/fabric combination for long-term durability and the need to fit it into a system which is deliverable (i.e. not too large or stiff), and which then allows easy, accurate deployment. As a result, the majority come preloaded into a purpose-built delivery system. The exception is the Gore Excluder, which is loaded onto a catheter with a separate delivery sheath.

Device configuration (Figure 4)

As explained previously, the absence of an adequate sealing zone in the distal aorta means that a bifurcated graft is used in the overwhelming majority of cases.

Bifurcated systems

The majority of these use the modular concept originally developed by Miahle. This consists of a main aortic body with a long and a short limb. The long limb is designed to engage in the common iliac artery on the ipsilateral side. The short limb is designed to open up in the aneurysm and is catheterised from the contralateral groin. The system is then completed by deployment of an appropriately sized contralateral iliac limb. Cannulation of the stump limb can be troublesome on occasion, especially in a large aneurysm with minimal thrombus. If direct cannulation from the groin proves difficult, it is usually possible to cross the bifurcation of the device from the ipsilateral side and snare a wire from the contralateral groin.

There are thus four sealing zones in this design: the infrarenal neck, both common iliacs and the stump overlap zone within the aneurysm. The modular approach has maintained popularity due to its simplicity, versatility and an established track record.

Only one system, the Powerlink (Edwards Lifesciences), is a single piece device, thus mimicking a surgical bifurcated graft. This has the attraction of reducing the number of sealing zones to three by avoiding the stump overlap zone in the aneurysm. The main problem with development of the single piece

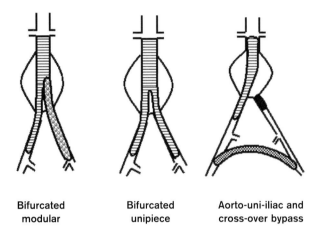

| Bifurcated modular | Bifurcated unipiece | Aorto-uni-iliac and cross-over bypass |

Figure 4. The range of options available for device configuration.

device has been overcoming the technical issues involved in safely deploying the contralateral iliac limb, without making it too complex for widespread use.

Aorto-uni-iliac (AUI) systems

A number of companies have an AUI variant as an option. This has the advantage of relative simplicity in terms of deployment, which can be fairly rapid since there is no need to cannulate the contralateral stump. The AUI approach can involve a single piece device sealing in the infrarenal neck and the common iliac. More versatility is afforded by a two-piece system, with a degree of overlap within the aneurysm, allowing one to deal with variable aortic anatomy. For this reason it has gained popularity in the emergency situation (see Chapter 3). The downside to the AUI approach is that it necessitates occlusion of the contralateral iliac system, usually with a short, blind ending stent graft, and a femorofemoral crossover in order to restore perfusion to the contralateral leg. It is for this reason that the AUI approach is not generally favoured for elective cases.

One indication for the AUI approach in the elective setting, albeit rare, is the presence of an occluded iliac system on one side.

Device fixation

This is crucial in order to maintain aneurysm exclusion, especially in the neck of the aneurysm. Fixation is, in the main, due to the radial expansion force of the stent frame in the sealing zones, and it is for this reason that a degree of oversizing is important, especially in the proximal neck. The current recommendation is for the aortic body to be oversized by 20% in respect of the neck diameter as measured on CT.

In addition to oversizing, proximal fixation can be improved by extending the length of apposition in the aorta and this is why a number of devices have a bare proximal stent which extends into the usually normal visceral segment. Initial concerns about impaired renal blood flow and late renal artery stenosis or occlusion have not been borne out in practice [16].

Another aid to fixation is the use of hooks or barbs which can embed into the aortic wall, providing further resistance to migration of the device.

Ease of use

This can be considered under two headings, the first relating to the percentage of cases in whom the device can be used and the second to issues around delivery and deployment.

Patient suitability

The first commercially available devices were made in a limited range of sizes of both length and diameter, and it was often difficult to find a case in which to fit them. This situation has improved considerably, with all devices coming in a much wider range of sizes than previously. The major advance has been the development of large diameter aortic bodies and iliac limbs, and as a consequence the percentage of cases deemed suitable for EVAR has risen dramatically from 25% to 60% or higher [17, 18]. The concept is now much more about putting together a system to fit the individual patient rather than the other way round.

The downside from the manufacturers' point of view is the need to produce a wide range of component pieces in order to fit varied anatomy, but this is more than offset by the increased proportion of cases which become suitable.

Delivery and deployment

The main issue with delivery is tracking a stiff delivery system through tortuous access vessels. Large diameter devices inevitably require a large sheath with an external diameter of up to 24 French, which require an external iliac artery of at least 8mm in diameter. To some extent, delivery of these large systems is considerably facilitated by the use of extra-stiff wires.

Once correctly positioned in relation to the renal arteries, deployment of the device needs to be accurate without being overly complicated. Each of the systems listed in Table 1 has a different means of deployment, some more complex than others, but all within the capability of an appropriately trained individual. Each of the companies involved in EVAR have a network of clinical specialists who provide training in device deployment and support during initial clinical use.

Which system to use?

In order to introduce an effective EVAR programme, it makes sense to include as large a proportion as possible of the elective AAA caseload. This dictates the use of a system with the versatility to fit most patients and for most this will be a modular system with a bare proximal stent (e.g. Talent or Zenith), as the principal device. Most centres with large experience will have used a number of different devices over the years (many of which are no longer in clinical use) and settled on one with which they have become very familiar with and achieve good results.

All of the other systems have their merits, however, and there is likely to be increasing diversity of use in established centres, with perhaps two or three systems used depending on the particular anatomical features of each individual case.

Conclusions

EVAR has now well and truly come of age and the next few years will see a considerable increase in the number of procedures being performed. Patient selection mandates careful assessment of anatomy, but the majority of cases will be found to be suitable for EVAR due to the availability of systems with appropriately large aortic and iliac diameters. Devices with an uncovered proximal stent predominate, currently due to the perceived need to assist fixation in the infrarenal neck. There is, in addition, a range of alternative devices, each with their own unique features, which will have a place to play as, with increasing experience, centres will look to select the best solution for each individual patient.

Summary

◆   EVAR is now firmly established as a therapeutic modality in the management of AAA.

◆   Multislice CT is the imaging modality of choice when assessing patient suitability.

◆   A relatively high proportion of cases (up to 80%) will be anatomically suitable for EVAR.

◆   Modular bifurcated systems predominate currently.

◆   Using a range of systems will allow the best option to be used for each case.

References

1. Powell JT, Brown LC. UK Small Aneurysm Trial: the natural history of abdominal aortic aneurysms and their risk of rupture. *Adv Surg* 2001; 35: 173-85.

2. Wolf YG, Fogarty TJ, Olcott CIV, *et al*. Endovascular repair of abdominal aortic aneurysm: elegibility rate and impact on the rate of open repair. *J Vasc Surg* 2000; 32: 519-23.

3. Zarins CK, Wolf YG, Hill BB, *et al*. Will endovascular repair replace open surgery for abdominal aortic aneurysm repair? *Ann Surg* 2000; 232: 501-7.

4. Parker MV, O'Donnel SD, Chang AS, *et al*. What imaging studies are necessary for abdominal aortic endograft sizing? A prospective blinded study using conventional computed tomography, aortography, and three-dimensional computed tomography. *J Vasc Surg* 2005; 41(2): 199-205.

5. Ingle H, Fiskwick G, Thompson MM, *et al*. Endovascular repair of wide neck AAA - preliminary report of feasibility and complications. *Eur J Vasc Endovasc Surg* 2002; 24: 123-7.

6. Gilling-Smith GL, Mc Williams RG, Brennan JA. Freedom from endoleak after endovascular aneurysm repair does not equal treatment success. *Eur J Vasc Endovasc Surg* 2000; 19(4): 421-5.

7. Vallabhaneni SR, Gilling-Smith GL, Brennan JA, *et al*. Can intrasac pressure monitoring reliably predict failure of endovascular aneurysm repair? *J Endovasc Ther* 2003; 10(3): 524-30.

8. Sampaio SM, Panneton JM, Mozez GI, *et al*. Proximal type I endoleak after endovascular aortic abdominal aneurysm repair: predictive factors. *Ann Vasc Surg* 2004; 18(6): 621-8.

9. Karmachaya J, Parmer SS, Antezana JN, *et al*. Outcomes of accessory renal artery occlusion during endovascular aneurysm repair. *J Vasc Surg* 2006; 43 (1): 8-13.

10. Malgari K, Brountzos E, Gougoulakis A, *et al*. Large diameter limbs for dilated common iliac arteries in endovascular aneurysm repair: is it safe? *Cardiovasc Intervent Radiol* 2004; 27(3): 237-42.

11. Timaran CH, Lipsitx EC, Veith FJ, *et al*. Endovascular aortic aneurysm repair with the Zenith endograft in patients with ectatic iliac arteries. *Ann Vasc Surg* 2005; 19(2): 161-6

12. Metha M, Veith FJ, Ohki T, *et al*. Unilateral and bilateral hyogastric artery interruption during aortoiliac aneurysm repair in 154 patients: a relatively innocuous procedure. *J Vasc Surg* 2001; 33 (Suppl): S27-S32.

13. Gelfand DV, White GH, Wilson SE. Clinical significance of type II endoleak after endovascular repair of abdominal aortic aneurysm. *Ann Vasc Surg* 2006; 20(1): 69-74.

14. Harris PL, Buth J, Van Marrewijk C, *et al*. Endoleaks during follow-up after endovascular repair of abdominal aortic aneurysm. Are they all dangerous? *J Cardiovasc Surg (Torino)* 2003; 44(4): 559-66.

15. May J, White GH, Waugh R, *et al*. Improved survival after endoluminal repair with second generation prosthesis compared with open repair in the treatment of abdominal aortic aneurysms: a five-year concurrent comparison using life-table method. *J Vasc Surg* 2001; 33: S21-26.

16. Parmer SS, Carpenter JP; Endologix Investigators. Endovascular aneurysm repair with suprarenal vs infrarenal fixation: a study of renal effects. *J Vasc Surg* 2006; 43(1): 19-25.

17. Armon MP, Yusuf SW, Latief K, *et al*. Anatomical suitability of abdominal aortic aneurysms for endovascular repair. *Br J Surg* 1999; 84: 178-80.

18. Carpenter JP, Baum RA, Backer CF, *et al*. Impact of exclusion criteria on patient selection for endovascular abdominal aortic aneurysm repair. *J Vasc Surg* 2001; 34: 1050-4.

Chapter 2

EVAR for short-necked aneurysms

Richard G McWilliams FRCS FRCR, Consultant Interventional Radiologist

Micheal Murphy FRCSI FRCR, Consultant Interventional Radiologist

Royal Liverpool University Hospital, Liverpool, UK

Introduction

The infrarenal aortic neck is the most critical anatomical area in the assessment of patients for EVAR. Poor case selection may result in primary proximal endoleak due to an inadequate seal or late proximal endoleak due to migration. Proximal Type 1 endoleaks after EVAR are known to carry a high risk of late conversion and aortic rupture [1, 2].

The pre-operative analysis must document the neck length, contour and quality. Standard endovascular grafts are generally reserved for patients with a neck length of at least 15mm. There is a small literature recording the use of standard endografts in patients with shorter necks. Alternative endovascular strategies for short-necked aneurysms include the use of fenestrated and branched grafts.

Hybrid procedures are described involving open surgical bypasses to the renal and mesenteric arteries before endografting, so that the perirenal segment may be used for fixation and seal [3]. These techniques have not gained much favour, most probably due to advances in endograft technology which allow for entirely endovascular repairs.

The purpose of this chapter is to outline the importance of the anatomy of the aortic neck and to review the literature on endovascular treatment of short-necked aneurysms.

The anatomy of the aortic neck

The infrarenal neck of an abdominal aortic aneurysm is defined as the segment of aorta between the lowermost renal artery and the beginning of the aneurysm. Many aortic necks gradually expand into aneurysm and the neck is considered by some authors to end at the point where the diameter increases by 3mm from the juxtarenal segment [4]. This is a contentious definition as the neck may increase by more than 3mm but then remain reasonably static in diameter for a long segment and this 'secondary aortic neck' may be a suitable landing zone for the proximal sealing stents of an endograft (Figure 1). In the authors' experience there are many aneurysms which have this neck anatomy. Sizing the endograft for the secondary neck allows for an adequate seal in this circumstance.

The lowermost renal artery may be an accessory renal vessel and the neck may on occasions be lengthened by sacrificing this. The decision will be based upon the size and estimated importance of such a vessel with reference to the patient's renal function and the volume of cortex supplied.

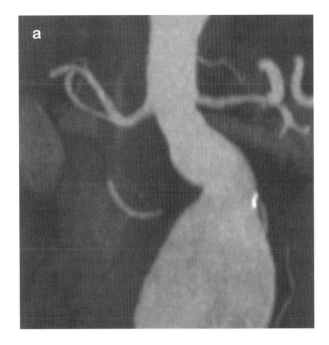

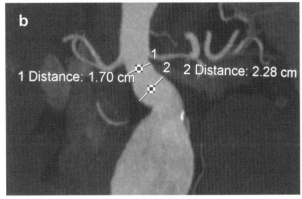

Figure 1. Reformatted oblique coronal CT image of an infrarenal abdominal aortic aneurysm. There is a short primary neck of less than 10mm length and 17mm diameter. Below this there is a secondary neck of 23mm diameter extending for another 2cm.

The required neck length for endovascular treatment with standard devices is 15mm. This figure has generally been accepted both in the medical literature and in the 'instructions for use' of most endovascular devices.

Favourable anatomical features of the aortic neck include limited angulation, minimal calcification, absence of neck atheroma and thrombus, and a non-conical shape.

The aortic neck angle is defined as the angle between the longitudinal axis of the aortic neck and the aneurysm sac. There is some confusion in how this is described; most studies record increasing angulation as an increase in the measured neck angle, while others choose the supplementary angle (one may recall from geometry that supplementary angles add up to 180 degrees) and hence, a decrease in this supplementary angle, is equivalent to increase in neck angle and therefore more complex neck anatomy [1].

Assessment of neck calcification requires the use of CT scanning and involves determining the percentage of the neck circumference that is calcified. Large exophytic plaques in the aortic neck may prevent adequate sealing at endovascular repair. Neck atheroma and thrombus are adverse features determined by review of CT data. Standard imaging protocols do not allow the distinction to be made between atheroma and mural thrombus.

A conical neck or reverse tapered neck has been defined as one where the distal diameter is ≥3mm wider than the proximal infrarenal diameter [1].

A posterior bulge in the aortic neck is best observed on sagittal reconstructions from CT datasets and, particularly when calcified this may compromise the proximal seal.

Complete pre-operative assessment demands high quality thin section CT scanning on a multi-slice scanner, with the opportunity to interrogate the data at a dedicated workstation with a suitable vascular software package. Multiplanar reformatting of the neck anatomy is essential. Final case selection and graft planning based on review of hard copy images is nowadays considered to be unacceptable.

Outcome data for standard endografts: relevance of neck anatomy

Sampaio *et al* reviewed their series of 202 patients to identify the anatomical risk factors predictive of proximal Type 1 endoleak. Patients with large aneurysms, short necks and heavily calcified necks were found to have an increased risk of proximal endoleak. Review of the post-deployment anatomy found that the most significant measurement was the length of the overlapped zone of the endograft in the aortic neck [1].

A review of the Australasian experience with the Zenith device recorded a 57% proximal endoleak rate for aneurysms with an infrarenal neck length of ≤10mm. They concluded that necks ≤10mm are unsuitable for the standard Zenith graft and that necks between 10-20mm long should be treated with caution, with regard to the additional risks associated with neck contour, angulation and neck diameter [5].

Midterm results have been reported with the use of the Talent endograft, with analysis of the results for complicated and uncomplicated aortic necks [4]. Complicated necks were defined as either short (≤15mm), very short (≤10mm), dilated (>28mm), angulated (≥45 degrees), calcified and thrombus-lined, with or without ulceration. A total of 237 consecutive patients were followed for a mean length of 620.5 days. In this study, 70% of patients had complicated necks, and overall, 32.3% had short necks and 19.3% had very short necks. There was no significant difference in endoleak rates between the groups and no difference in migration rates. Migration in this study was defined as displacement of 10mm or greater or any movement that necessitated a secondary procedure. Freedom from migration was 87.0% and 86.9% at 24 months in the complicated and uncomplicated neck groups respectively. Adverse renal events were more common in the group with complicated necks, especially in patients with calcified or angulated necks. The authors concluded that the Talent LPS system may be used successfully in treating patients with complicated neck anatomy as defined in their methodology.

An audit of Australian cases of EVAR submitted to a national register between 1999 and 2001 reported that 10% of treated patients (84/872 cases) had a neck length of <15mm. Outcome data record that patients with Type 1 endoleaks had significantly shorter necks than those without endoleaks. Significant factors in the development of Type 1 endoleak were a large pre-operative aneurysm diameter, aortic neck angle >45 degrees and a short infrarenal neck length [6].

Endovascular repair

Endovascular options for short-necked aneurysms may involve the judicious use of standard devices or alternatively, more complex endografts, which incorporate fenestrations or branches that allow the sealing zone to be extended across the visceral vessels. Hybrid procedures combining open bypass surgery to the renal and mesenteric vessels also allow proximal extension of the sealing zone.

In the presence of adverse anatomical features for endovascular repair, it is essential that the case against open aneurysm repair is strong.

Standard devices

Few operators would treat neck lengths of less than 10mm with a standard device and the grey area in this context relates to aneurysms with borderline necks of between 10-15mm. When choosing a standard device in this scenario we feel that suprarenal fixation is essential. It has been shown from previous literature that devices which incorporate hooks and barbs are associated with a decreased risk of migration, which is a known risk for EVAR in this setting [7].

If a standard device is being considered in a patient with a short neck then it is imperative that the operators are able to maximise the engagement of the endograft in the available neck. This requires adequate imaging during the procedure, with the facility to angle the C-arm in the craniocaudal and oblique planes so that the ostium of the lowermost renal artery is profiled optimally. Some operators place a catheter in the lowermost renal artery to ensure that this vessel is continuously monitored. Placing the renal arteries in the centre of the image also reduces the potential for parallax errors. Our own practice is to retain a radio-opaque tipped pigtail catheter alongside the endograft and to perform repeated check angiograms on magnified views during gradual release of the proximal endograft. This can be achieved using low volumes at high flow rates, typically 10ml at 20ml/sec, to minimise the contrast medium load. This catheter can easily be removed post-deployment by straightening the pigtail with a guidewire before it is withdrawn alongside the supra-renal barbed stent.

When attempting to optimise the engagement of the sealing stent in a short aortic neck, there is a risk of partially compromising renal blood flow. It is important to recognise this partial renal coverage, which may lead to subsequent renal artery occlusion. Recovery options in this situation include attempts to carefully move the fabric inferiorly with downward traction on the endograft or to stent the partially covered renal artery (Figure 2).

speed of this evolution indicates the perceived need to incorporate the perirenal segment in the endovascular repair of short-necked aneurysms.

The basis of this graft design is the incorporation of the perirenal aortic segment into the sealing zone, thus increasing the available neck length. Fenestrations in the graft fabric preserve blood flow to the visceral arteries. Each fenestrated stent graft is customised for the patient's anatomy based on the number, height and circumferential position of the visceral arteries which need to be incorporated in the

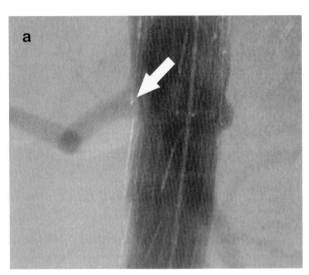 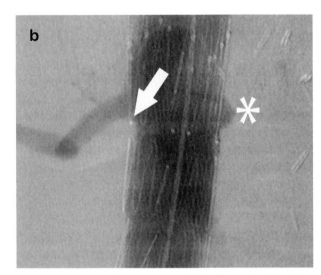

Figure 2. a) Angiographic image during EVAR with a standard device with suprarenal fixation showing the fabric markers (white arrow) across the ostium of the right renal artery. **b)** There has been previous left nephrectomy (asterisk). Downward traction on the device to engage the barbs results in resolution of the renal coverage.

Primary proximal endoleaks with standard endografts may be treated with balloon dilatation, the use of cuff extensions or the adjunctive use of large Palmaz stents.

Fenestrated endografts

Fenestrated endografts were developed to allow the endovascular treatment of short-necked aneurysms. The first report of the use of fenestrated grafts was in 1999, less than a decade after the original paper by Parodi [8] on the use of an endograft for the repair of an abdominal aortic aneurysm [9]. The

repair. Pre-operative planning necessitates thin section multi-slice CT reviewed at a dedicated workstation. The fenestrations are planned from images reconstructed at right angles to the longitudinal axis of the perirenal aorta. Graft planning and deployment are more difficult if there is significant neck angulation, which is a relative contraindication to the use of fenestrated grafts.

The commercially available fenestrated endograft is based on the Zenith platform, but there are several differences from the standard three-part modular endovascular device. The fenestrated graft comprises a composite body and the straight, proximal

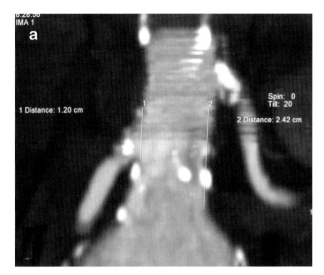
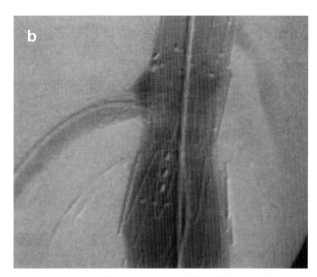

Figure 3. a) Reformatted coronal CT image of an infrarenal abdominal aortic aneurysm with a 12mm infrarenal neck below an asymmetrically placed right renal artery. b) Intra-operative angiographic image of a fenestrated device, with a single stented scallop for this renal artery, allowing the entire sealing stent to lie in the parallel perirenal segment.

fenestrated portion of this composite body is inserted first. This is partially deployed with the fenestrations at the level of the target vessel ostia and with the device in the correct antero-posterior orientation as judged by markers on the endograft. Rotation of this partially opened portion is facilitated by a restricting or diameter-reducing tie, which is not released until the target vessels are cannulated. Without this adjunct, this procedure would be technically more difficult and almost certainly much more hazardous.

The distal end of the partially deployed proximal body section is catheterised from the contralateral femoral artery and each target vessel is cannulated. Introducer sheaths or guiding catheters are passed into the target vessels before final deployment of the fenestrated segment. This guides the fenestrations down onto the ostia and allows subsequent stenting of the fenestrations which maintains the stability of the graft and patency of the target vessels. The graft is completed with a distal bifurcated body and appropriate limb extensions.

There are three distinct types of fenestration which may be used and these are dictated by the Gianturco stent design of the Zenith endograft. A scallop describes a U-shaped gap in the fabric at the top of

the endograft. This may be used as a single fenestration to accommodate the lowermost of asymmetrically positioned renal arteries (Figure 3) or as part of a more complex endograft with combinations of fenestrations. In this more complex graft, the scallop is usually placed anteriorly to protect the superior mesenteric supply. Single scallops are nowadays routinely stented, as experience has recorded an incidence of renal artery loss, due to presumed graft realignment post-deployment.

Other types of fenestrations are below the superior fabric margin and either have stent struts across them (large fenestrations) or reside between the struts (small fenestrations). Small fenestrations are routinely stented to avoid partial shuttering of target vessel ostia by fabric (Figure 4). Large fenestrations are not intended to be secondarily stented.

There are several case series now published in the literature on the use of fenestrated grafts. The initial technical success rates are high and this reflects our own practice. Primary proximal endoleak rates are very low and the evolution of the aortic sac is generally good. There are some problems which arise from the use of renal stents with some reported vessel loss in most series. Renal artery stenosis and occlusion may

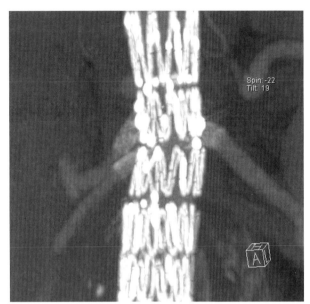

Figure 4. CT image following fenestrated repair of a juxtarenal aneurysm with three small fenestrations for renal arteries which have all been stented.

occur, as may stent deformation, due to longitudinal and rotatory movements of the endograft causing shear forces on the visceral artery stents.

Movement of the overlap zone of the composite body may occur and this has been recorded to cause Type 3 endoleak and prophylactic re-intervention may be required if modular movement is seen during surveillance.

Deployment of the endograft requires accurate positioning both in terms of the height of the fabric and the rotation of the endograft. In some patients it may require considerable effort to achieve satisfactory rotation. The catheterisation of the renal arteries involves additional manipulation in the region of the aortic wall and these combined events probably result in an increased incidence of micro-embolisation. Significant aortic wall disease should be considered an adverse feature for fenestrated endografting. Anecdotally, we have seen cholesterol embolisation in this setting and the Cleveland series also records this [10].

The ideal renal stent for use in this setting probably differs from renal stents used for isolated stenotic disease. Nowadays the emphasis for stenotic disease

is for low-profile stents which are flexible and trackable. These attributes are often achieved with overall loss of metal and a reduction in the connections between the struts and crowns of the stent. This may result in a stent with limited resistance to shear forces which are encountered at the interface between the fenestration and the renal stent. The ideal stent does not yet exist but it is important to remember the different demands on the stent when choosing adjunctive stents during fenestrated endografting.

Covered renal stents are now available which will effectively create a branched graft when used in combination with fenestrations. These allow aneurysms to be treated that have no infrarenal neck; however, the patency rates for covered renal stents are probably not as good as for uncovered stents and, if there is a short sealing zone below the renal arteries, then we would generally opt for an uncovered stent.

The increased labour and technical challenges in manufacturing fenestrated grafts increases the delivery time and costs. This must be factored into the decision-making process and currently precludes the treatment of some patients.

Outcome data for fenestrated grafts

Thus far the literature on fenestrated grafts includes only small, single-centre series with early outcome data [10-13].

John Anderson who has been one of the Australian pioneers of fenestrated endografts reported his experience of 13 patients treated from 1998 to 2000. The median neck length in this group was 4mm and the procedural success was 100% with all 33 targeted vessels preserved and no proximal endoleaks. Follow-up ranging from three to 24 months revealed no delayed proximal or distal endoleaks, but one stented renal artery occluded [11].

Eric Verhoeven reported his experience of 18 cases of fenestrated endografting. The median neck length was 8mm and the mean procedure time was 166 minutes. The need for pulsed fluoroscopy to reduce the radiation exposure was stressed by these authors. At completion of the procedure, 45 of 46 targeted vessels remained patent and one accessory renal artery was occluded by the endograft. There were no primary or delayed proximal endoleaks at mean follow-up of 9.4 months. In addition, there was one case of delayed renal artery occlusion[13].

The largest published series have been from the Cleveland Clinic. In 2004, a series of 32 patients was reported. This group comprised 24 patients with aortic neck length <10mm and eight patients with a neck length of between 10-16mm, but with additional adverse neck anatomy due to angulation or thrombus. All devices were successfully implanted with no immediate loss of the 83 targeted vessels. There were no primary or delayed proximal endoleaks and only one case of sac growth thought due to a Type 2 endoleak. At mean follow-up of 9.2 months there was impairment of flow to 6/83 targeted vessels, three of which were successfully managed endovascularly. There were three delayed target vessel occlusions [12].

A larger series of 72 patients treated with fenestrated endografts at the Cleveland clinic was reported in 2005 [10]. The emphasis in this paper was a review of the renal complications associated with this technique. There were 142 targeted renal arteries in this series. During follow-up, ranging from one to 24 months, there were ten renal artery stenoses, five renal artery occlusions and four patients who required haemodialysis, for two of whom this was permanent

dialysis. Renal events were more common in those with pre-existing renal dysfunction and all those patients who required dialysis had pre-existing renal dysfunction. The authors stress the need for post-procedural surveillance to screen for renal artery stenosis and combine renal duplex ultrasound and CT in their surveillance protocol.

Conclusions

Pre-operative assessment of the aortic neck is crucial for successful endovascular repair. A neck length of 15mm is required for standard devices. Borderline necks of 10-15mm, in the absence of additional adverse features, may be considered for a standard device, but the operating team must be able to fully utilise the available neck. Physicians must be aware of the increased risk of Type 1 endoleak when shorter necks are treated with standard devices. Fenestrated grafts are now commercially available with promising early results for the endovascular management of short-necked aneurysms. The level of evidence for fenestrated grafts is currently low with only single centre case series reported. The primary technical success rates in experienced centres are high and the short-term complication rates are low. There is an expected attrition rate for the target vessels and long-term data are needed to fully understand the role of fenestrated grafts.

Summary

◆ The aortic neck anatomy is the most crucial factor in the success or failure of endovascular aneurysm repair.

◆ Proximal endoleaks are associated with short, conical and angulated necks.

◆ Standard endovascular devices require a minimum neck length of 15mm.

◆ The early results with fenestrated grafts for short-necked aneurysms are encouraging; however, there is an incidence of target vessel stenosis and occlusion.

◆ The longer-term results of fenestrated grafts are awaited.

References

1. Sampaio SM, Panneton JM, Mozes GI, Andrews JC, Bower TC, Karla M, *et al*. Proximal type I endoleak after endovascular abdominal aortic aneurysm repair: predictive factors. *Ann Vasc Surg* 2004; 18: 621-8.

2. Harris PL, Vallabhaneni SR, Desgranges P, Becquemin JP, van Marrewijk C, Laheij RJ. Incidence and risk factors of late rupture, conversion, and death after endovascular repair of infrarenal aortic aneurysms: the EUROSTAR experience. European Collaborators on stent/graft techniques for aortic aneurysm repair. *J Vasc Surg* 2000; 32: 739-49.

3. Becquemin JP. EVAR: new developments and extended applicability. *Eur J Vasc Endovasc Surg* 2004; 27: 453-55.

4. Fairman RM, Velazquez OC, Carpenter JP, Woo E, Baum RA, Golden MA, *et al*. Midterm pivotal trial results of the Talent Low Profile System for repair of abdominal aortic aneurysm: analysis of complicated versus uncomplicated aortic necks. *J Vasc Surg* 2004; 40: 1074-82.

5. Stanley BM, Semmens JB, Mai Q, Goodman MA, Hartley DE, Wilkinson C, *et al*. Evaluation of patient selection guidelines for endoluminal AAA repair with the Zenith Stent-Graft: the Australasian experience. *J Endovasc Ther* 2001; 8: 457-64.

6. Boult M, Babidge W, Maddern G, Barnes M, Fitridge R, on behalf of The Audit Reference Group. Predictors of success following endovascular aneurysm repair: mid-term results. *Eur J Vasc Endovasc Surg* 2006; 31: 123-29.

7. van Marrewijk CJ, Leurs LJ, Vallabhaneni SR, Harris PL, Buth J, Laheij RJ. Risk-adjusted outcome analysis of endovascular abdominal aortic aneurysm repair in a large population: how do stent-grafts compare? *J Endovasc Ther* 2005; 12: 417-29.

8. Parodi JC, Palmaz JC, Barone HD. Transfemoral intraluminal graft implantation for abdominal aortic aneurysms. *Ann Vasc Surg* 1991; 5: 491-99.

9. Browne TF, Hartley D, Purchas S, Rosenberg M, Van Schie G, Lawrence-Brown M. A fenestrated covered suprarenal aortic stent. *Eur J Vasc Endovasc Surg* 1999; 18: 445-49.

10. Haddad F, Greenberg RK, Walker E, Nally J, O'Neill S, Kolin G, *et al*. Fenestrated endovascular grafting: the renal side of the story. *J Vasc Surg* 2005; 41: 181-90.

11. Anderson JL, Berce M, Hartley DE. Endoluminal aortic grafting with renal and superior mesenteric artery incorporation by graft fenestration. *J Endovasc Ther* 2001; 8: 3-15.

12. Greenberg RK, Haulon S, O'Neill S, Lyden S, Ouriel K. Primary endovascular repair of juxtarenal aneurysms with fenestrated endovascular grafting. *Eur J Vasc Endovasc Surg* 2004; 27: 484-91.

13. Verhoeven EL, Prins TR, Tielliu IF, van den Dungen JJ, Zeebregts CJ, Hulsebos RG, *et al*. Treatment of short-necked infrarenal aortic aneurysms with fenestrated stent-grafts: short-term results. *Eur J Vasc Endovasc Surg* 2004; 27: 477-83.

Chapter 3

Recommendations for EVAR in ruptured aneurysms

Chee V Soong MD FRCS, Consultant Vascular Surgeon
William Loan FRCR, Consultant Radiologist
Bernard Lee FRCS, Consultant Vascular Surgeon
Belfast City Hospital, Belfast, Ireland

Introduction

The mortality rate of conventional open repair (OR) of ruptured abdominal aortic aneurysm (rAAA) varies from centre to centre, with most published outcomes subject to the selection or reporting bias particular to individual institutions. The overall operative mortality for unselected ruptures still remains over 40%, despite the gradual improvement over the years [1]. Patient selection may account for some of the improvement in survival, although a meta-analysis by Bown et al [1] on operative mortality of rAAA repair was unable to determine that any improvement was related to pre-operative selection, intra-operative or postoperative factors. In addition to this high mortality, recovery amongst the survivors may be protracted with prolonged stay in the intensive therapy unit (ITU), placing a significant burden on an already overstretched ITU service in UK hospitals.

Single centre case series and anecdotal reports from enthusiastic centres have demonstrated both the feasibility and potential benefits of emergency endovascular repair (eEVAR) in rAAA [2-6]. Reflecting the pattern for open repair, mortality rates for eEVAR differ widely amongst reporting institutions. A worldwide series from 48 centres involving 442 patients reported an average mortality of 18% [7].

There was, however, selective usage of eEVAR, and the proportion of stented patients ranged between 18%-76%. This again illustrates the role of reporting bias and patient selection, especially when most reports were based on patients who were haemodynamically stable and who may otherwise have done just as well with OR.

An international multicentre trial evaluating the use of eEVAR in rAAA failed to demonstrate a significant difference in mortality rates between EVAR and OR, and has only served to fuel the controversy [5]. The undoubted theoretical attractions of eEVAR for ruptured aneurysms have still to be confirmed in practice, and even accepting a possible reduction in mortality rates, few endovascular practitioners would currently argue that the postoperative recovery following eEVAR is any shorter than that following OR, although the ITU stay may be reduced [5]. Unfortunately, even if the results were to demonstrate a clear advantage of eEVAR over OR, not many vascular units are in a position to provide a round-the-clock emergency endovascular service. The establishment of an eEVAR service is logistically challenging, wholly dependent on enthusiastic and committed personnel, requires specific equipment and a rigorous attention to protocols and technique.

Logistics of setting up an emergency endovascular service

Pre-operative imaging and patient selection

The assessment of suitability for endovascular repair requires some form of imaging. If the patient is sufficiently stable, CT provides information, which can allow detailed planning and will confirm the diagnosis. The use of angiography alone has been shown to be feasible by some workers, while others are sceptical of its accuracy in sizing stent grafts [8]. Angiographic measurements are based on 'intima-to-intima', while CT measurements are made from 'adventitia-to-adventitia'. In addition, the presence of thrombus within the lumen may further compromise the accuracy of angiography. It can be argued that accuracy may not be as important in a life-and-death situation, and if angiography were to be used, then slightly more over-sizing may be all that is required, and a thin concentric lining of thrombus does not always signify unsuitability. A reasonable approach is to proceed directly to angiography for those patients who are markedly unstable and use CT for the more stable. Lloyd et al [9] have demonstrated that in patients with rAAA, who do not undergo surgery, the median survival from the time of admission is ten hours and nearly 90% survived more than two hours after admission. Based on these data, pre-operative CT should be feasible for most patients with rAAA.

Equipment and venue

Whether eEVAR is peformed in a purpose-built endovascular suite, or in theatre with a mobile C-arm, is probably irrelevant. There are, however, certain prerequisites for eEVAR to be carried out safely and effectively. Appropriate positioning of the graft and the ability to identify and characterise any endoleak accurately and rapidly, requires high quality imaging systems and good angiographic techniques.

The operating light must be adequate, because of the need to perform a femoro-femoral bypass if an aorto-uni-liac (AUI) device was to be used. In addition, the potential for adjunctive surgical procedures is much greater than in elective EVAR. Conversion to OR will be required if the aneurysm cannot be excluded and the patient fails to stabilise. Some patients will develop a tense abdomen and necessitate prophylactic decompression to prevent abdominal compartment syndrome.

Type of graft

There is still much debate about whether a bifurcated or an AUI stent graft system is better for rAAA. The overriding requirement for any graft system is that it must be simple to use and will allow rapid exclusion of the aneurysm. An AUI system fulfils these requirements, and typically requires a smaller shelf stock to allow management of an adequate range of patient anatomy. The more promising AUI devices comprise two separate components with a universal joint that will allow the length to be adjusted by tromboning the distal portion into the proximal portion as necessary. A minimum stock of grafts should include:

- three proximal components with top diameters measuring 28mm, 32mm and 36mm;
- three distal components with bottom diameter of 16mm, 20mm and 24mm;
- one extension piece that will allow the length of the device to be adjusted as necessary between 150mm to 200mm; and
- two occluders measuring 18mm and 26mm. The precision in sizing the occluder is arguable, as occlusion of any contralateral iliac artery smaller than 24mm can be achieved with a 26mm device, the largest commercially available off-the-shelf device.

The need for a femoro-femoral crossover bypass graft to revascularise the contralateral leg adds to the procedure time, but is performed when the aneurysm is already excluded. Bifurcated systems are preferred by some workers and certainly, in the more stable patient, there is unlikely to be any difficulty in this approach [10]. Unfortunately, with the volatile nature of rAAA, any delays in cannulating the contralateral limb will risk loss of haemostasis. To minimise this risk, Jongkind et al [11] have described a bifurcated graft with a haemostatic valve in the contralateral limb stump, which will maintain exclusion of the aneurysm until it is cannulated. This will permit rapid exclusion of the aneurysm and at the same time avoid the need for an extra-anatomical bypass.

Personnel

The emergency treatment of rAAA requires all the appropriate personnel to be assembled within a short time frame. The members of this emergency endovascular team will vary from institution to institution, but should include all the usual staff involved in OR and, depending on local set-up, an interventional radiologist, radiographer and radiology nurse. Although surgical teams have always been involved in the management of rAAA, participation in such an onerous emergency service may stretch the resources of even the most supportive interventional radiology departments. Nevertheless, the successful provision of an emergency endovascular service will depend on a good working relationship within an enthusiastic group, which must be established from the outset. Training of nursing staff, some of whom may only work night shifts, is vital in order that they are *au fait* with all the devices and endovascular techniques. The anaesthetist should be aware of resuscitation and anaesthetic protocols for eEVAR, as this will differ from elective and OR cases. The CT scan staff will inevitably form part of the eEVAR team. Their co-operation is vital in the initial assessment, as the relative risk of the patient dying while undergoing a CT scan may be unacceptable to some.

Patient suitability

There are many factors to consider when deciding whether a patient is suitable for eEVAR. Conventional vascular teaching has always been to operate on rAAA as soon as the diagnosis is made, based on clinical findings of abdominal pain with or without back pain, hypotension and collapse. eEVAR defies this traditional practice by delaying surgery in order to allow further investigations to assess for suitability. In the stable patient, this delay may be acceptable, but in the unstable patient any delay in treatment may be difficult to fathom and justify, especially when there is a likelihood that the patient may be morphologically unsuitable.

Anatomical suitability

CT scan criteria for elective EVAR suitability are generally similar for most of the commercially available graft systems. If these criteria were to be applied to the emergency situation, only about 20% of rAAA patients will be suitable for EVAR, the largest limiting factor being proximal neck length of <1.5cm [12]. However, the proportion of patients reported to be suitable appears to be higher, as most practitioners are more tolerant of adverse anatomical features that would normally prejudice against EVAR in the elective setting. Neck diameter of up to 32mm and iliac diameter of 22mm are probably still acceptable, as there are commercially available off-the-shelf devices of 36mm and of 24mm, allowing for an oversize of approximately 10% respectively. Although some workers have treated neck lengths <1cm and achieved haemostatic seal, necks this short should only be attempted in the absence of other unfavourable features, and might require an adjunctive procedure, such as placement of a balloon expandable stent (Palmaz, Cordis Corp, Miami Florida USA) at the time of surgery or later during follow-up.

While the neck of the aneurysm is the most critical area, at least one iliac system needs to be suitable for delivery of the stent graft. Likewise, the presence of one unfavourable factor in the iliac artery alone may not rule out EVAR, but any combination of wall calcification, diameter of 7mm and tortuosity should deter any attempts at stenting. The presence of a unilateral iliac artery aneurysm does not preclude eEVAR if the contralateral iliac is suitable, but if the aneurysm involves both iliac systems to their bifurcation, exclusion of the aneurysm complex will be difficult. Coiling of the internal iliac arteries and extending the stent graft beyond the aneurysmal segments to the external iliac artery can be performed, except that this will lead to long delays in excluding the aneurysm.

Pre-operative preparation and intra-operative considerations

An advantage of working in a team, consisting of surgeons and radiologists, is the ability to divide up the task of assessing and resuscitating the patient, evaluating the CT scan and planning the device, and preparing the operating room. The latter should preferably be prepared to deal with either open or endovascular repair. It is advisable to have an emergency endovascular box, stocked with all the wires, catheters and other angiographic equipment likely to be needed for eEVAR. This allows out of hours theatre nurses with relatively limited experience of EVAR procedures to set up a comprehensive trolley.

Patient resuscitation

Regardless of the decision, patient resuscitation and preparation should commence as soon as the diagnosis is suspected. Any attempts at aggressive fluid resuscitation of patients with rAAA must be resisted. The blood pressure should be kept stable, rather than raised above that at presentation, unless the patient's level of consciousness is affected. The exact criteria for stability remain to be defined, but the level of consciousness and a systolic blood pressure of >50mmHg is usually a good guide [8]. There is compelling evidence in animal studies and in trauma patients that the use of 'hypotensive resuscitation' or 'permissive hypotension' leads to improved survival compared to normotensive or immediate resuscitation [13,14]. Permissive hypotension is believed to allow clot formation and avoid coagulopathy which are vital determinants in the outcome of patients with rAAA.

Type of anaesthesia and patient preparation

Patients with rAAA are in a state of compensated shock with maximal vasoconstriction. Induction of general anaesthesia is associated with a loss of arterial sympathetic tone and relaxation of the abdominal wall musculature. This causes loss of tamponade, frequently causing complete circulatory collapse and a significant increase in mortality. Most of the patients with rAAA treated by eEVAR are operated under regional anaesthesia [3]. In a series by Peppelenbosch et al [3], 58% of patients had local or regional anaesthesia.

The entire eEVAR procedure, including femoro-femoral cross-over, may be performed under local anaesthesia and an appropriate level of sedation, avoiding the precipitous hypotension associated with general anaesthesia [10]. Sedation should be just adequate to enable the patient to be comfortable and serene, but still compliant. Unfortunately, some patients can become agitated and restless and may require general anaesthesia. In most cases, induction of general anaesthesia may be deferred until the stent graft has been deployed and the aneurysm excluded [6].

The patient is always prepared and draped as for open repair, with access to both groins, allowing rapid conversion to OR if required. With experience, it is feasible to perform percutaneous access even in hypotensive patients with the aide of an ultrasound machine and closure devices [15]. However, at present, the closure devices available require placement prior to introduction of any large device, introducing a delay when surgical exposure of the common femoral arteries is necessary for femoro-femoral cross-over anastomoses, if an AUI system is used.

Aortic occlusion

This is only necessary when the patient becomes unstable. An occlusion balloon may be passed into the descending aorta via a transbrachial or transfemoral approach and many different techniques have been proposed. Unfortunately, maintaining the position of the occluding balloon passed through the femoral approach remains a problem due to its tendency to be expelled by the force of pulsatile blood within the abdominal aorta. Passing the balloon over a stiff wire may help but this alone is usually ineffective.

Matsuda et al [16] described a technique of passing the occlusion balloon into the aneurysm sack via the brachial artery and pulling back until the balloon is lodged in the neck from below [8,16]. This approach has advantages as it does not interfere with the passage of devices from the groin and the balloon can be moved to supra or infracoeliac positions as required. However, there are problems associated with this technique, such as:

◆ the balloon bursting and arterial embolism during manipulation around the aortic arch;
◆ difficulty in puncturing and exposing the artery in hypotensive patients;

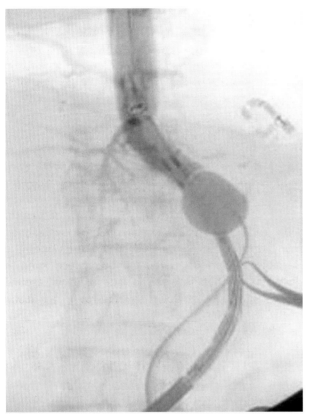

Figure 1. An occlusion balloon inflated in the aneurysm and wedged against the neck of the aneurysm in the infrarenal position.

♦ the artery being too small to accommodate the 14 to 16 French introducer sheaths, which are required for the insertion of the large balloon catheter; and

♦ manpower implications, as maintenance of the transbrachial balloon requires a surgeon or radiologist at the left upper limb.

Supracoeliac occlusion of the aorta should be avoided as much as possible to lessen the mass of tissue exposed to ischaemia/reperfusion injury. Infra-renal occlusion may be achieved through a femoral approach without detailed angiography by firstly passing a balloon over a guidewire through a long 14 French introducer sheath into the aneurysm sac. The balloon can then be inflated within the aneurysm and advanced with the sheath so that it wedges in the aneurysm neck from below. With the balloon in this position a second guidewire may be passed from the other groin and a graft delivered into position without having to deflate the balloon (Figure 1). Unfortunately,

the balloon requires deflation during deployment of the graft, but if required, occlusion can be maintained by moving it to the supracoeliac segment.

Trouble-shooting

As with elective EVAR, endoleaks remain the Achilles heel of this procedure. The checklist should be methodical, starting at the proximal neck with antero-posterior and lateral views. It is worth emphasising that many rAAA patients have less favourable necks than their elective counterparts and Type 1 endoleaks will be more common than in elective patients. As a result, the use of a balloon expandable Palmaz stent (Cordis Corp, Miami, Florida, USA), as an adjunctive measure, is a reasonable proposition to resolve any proximal endoleaks. These giant stents are crimped onto large balloons (Cristal Valvoplasty, Balt, Montmorency, France), but can easily be dislodged during its passage through artery and graft, unless it is passed through a long, large bore (16 French) sheath to its deployment position.

If there is difficulty identifying the site of the endoleak, it is advisable to perform a low injection rate run within the stent graft. If no contrast refluxes to the top of the graft, a proximal Type 1 endoleak is excluded or confirmed depending on whether the leak persists. A Type 2 and 4 endoleak may be left if the patient remains stable. Type 3 leaks are unusual, unless the overlap between the two components of the stent graft is inadequate. After the above checklist has been exhausted and a small endoleak is still visible, it is acceptable to speculate a degree of graft porosity. The latter is probably more commonly seen in rAAA than in elective cases, because of heamodilution and coagulopathy, which tend to be associated with large volumes of blood loss and fluid given for resuscitation. If the patient remains stable, it is reasonable to complete the procedure and re-image a couple of days postoperatively, using a duplex ultrasound or CT scan. However, re-intervention including conversion to OR, may be necessary if the patient becomes unstable.

In the presence of instability, it is possible to re-inflate an occlusion balloon in the proximal neck of the graft, preserving renal and mesenteric perfusion. A systematic approach to investigating continuing blood loss should be adopted and include a check of the rest of the aortic segments. Nevertheless, it is important to bear in mind that the risk of failure will be greater than in elective cases, especially when patients with less than ideal anatomy are to be offered eEVAR. In these situations, it might be best to convert to open repair earlier rather than later.

Postoperative recovery and complications

The image of a patient able to eat and mobilise the day after surgery has been used to champion eEVAR as a better technique of repairing rAAA than OR. Although there are many anecdotal reports of patients recovering rapidly following eEVAR without the need to stay in ICU, the physiological stress suffered by these patients must not be taken lightly. The amount of blood lost by patients undergoing eEVAR is often underestimated by the immeasurable volume concealed within the abdomen. The hypotension during induction of general anaesthesia for OR, which indicates the presence of significant hypovolaemia, may not occur during eEVAR, if this is performed under local anaesthesia. Nevertheless, the physiological stress that accompanies rAAA, even if repaired endovascularly, may still lead to the spectrum of complications that is often associated with OR. In addition, there are also potential problems that are unique to eEVAR that must be recognized.

Early complications

One obvious drawback of eEVAR is failure to successfully exclude the aneurysm sac, resulting in continued blood loss. If this is subtle, it can be difficult to detect at the time of surgery and only manifests as an inability to maintain a stable blood pressure during the recovery phase. Blood lost may be exacerbated by the presence of coagulopathy, which can also perpetuate the endoleak [3]. The importance of ensuring a homeostatic coagulation cannot be overemphasised. The prophylactic use of clotting factors and fresh frozen plasma should be considered in patients who require large volumes of fluid and blood replacement.

Organ failure

Most patients presenting with rAAA are elderly and often have other comorbidities that may be unknown even to the patient. The presence of these comorbid conditions will serve to delay recovery and lead to a poorer outcome, and may account for the 45% mortality rate quoted by Hinchliffe *et al* [4]. Many of their patients were unfit for OR and this is reflected by the number of patients who died from failure of various organs. Renal impairment has been reported in over a quarter of patients following eEVAR. It is likely that the hypotensive insult, large doses of contrast and inadvertent coverage of the renal arteries have aggravated latent renal impairment. Some may require renal support during the initial recovery phase, but very few end up requiring long-term renal dialysis [17].

Although bowel function is better preserved following eEVAR, the presence of a large retroperitoneal haematoma and free intraperitoneal blood can lead to impaired intestinal motility and function. A slow introduction to oral diet is recommended, even in patients who may appear to have tolerated the insult of rAAA and eEVAR favourably. In addition, the combination of hypotension, occlusion of the internal iliac arteries in some patients and increased abdominal compartment pressure can compromise mesenteric blood flow with the subsequent development of bowel ischaemia [3, 4].

Abdominal compartment syndrome

Another complication that may occur following eEVAR, but is likely to be underdiagnosed, is abdominal compartment syndrome (ACS) [17]. The increased intra-abdominal compartment pressure is due to the presence of blood within the abdomen, oedema of the viscera and distension of the intestine, the latter precipitated by the large amount of fluid given during resuscitation and ischaemia/reperfusion injury. Failure to recognise and treat ACS will result in increased risk of renal impairment, visceral and intestinal ischaemia, respiratory failure and death.

The possibility of acute ACS should be assumed if intra-abdominal pressure is ≥20mmHg, associated with diminishing urinary output and increasing airways pressure. If this is suspected abdominal decompression must be considered [18]. Decompression should take the form of haematoma evacuation and temporary abdominal closure to allow further decompression as required. The abdominal wound can be closed when it is feasible to approximate the wound edges without tension.

Perigraft collection and infection

Another complication which often occurs is the development of a perigraft collection in the tract of the femoro-femoral bypass (Figure 2). It is most probably multifactorial in origin and may be prevented by leaving a low-grade suction drain in the tract of the

bypass graft for 48 hours or more. The majority of perigraft collections are sterile, but infection of the femoro-femoral cross-over graft can develop [3]. The incidence of this is unknown, but with all the compounding factors that accompany rAAA, a course of prophylactic antibiotics should be considered.

Late complications

Organ failure

Failure of the various organs at midterm follow-up is also more common after eEVAR compared to OR. This may be due to the fact that patients with significant comorbidities, who may have died if OR were performed, have survived with eEVAR [3]. However, unlike elective EVAR, there is no catch-up of the initial survival advantage of eEVAR over OR.

Graft migration

The more unfavourable anatomy of rAAA will predispose to stent graft complications [3, 19]. In addition, the aneurysm neck of rAAA has been found to dilate at a greater rate than elective AAA [20] (Figure 3). As a result, the cumulative risk of secondary procedures was found to be around 35% at two years, with a late conversion rate to OR of 9% due to migration. Consequently, there is a temptation to counter these potential complications by increasing the percentage oversize of the stent graft [20]. However,

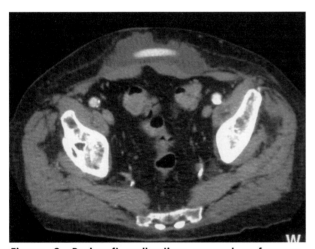

Figure 2. Perigraft collection around a femoro-femoral bypass graft.

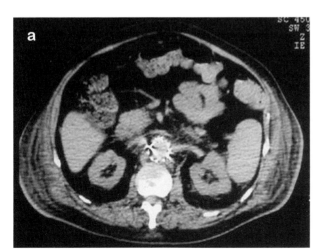
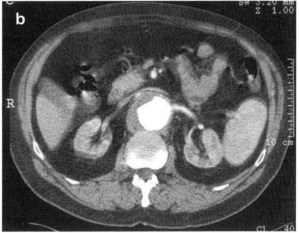

Figure 3. Rapid neck dilatation post-endovascular repair in a patient with a ruptured aneurysm. a) Measured 2.9cm at two months. b) Measured 3.7cm at six months post-repair.

greater oversizing may cause more dilatation as the radial force of self-expanding stents is proportional to the percentage of oversize.

In view of the adverse anatomy and high incidence of complications, it has been proposed that eEVAR should be considered a temporising procedure, used to convert an acute unstable situation to a controlled stable one, to allow the patient to be optimised for late open conversion if necessary [19]. Although this contentious practice may be a logical proposal in fit patients who have evidence of irredeemable stent graft complication and adverse anatomy, it may be difficult in those who have multiple comorbidities. Nevertheless, in patients who are unfit, it is possible to limit the extent of open conversion by using the stent graft as the conduit and suturing the graft to the neck of the aneurysm and securing the junction of the different components. This will avoid the need to cross-clamp the aorta and replace the stent graft, even though it is mandatory to have control of the aneurysm neck in case the graft were to be displaced accidentally.

Conclusions

There is no doubt that eEVAR is a feasible alternative of repairing rAAA. However, the provision of an emergency endovascular service is logistically difficult and will challenge even the most enthusiastic of centres. Although current non-randomised data would indicate a survival advantage in eEVAR over OR in selected patients, there is no convincing evidence that it offers the same benefit in unstable patients. Unfortunately, it is in this unstable group of patients that eEVAR needs to show better outcome before it will appeal to the majority of endovascular teams.

Summary

◆ EVAR for rAAA is feasible, but logistically challenging.

◆ Factors necessary to establish an eEVAR service include an enthusiastic team, a stock of devices and good imaging facilities in a sterile room with adequate lighting.

◆ Fluid resuscitation should be restricted to allow permissive hypotension.

◆ Local anaesthesia is preferable to general anaesthesia.

◆ Raised intra-abdominal pressure should be relieved if abdominal compartment syndrome is suspected.

◆ Complications are frequent and a good knowledge of endovascular techniques is required to deal with them.

◆ eEVAR should be viewed as a temporising procedure.

◆ Benefit of eEVAR is still unproven in unstable patients.

References

1. Bown MJ, Sutton AJ, Bell PRF, *et al*. A meta-analysis of 50 years of ruptured abdominal aortic aneurysm repair. *Br J Surg* 2002; 89: 714-30.
2. Yusuf SW, Whitaker SC, Chuter TAM, *et al*. Emergency endovascular repair of leaking aortic aneurysm. *Lancet* 1994; 344: 1645.
3. Peppelenbosch N, Yilamz N, van Marrewijk M, *et al*. Emergency treatment of acute symptomatic or ruptured abdominal aortic aneurysm. Outcome of a prospective intent-to-treat by EVAR protocol. *Eur J Vasc Endovasc Surg* 2003; 26: 303-10.
4. Hinchliffe RJ, Yusuf SW, Macierewicz JA, *et al*. Endovascular repair of ruptured abdominal aortic aneurysm - a challenge to open repair? Results of a single centre experience in 20 patients. *Eur J Vasc Endovasc Surg* 2001; 22: 528-34.
5. Peppelenbosch N, Geelkerkeen RH, Soong C, *et al*. Endograft treatment of ruptured abdominal aortic aneurysm using the Talent AUI system. International multicenter study. Abstract Book. Annual Meeting of the American Society for Vascular Surgery, 2005.
6. Hinchcliffe RJ, Braithwaite BD, Hopkinson BR. The endovacular management of ruptured abdominal aortic aneurysms. *Eur J Vasc Endovasc Surg* 2003; 25: 191-201.
7. Veith FJ for the EVAR ruptured aortic aneurysm investigators. Update on endovascular repair of ruptured abdominal aortic and thoracic aneurysms: the collected world experience. 2005; 13: S38-39.
8. Ohki T, Veith FJ. Endovascular grafts and other image-guided catheter-based adjuncts to improve the treatment of ruptured aortoiliac aneurysms. *Ann Surg* 2000; 232: 466-79.
9. Lloyd GM, Brown MJ, Norwood MG, *et al*. Feasibility of preoperative computer tomography in patients with ruptured abdominal aortic aneurysm: a time-to-death study in patients without operation. *J Vasc Surg* 2004; 39(4): 788-91.
10. Verhoeven EL, Prins TR, van den Dungen JJ, *et al*. Endovascular repair of acute AAAs under local anesthesia with bifurcated endografts: a feasibility study. *J Endovasc Ther* 2002; 9(2): 158-64.
11. Jongkind V, Diks J, Linsen MA, *et al*. A temporary hemostatic valve in the short limb of a bifurcated stent-graft to facilitate endovascular repair of ruptured aortic aneurysm: experimental findings. *J Endovasc Ther* 2005; 12(1): 66-9.
12. Rose DF, Davidson JR, Hinchcliffe RJ, *et al*. Anatomical suitability or ruptured abdominal aortic aneurysms for endovascular repair. *J Endovasc Ther* 2003; 10(3): 453-7.
13. Owens T, Watson WT, Prough MD, *et al*. Limiting initial resuscitation of uncontrolled haemorrhage reduces internal bleeding and subsequent volume requirements. *J Trauma* 1995; 39: 200-9.
14. Bickell WH, Wall MJ Jr, Pepe PE, *et al*. Immediate versus delayed fluid resuscitation for hypotensive patients with penetrating torso injuries. *N Engl J Med* 1994; 331: 1105-9.
15. Howell M, Villarel R, Krajcer Z. Percutaneous access and closure of femoral artery access sites associated with endoluminal repair of abdominal aortic aneurysms. *J Endovasc Ther* 2001; 8(1): 68-74.
16. Matsuda H, Tanaka Y, Hino Y, *et al*. Transbrachial arterial insertion of aortic occlusion balloon in patients with shock from ruptured abdominal aortic aneurysm. *J Vasc Surg* 2003; 38: 1293-6.
17. Lachat ML, Pfammatter Th, Witzke HJ, *et al*. Endovascular repair with bifurcated stent grafts under local anaesthesia to improve outcome of ruptured aortoiliac aneurysms. *Eur J Vasc Endovasc Surg* 2002; 23: 528-36.
18. Meldrum DR, Moore FA, Moore EE, *et al*. Prospective characterization and selective management of the abdominal compartment syndrome. *Am J Surg* 1997; 174: 667072.
19. Hechelhammer L, Lachat ML, Wildermuth S, *et al*. Midterm outcome of endovascular repair of ruptured abdominal aortic aneurysms. *J Vasc Surg* 2005; 41: 752-57.
20. Badger SA, O'Donnell ME, Makar R, *et al*. Aortic necks of ruptured abdominal aneurysms dilate more than asymptomatic aneurysms following endovascular repair. Annual Meeting of the Vascular Society of Great Britain and Ireland, Yearbook 2005: 56.

Chapter 4

EVAR for fit patients: evidence from the randomised trials

Jonathan D Beard ChM MEd FRCS, Consultant Vascular Surgeon

Sheffield Vascular Institute, The Northern General Hospital, Sheffield, UK

Introduction

Elective repair of abdominal aortic aneurysm (AAA) is undertaken to prevent subsequent rupture, which carries a mortality of 80%. Open surgical repair has been used for more than 50 years and has proved remarkably durable, with a graft failure rate of about 0.3% per year [1]. However, this is major surgery that is often required in elderly patients with significant cardiac, respiratory and renal comorbidity. Unsurprisingly, it carries significant peri-operative mortality and morbidity, plus a recovery time of several months. Therefore, the dilemma is whether to risk an open repair in an asymptomatic patient, whose individual risk of rupture is largely a matter of guesswork.

Endovascular repair of abdominal aortic aneurysm (EVAR) was developed to provide a less traumatic alternative to open repair. Over the last ten years EVAR has mushroomed from a technique that was performed only by a few early pioneers to one that is routinely practised by many vascular centres. A recent systematic literature review has found nearly 20,000 reported cases of EVAR [2]. During this developmental phase, most information came from registries such as RETA and EUROSTAR [3,4], and these registries helped to inform the design of the subsequent randomised trials. Two such trials of EVAR versus open repair have now been published and this chapter concentrates on the evidence from these trials.

Trial design

The two published randomised trials of open versus endovascular AAA repair are the UK EVAR 1 trial [5] and the Dutch Randomised Endovascular Aneurysm Management (DREAM) trial [6]. The detailed methodology of the EVAR 1 trial has been published previously [7]. Centres were required to have submitted data on 20 EVAR procedures to the RETA registry before entry into the trial. All patients being considered for AAA repair were registered to provide data on generalisability.

Entry criteria were patients over 60 years with a non-ruptured AAA (CT diameter 5.5cm or more in any plane), who were deemed fit enough for open repair and morphologically suitable for EVAR. Fitness for surgery was determined locally, according to guidelines for cardiac, respiratory and renal status. Morphological suitability for EVAR and choice of stent-graft was also decided locally. Patients deemed unfit for open repair were entered into the EVAR 2 trial (see Chapter 5).

The primary outcome for EVAR 1 was long-term mortality and the recruitment target was 900 patients to provide an 80% power for detecting at the 5% significance level a reduction in total mortality from 7.5% to 5% per year. Aneurysm-related mortality (deaths occurring within 30 days of surgery and late complications of aneurysm repair, such as aortoduodenal fistula or aortic rupture after endografting) was also estimated. Secondary outcomes included the incidence of postoperative complications of aneurysm repair and secondary interventions, Health Related Quality of Life (HRQL) and hospital costs. To monitor graft durability, CT scan data were collected annually for all patients in both treatment groups with EVAR patients having additional CT scans at one and three months post-procedure. Analysis was on an intention to treat basis.

The DREAM Trial had a similar protocol to the EVAR 1 trial, apart from a lower AAA diameter threshold of 5cm or greater, and a primary endpoint that was a composite of operative mortality and complications. Ongoing trials with a similar protocol are being performed in France: Aneurisme de l'aorte abdominale Chirugie versus Endoprosthese (ACE) and the United States: veterans affairs Open Versus Endovascular Repair (OVER).

Short-term results

Between 1999 and 2003, 1082 elective patients with an AAA ≥5.5cm, from 34 centres in the UK, were randomised to EVAR (n=543) or open repair (n=539). The trial, therefore, exceeded its recruitment target by a considerable margin and 94% of patients complied with the allocated treatment. During a similar time-period, 345 elective patients with an AAA ≥5cm, from 24 centres in the Netherlands and four centres in Belgium, were randomised to EVAR (n=171) or open repair (n=174). Because of the smaller minimum AAA diameter in the DREAM trial, the baseline characteristics of the two trials differed slightly, with a lower mean AAA diameter of 6cm compared to 6.5cm and a lower mean age of 70 compared to 74 years in the Dream and EVAR 1 trials respectively.

The data from the UK RETA and European EUROSTAR registries suggested that EVAR had an early mortality of about 1-2% for patients who were deemed fit for open repair [3,4]. This compared favourably with the higher mortality of 3-6% from open repair in the previous trials in the UK and the USA of surveillance versus open repair in small aneurysms >5.5cm diameter [8,9]. A study of the 2001 Nationwide Inpatient Sample in the USA found a similar mortality of 3.8% for open repair and 1.3% for EVAR [10].

The short-term efficacy of EVAR was confirmed by both randomised trials, both of which produced results that were almost identical to the registry and US data. The UK EVAR 1 trial reported a 30-day mortality for EVAR of 1.7% compared with 4.7% for open repair [5] and the DREAM trial results were 1.2% and 4.6% respectively [6]. The difference in mortality was significant in the EVAR 1 trial (p=0.009), but neither operative mortality nor the combined endpoint achieved statistical significance in the DREAM trial, probably because of the small sample size. Despite this, the DREAM authors rashly concluded that "endovascular repair is preferable to open repair", whereas the EVAR 1 authors were more cautious, stating that their findings "were a license to continue scientific evaluation but not to change clinical practice".

Nevertheless, we now have data from two registries and two trials that show remarkable agreement in terms of operative mortality. This equates to level I evidence that EVAR more than halves the operative mortality rate from elective AAA repair. This is a difference that many patients will find irresistible, whatever worries there are about long-term durability.

Applicability

During the course of the EVAR trials, the 34 centres registered 4799 patients for consideration for entry into either EVAR 1 or 2 trials. Three thousand nine hundred and twenty-seven (82%) of these patients consented to have a CT scan that was reviewed for EVAR suitability and to confirm that the aneurysm measured at least 5.5cm in diameter. Of these, 2132 (54%) were considered anatomically suitable for EVAR, but the suitability for EVAR ranged dramatically between centres from 6-100%. The reasons for this are currently being investigated, as it has been suggested that centres with a high rate of EVAR applicability might have a higher device-related complication rate (see next section). A consequence of the substantial percentage of patients found anatomically unsuitable for EVAR is that vascular surgeons will still need to perform open repair in the future. In fact, open repair is likely to become more difficult as the 'easy' cases with long infrarenal necks will be treated by EVAR, leaving those with a short or no neck to the vascular surgeon. We should, therefore, be careful to ensure that outcomes are based on results by centre rather than results by technique.

Long-term results

The RETA and EUROSTAR registries indicated a need for close surveillance of endografts for many years, as procedure-related complications occurred at a rate of 10-15% per annum [3, 4]. These complications included: neck dilatation and/or dislodgement of the graft; stent fractures, fabric tears or component separation; secondary endoleaks from patent lumbar arteries; aneurysm rupture due to endotension from endoleaks; and kinking of the endograft as the aneurysm sac shrank. Such complications could usually be treated by further endovascular intervention, but the concern was that the need for continued surveillance and subsequent intervention would increase the costs of EVAR and adversely affect the long-term mortality [11].

As the technology of EVAR developed, it was anticipated that graft durability would improve and the number of complications reported would diminish. The EUROSTAR registry analysed the long-term complications of 1428 'current' second-generation devices and 2777 older first-generation devices that had been withdrawn. There was a significant reduction of almost 10% in the number of device-related complications at three years in the current second-generation devices (p=0.0008) [12]. A more recent report from the EUROSTAR registry has compared the rate of complications in second generation devices (Stentor and Vanguard) with third generation devices (Excluder, Talent and Zenith). The all-cause mortality, aneurysm-related mortality and procedure-related complications were all significantly

lower in the newer devices, as was the rate of secondary interventions (12.9% vs 4.4%) [14]. The devices used in the EVAR 1 and DREAM trials were mainly second-generation devices plus some third-generation endografts. Randomisation continued after the formal end of the EVAR 1 trial to enable more of these third generation devices to be subsequently analysed on the basis of temporal (tracker trial) stratification in the anticipation that there might be a further improvement in endograft durability [13]. Only the EVAR 1 trial has reported long-term results thus far [15].

Mortality

By 31st December 2004, the proportion of patients in the EVAR 1 trial who had the potential to be followed-up for at least at one, two, three and four years was 100%, 70%, 47% and 24% respectively (median follow-up 2.9 years). There were 209 deaths: 53 from aneurysm-related causes and 68 from cardiovascular disorders. All-cause mortality at four years after randomisation was similar in the two groups (around 28%) and the survival curves to four years showed no difference between the groups: crude hazard ratio 0.90 (95% CI 0.69-1.18), p=0.46 (Figure 1). However, there was a persistent difference in aneurysm-related mortality of 4% for the EVAR group and 7% for the open repair group by four years: crude hazard ratio 0.55 (95% CI 0.31-0.96), p=0.04 (Figure 1). However, aneurysm-related mortality was an estimate, as only 16% of those who died had a post mortem to confirm the cause of death. There were no significant interactions, for either total or aneurysm-related mortality, with age, sex, aneurysm diameter or creatinine.

Complications

During the first four years of follow-up, the overall rates of complications and re-interventions appeared to decrease as well as diverge between the two groups (Figure 2). By 31st December 2004, the proportion of patients with at least one postoperative complication was 41% (95% CI 36-46) in the EVAR group, compared to 9% (95% CI 7-13) in the open repair group. Similarly, the proportion of patients with at least one re-intervention by four years was 20%

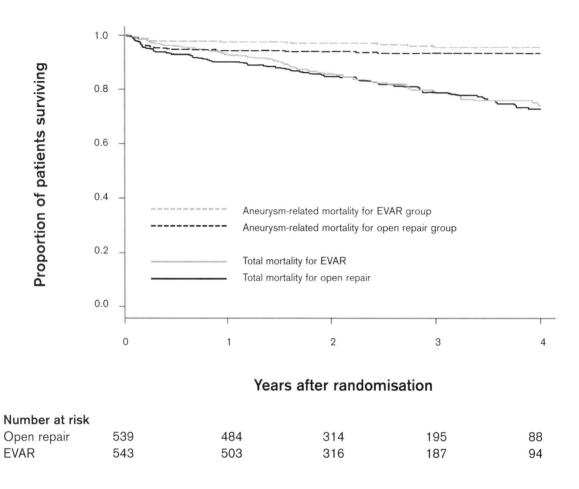

Number at risk					
Open repair	539	484	314	195	88
EVAR	543	503	316	187	94

Figure 1. Survival and survival free from aneurysm-related death by randomised group for up to 4 years from randomisation. At 4 years, all-cause mortality was 26% for the EVAR group and 29% for the open repair group, crude hazard ratio=0.90 (95% CI 0.69-1.18), p=0.46. At 4 years, aneurysm-related mortality was 4% for the EVAR group and 7% for the open repair group, crude hazard ratio=0.55 (95% CI 0.31-0.96), p=0.04. *Reproduced with permission from Elsevier* [15].

(95% CI 16-26) in the EVAR group and 6% (95% CI 4-8) in the open repair group (Figure 2). There were 14 conversions to open repair following EVAR; four during the primary procedure, two more during the primary admission and eight after initial discharge from hospital. The annual complication rate of about 10% per annum matches the registry data, although the decrease in complications with time is encouraging. It is also encouraging that the early mortality advantage from EVAR seems to have been maintained, despite the need for secondary intervention due to device-related complications.

Quality of life

The HRQL scores were similar to age and sex-matched population norms and between EVAR and open repair in both the EVAR 1 and DREAM trial. Both trials showed a diminished HRQL in the open repair group at one month. However, this rapidly recovered and the DREAM trial actually reported an improved HRQL for the open repair group by six months[16]. This trial also found that the risk of post-procedure impotence in male patients was not decreased by EVAR. This may be due to the need to embolise one

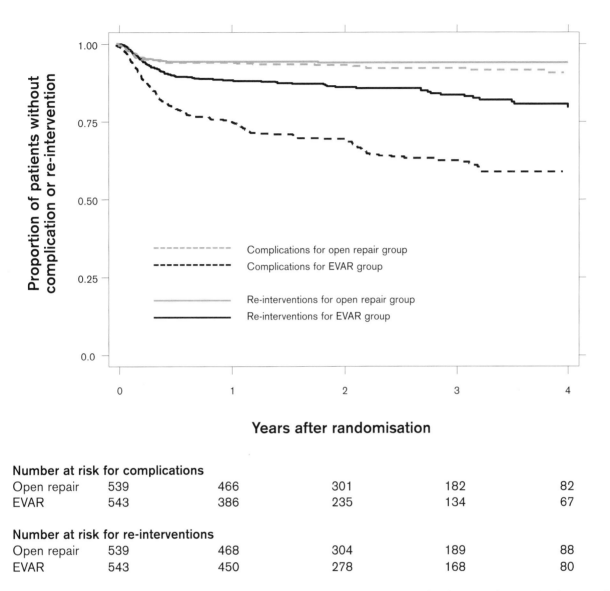

Number at risk for complications

Open repair	539	466	301	182	82
EVAR	543	386	235	134	67

Number at risk for re-interventions

Open repair	539	468	304	189	88
EVAR	543	450	278	168	80

Figure 2. Postoperative complications and re-interventions by randomised group for up to 4 years from randomisation. At 4 years, complications had occurred in 41% of patients in the EVAR group and 9% in the open repair group, crude hazard ratio=4.9 (95% CI 3.5-6.8), p<0.0001. At 4 years, re-interventions had occurred in 20% of patients in the EVAR group and 6% in the open repair group, crude hazard ratio=2.7 (95% CI 1.8-4.1), p<0.0001. *Reproduced with permission from Elsevier* [15].

or both internal iliac arteries to prevent distal endoleak in over 10% of patients. The EVAR 1 trial found no difference in HRQL between the two groups at either 3-12 or 12-24 months.

Costs

The costs for the primary procedure and hospitalisation were £10,818 and £9,204 for the EVAR and open repair groups respectively, a mean difference £1,613 (SE 607). The mean estimated costs per patient over four years were £13,258 for the

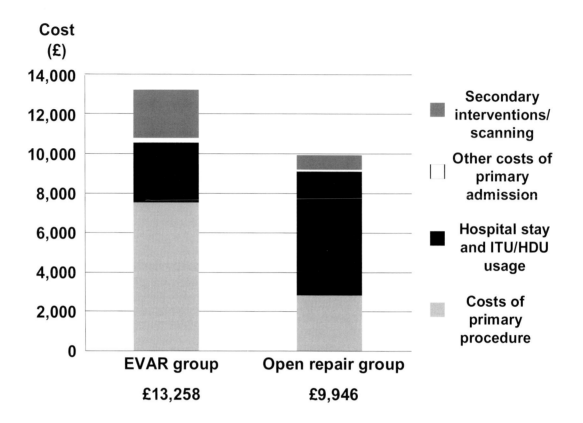

Figure 3. The mean estimated costs per patient over 4 years were £13,258 for the EVAR group and £9,946 for the open repair group, a mean difference of £3,311 (SE 690). The shorter ITU and hospital stay in the EVAR group does not compensate for the initial cost of the endograft and the subsequent cost of secondary interventions.

EVAR group and £9,946 for the open repair group, a mean difference of £3,311 (SE 690). The shorter ITU and hospital stay in the EVAR group did not compensate for the initial cost of the endograft and the subsequent cost of surveillance and secondary interventions (Figure 3).

The future for EVAR

There are some clear messages from the results of the randomised trials that are reinforced by similar results from the registries. EVAR has a significant benefit in terms of early mortality, but this is offset by the high rate of device-related complications that requires regular surveillance and re-intervention. Although this

did not result in any increased mortality in the EVAR 1 trial, concern remains about any long-term benefit in overall mortality. EVAR is also more expensive with no long-term advantage in quality of life. Economic modelling suggests that both the cost of the endograft and the re-intervention rate will need to be reduced for the procedure to become cost-effective [17].

It has been postulated that suprarenal fixation, fenestrated grafts, endovascular sutures and laparoscopic 'assist' will reduce the risk of endoleaks, but there is no good evidence for these claims at present. However, technology continues to evolve rapidly and new endograft materials, including polymers and ceramics, are under development. These are likely to supplant the existing 'wire and fabric' technology that is reminiscent of the first aeroplanes. If the current regulations were applied to the first generation of aeroplanes, it seems unlikely that any of us would be flying regularly today!

The conclusion at present must be that EVAR has still to be regarded as an experimental procedure. Therefore, it seems essential that patients are fully informed of its limitations and uncertainties, as well as the early benefits. The National Institute for Health and Clinical Excellence in the UK has recommended that EVAR be carried out only as part of a clinical trial or with appropriate data submission to a registry [18]. In the absence of another trial, all clinicians in the UK have a duty to submit their data to the RETA Registry. This registry, like EUROSTAR, is voluntary and there has been a large fall-off in data submission since the end of the EVAR 1 trial. Registry data have been shown to accurately predict the results of subsequent trials, and so one solution for the future would be a compulsory national registry. This could be supported by industry (as at present), linked to re-imbursement to ensure compliance, and the results used to track new developments in endograft technology. Registry data could become even more powerful if national results were combined into a central European registry.

Summary

◆ EVAR more than halves operative mortality from about 4-5% to 1-2% in fit patients with AAA >5cm.

◆ Patients must be fully informed of the long-term uncertainties as well as the short-term benefits of EVAR, compared to open repair, as it remains an experimental procedure.

◆ There is no difference in long-term overall mortality between EVAR and open repair and EVAR does not result in any long-term improvement in quality of life.

◆ EVAR is associated with a 10% risk of aneurysm-related complications per annum but most complications can be dealt with by further endovascular re-intervention.

◆ The costs of the endograft, combined with the costs of surveillance and re-intervention, outweigh the savings in hospital stay and ITU usage.

◆ The durability of endografts must be improved for them to become cost-effective.

◆ Compulsory national registries are required to monitor the development of new endograft technology.

References

1. Hallett JW Jr, Marshall DM, Petterson TM, *et al*. Graft-related complications after abdominal aortic aneurysm repair: reassurance from a 36-year population-based experience. *J Vasc Surg* 1997; 25: 277-86.

2. Drury D, Michaels JA, Jones L, Ayiku L. Systematic review of recent evidence for the safety and efficacy of elective endovascular repair in the management of infra-renal abdominal aortic aneurysms. *Br J Surg* 2005; 92: 937-46.

3. Thomas SM, Gaines PA, Beard JD, on behalf of the Vascular Surgical Society of Great Britain & Ireland and the British Society of Interventional Radiology. Short-term (30-day outcome of endovascular treatment of abdominal aortic aneurysms: results from the prospective Registry of Endovascular Treatment of Abdominal Aortic Aneurysms (RETA). *Eur J Vasc Endovasc Surg* 2001; 21: 57-64.

4. Harris PL, Vallabhaneni SR, Desgranges P, Becquemin JP, Van Marrewijk C, Laheij RJF. Incidence and risk factors of late rupture, conversion and death after endovascular repair of

infrarenal aortic aneurysms: the EUROSTAR experience. *J Vasc Surg* 2000; 32: 739-49.

5.   The EVAR trial participants. Comparison of endovascular aneurysm repair with open repair in patients with abdominal aortic aneurysm (EVAR trial 1), 30-day operative mortality results: randomised controlled trial. *Lancet* 2004; 364: 843-48.

6.   Prinssen M, Verhoeven EL, Buth J, *et al.* A randomised trial comparing conventional and endovascular repair of abdominal aortic aneurysms. *New Engl J Med* 2004; 351: 1607-18.

7.   Brown LC, Epstein D, Manca A, Beard JD, Powell JT, Greenhalgh RM. The UK EndoVascular Aneurysm Repair (EVAR) Trials: design, methodology and progress. *Eur J Vasc Endovasc Surg* 2004; 27: 372-81.

8.   The UK small aneurysm trial participants. Long-term outcomes of immediate repair compared with surveillance of small abdominal aortic aneurysms. *Lancet* 1998; 352: 1649-55.

9.   Lederle FA, Wilson SE, Johnson GR, *et al.* Immediate repair compared with surveillance of small abdominal aortic aneurysms. *N Engl J Med* 2002; 346: 1437-44.

10. Lee WA, Carter JW, Upchurch G, Seeger JM, Huber TS. Perioperative outcomes after open and endovascular repair of intact abdominal aortic aneurysms in the United States during 2001. *J Vasc Surg* 2004; 39: 491-6.

11. Thomas SM, Beard JD, Ireland M, Ayers S, on behalf of the Vascular Society of Great Britain & Ireland and the British Society of Interventional Radiology. Results from the Prospective Registry of Endovascular Treatment of Abdominal Aortic Aneurysms (RETA): midterm results to five years. *Eur J Vasc Endovasc Surg* 2005; 29 (6): 563-70.

12. Torella F and EUROSTAR collaborators. Effect of improved design on outcome of endovascular aneurysm repair. *J Vasc Surg* 2004; 40: 216-21.

13. Lilford RJ, Braunholz DA, Greenhalgh R, Edwards SJ. Trials and fast changing technologies: the case for tracker studies. *Br Med J* 2000; 320: 43-6.

14. Leurs LJ, Buth J, on behalf of the EUROSTAR collaborators. Annual risk of adverse events after endovascular abdominal aortic aneurysm repair. A comparison between the second and third generation stent-grafts. *Eur J Vasc Endovasc Surg* 2006: in press.

15. The EVAR Trial Participants. Endovascular aneurysm repair versus open repair in patients with abdominal aortic aneurysm (EVAR Trial 1): randomised controlled trial. *Lancet* 2005; 365: 2179-86.

16. Prinssen M, Buskens E, Blankensteijn JD and DREAM trial participants. Quality of life after endovascular and open AAA repair. Results of a randomised trial. *Eur J Vasc Endovasc Surg* 2002; 27: 121-27.

17. Michaels JA, Drury D, Thomas SM. Cost-effectiveness of endovascular abdominal aortic aneurysm repair (EVAR): an economic model to inform clinical practice and research. *Br J Surg* 2005; 92: 960-67.

18. National Institute for Clinical Excellence (Great Britain). Stent-graft placement in abdominal aortic aneurysm, guidance (IPG010), London, UK, 2003.

Chapter 5

EVAR for unfit patients: evidence from the randomised trials

Robert K Fisher MD FRCS, Endovascular Fellow

John Rose FRCP FRCR, Consultant Interventional Radiologist

Northern Vascular Centre, Freeman Hospital, Newcastle upon Tyne, UK

Introduction

The presence of an abdominal aortic aneurysm (AAA) may be considered as a surrogate marker for other systemic diseases. A recent study reported that, across a population of patients with AAA, 67% had coronary artery occlusive disease, 63% hypertension, 24% peripheral vascular disease, 22% chronic obstructive pulmonary disease, 10% diabetes, and 7.3% renal failure [1]. The prevalence of these comorbidities will, by definition, be greater in patients considered 'high risk'. Since its introduction in 1991, there has been a perception that EVAR would especially benefit the unfit patient requiring AAA repair. Indeed, studies have indicated that the stress response to EVAR is significantly less than to open AAA repair. Pearson et al compared neuroendocrine responses in patients undergoing open AAA repair with those receiving EVAR [2]. They reported a significantly reduced cortisol response in patients undergoing EVAR, as well as a significantly lower incidence of systemic inflammatory response syndrome, sepsis and all complications. Such potential benefit has been attributed to several factors. The minimal access associated with EVAR imparts an obvious surgical advantage. As techniques have continued to be refined, as superior generations of devices have been introduced and as surgical and radiological experiences have increased, the

operation times for routine stent placement have been reported as shorter than open procedure [1]. There is additional benefit with EVAR in terms of reduced blood loss, improved postoperative respiratory function, early mobilisation and introduction of oral diet. In appropriate cases, the minimal access endovascular technique also enables the use of local anaesthesia instead of general or spinal anaesthesia. Considering all of these potential advantages, it would appear reasonable to deem EVAR as the procedure of choice for high-risk patients compared to open operation.

Furthermore, since untreated rupture is usually fatal, there would appear to be a strong indication for EVAR over conservative management, in those patients considered unfit for open surgical repair. However, since the risk of rupture cannot be calculated precisely, our poor understanding of the natural history of AAA may actually distort clinical judgement in such cases. Studies suggest an average rupture rate of 11% per annum for AAA greater than 5cm, but there remains a degree of subjectivity in balancing the rupture risk against the risk of intervention. Reports have correlated aneurysm expansion rates with diameter and smoking status [3], which may help to estimate an approximate risk. But these results are derived from data from trial populations and may not represent a standard surveillance cohort, nor a population of high-risk patients, whose disease progression may be accelerated.

Therefore, a patient unfit for open repair has the option of EVAR or conservative management. Whilst one may accept that the comorbidities will significantly reduce life expectancy in this population, the dilemma presenting itself is: will EVAR sufficiently reduce the all-cause mortality to justify its use? Clarification has been sought through interrogation of registries, such as the EUROpean collaborators on Stent-graft Techniques for abdominal aortic Aneurysm Repair (EUROSTAR) [4], and a (single) randomised trial [5].

Definition of the unfit patient

The precise definition of a patient unsuitable for open AAA repair is impossible and subjective opinion inevitably influences the clinical judgement of the surgeon, anaesthetist and potentially even the primary care physician making the initial referral. Comorbidities, such as cardiac, respiratory, renal and metabolic diseases, must be considered alongside the patient's age and body mass index. The individual and combined influences of each on the outcome after open and endovascular repair are difficult to quantify and evidence remains sparse.

Cardiac disease

Coronary artery occlusive disease is the commonest comorbidity in patients presenting with AAA, affecting up to two thirds. High peri-operative mortality in this group of patients is often due to myocardial ischaemia, induced by exceeding the anaerobic threshold (AT). The combination of cardiac and pulmonary disease is common and represents a potentially lethal union whose pre-operative identification may predict adverse outcome. Older *et al* reported on cardiopulmonary exercise testing (CPX), a method by which high risk surgical patients can be objectively identified [6]. They found that patients with cardiopulmonary disease resulting in an AT <11ml/min/kg had an 18% peri-operative mortality compared to that of 0.8% in patients with an AT >11ml/min/kg (p<0.001). Furthermore, they reported

that in the presence of pre-operative ischaemia, patients with a low threshold had a significantly higher mortality (42% versus 4% in those with high AT). They concluded that pre-operative ischaemia and pre-operative cardiac failure are independent risk factors for peri-operative mortality in the elderly. The quantification of anaerobic threshold through CPX alerts the clinician to those susceptible to adverse peri-operative events and may direct pre-operative management in an attempt to optimise the patient.

Respiratory disease

Chronic obstructive pulmonary disease (COPD) is known to be associated with an increased prevalence of AAA and acts as an independent predictor of rupture. Compton *et al* reported on the outcome of aneurysm repair in this group of oxygen-dependent COPD patients whose disease may be considered to preclude surgery [7]. They retrospectively studied 44 patients, 24 undergoing EVAR and 20 open repair. Hospital stay and postoperative morbidity was less in patients receiving EVAR, but there was no advantage in peri-operative or long-term mortality (0%) compared to open repair. Comparison with historical data indicated a survival benefit compared to untreated AAA greater than 6cm. These results suggest a potential advantage of EVAR over open and conservative management in the treatment of large aneurysms in COPD patients. However, no robust data exist to provide definitive conclusions.

Age

Atheromatous aneurysm formation in the abdominal aorta is an age-related disease, and whilst chronological age does not represent an absolute contraindication, it must be considered in conjunction with physiological status when determining suitability for EVAR. There is an acceptance that with progress through the ninth decade there is a diminishing physiological reserve irrespective of comorbidity, and the clinician may be reluctant to intervene. However, acceptable results following open and endovascular AAA repair in elderly patients have been reported [8, 9], although these are results from a single centre.

A recent interrogation of the EUROSTAR database has provided more robust results [10]. Lange *et al* reported early and late outcomes after EVAR, comparing 697 octogenarians with 4198 patients <80 years. The proportion of patients >80years undergoing EVAR rose during the study period from 11% in 1996 to 18% in 2004. There was a significantly higher incidence of cardiac, pulmonary and renal disease in the octogenarians, 32% of whom were deemed unfit for open repair, compared to 22% in the younger patients. Combined 30-day and in-hospital mortality was significantly higher in the older age group (5% vs. 2%) as were device-related and systemic complications (7% vs. 5% and 19% vs. 11% respectively). There was no observed difference in conversion or late rupture rate. Late all-cause mortality and aneurysm-related deaths were also significantly higher in the octogenarians (10% vs. 7%, and 7% vs. 3% respectively). They concluded that the results support the consideration of EVAR in elderly patients, and that the benefits of lower peri-operative complications and mortality may outweigh the late complication risks when compared to open AAA repair. It is evident from these results, however, that age does act as a significant morbidity, nearly doubling the risk of complication and mortality, compared with a younger age group. Indeed, the report states that multivariate analysis identified age >80 years as an independent risk factor for late mortality and endoleak.

Pre-assessment

In making the decision regarding suitability for open AAA repair, appropriate investigations are required to explore the physiological reserve. Although standard pre-operative 'work-up' protocols are widely adopted, there remains variation depending on local facilities, service provision and budgets; hence a degree of heterogeneity between institutions. Similarly, departmental caseload has been shown to influence results and may affect judgement. Variation in open techniques, such as mid-line, mini-laparotomy and transverse incisions, as well as postoperative critical care facilities, may further influence a patient's exclusion for AAA repair.

The issue of disease reversibility may complicate the definition of an 'unfit' patient. An initial contra-indication to open AAA surgery does not represent absolute exclusion, but rather an opportunity for the clinician to optimise the patient's treatment, with the potential for improvement. Appropriate referral to specialties such as cardiology, nephrology, diabetology and general and respiratory medicine may result in an improvement in the patient's baseline status. Therefore, re-assessment of a patient's operative risk, particularly in the event of continuing AAA expansion, is essential if the appropriate management decision is to be made. The case demonstrated in Figure 1 illustrates some of the difficulties associated with such decisions.

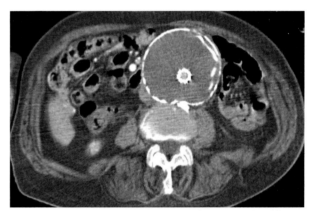

Figure 1. A CT scan three months post-EVAR showing a patent aorto-mono-iliac stent graft and no endoleak. The patient was a 92-year-old man with a tender 9.5cm AAA, renal dysfunction and severe cardio-respiratory comorbidities (ASA 4). He underwent successful EVAR under GA, but died at home of a non-aneurysm-related illness six months later.

Scoring systems

There are many scoring modalities aimed at determining whether a patient is suitable for AAA repair. The American Society of Anaesthesiology score is universally employed by anaesthetists and can act as a crude measure of suitability, although it does not represent a quantitative assessment of the patient's physiological condition [11]. There is evidence suggesting the potential predictive benefit of many of the scoring systems, and disease-specific scores have been devised such as V-POSSUM and rAAA-

POSSUM. The POSSUM was devised as an audit tool, solely for retrospective prediction of mortality, and criticism may be levelled at those methods that have developed the original equation into prospective, disease-specific scoring systems. A scoring system proposed by the Society of Vascular Surgery and the International Society of Cardiovascular Surgery - North American Chapter (SVS/ISCVS-NA), has been adopted by many vascular studies in order to assess operative risk, the key elements of which are the presence of diabetes, smoking, hypertension, hyperlipidaemia, cardiac disease, carotid disease, renal impairment, and pulmonary disease [12]. This system was developed for operative risk assessment in ischaemic limbs, and its application to other diseases and specific treatment modalities such as EVAR may detract from its efficacy.

The EVAR 2 trial recognised the limitations of scoring systems, and particularly the subjectivity of ASA [13]. This study deemed myocardial infarction or new onset angina within three months, and unstable angina at night as absolute contraindications for any surgical interventions. Beyond that, broad categories of cardiac, respiratory and renal disease acted as relative exclusion criteria at the discretion of the local institution, reflecting the complexity of accurate pre-operative prediction of patient outcome based on health parameters.

The Glasgow Aneurysm Score (GAS) has been devised more recently, and has undergone evaluation as to its efficacy in predicting the survival of patients after EVAR [14]. Biancari et al studied 5498 EVAR patients enrolled in EUROSTAR between 1996 and 2005, and correlated the GAS to outcome measurements. Thirty-day mortality was significantly different between tertiles: 1.1% in patients with GAS <74.4; 2.1% for those with scores between 74.4 and 83.6; and 5.3% for those scoring >83.6 (median GAS was 78.8 across the whole group). Receiver-operator characteristic curve indicated that GAS accurately predicted immediate postoperative death (p<0.001 for area under the curve of 0.70; 95% CI 0.66-0.74). Overall survival was also significantly different among tertiles of GAS on multivariate analysis.

Scoring systems are not infallible, however, and can be cumbersome to use in the clinical setting. Used as an aid they can act as important indicators of suitability for procedures and their use is likely to become more commonplace.

The evidence for EVAR in high-risk patients

There is a paucity of robust clinical data to provide evidence for EVAR in surgically unfit patients. There are many small, retrospective, single centre series advocating its use [15]; however, only two reports represent level II evidence or better.

The EUROSTAR experience [16]

The EUROSTAR registry represents the largest prospective registry of EVAR patients, and has generated an enormous amount of information on many areas relating to EVAR. One such study has evaluated the risk factors taken into account for the definition of a patient unfit for open surgery or general anaesthesia, and assessed the outcome of interventions [16]. A patient's operative risk was assessed using ASA, SVS/ISCVS-NA, and the physician's own assessment according to the broad categories A: normal medical condition; B: condition unfit for open surgical repair of AAA; and C: condition unfit for general anaesthesia. Retrospective analysis defined the conditions that categorised patients into groups B or C (Table 1). Of 3075 EVAR patients, 2525 were considered normal operative risk (group A), 399 (13%) fell into category B, and 151 (5%) were categorised into group C. Unsurprisingly, patients in groups B and C were significantly older, had a higher prevalence of ASA III or IV, and had higher individual systemic risk scores than those in group A. They also had less favourable anatomical and procedural factors, requiring significantly more adjunct procedures. Pulmonary conditions were most prevalent in groups C. Groups B and C were combined, representing the high-risk surgical group for subsequent analyses. Various factors were not considered when categorising patients, and multivariate analysis of these correlated age, diabetes, obesity and ankle-brachial pressure index with classification into groups B or C.

Table 1. Factors categorising patients into groups B or C [16].

Factor	Examples
Cardiovascular	Ischaemic heart disease, cerebrovascular disease, post-heart transplant
Pulmonary disorders	COPD, bronchiectasis, fibrosing alveolitis
Combined cardiac and pulmonary disorders	As above
Malignant disease	
Abdominal approach/ local anatomical factors	Previous laparotomies, hostile abdomen, obesity, retroperitoneal fibrosis, inflammatory aneurysm, aortitis, dissection, stoma, peritoneal dialysis, renal/liver transplant, pancreatitis etc.
Specified general disorders	Rheumatoid arthritis, connective tissue disease, chronic renal failure, liver disorders, neurological disorders, Parkinson's disease, muscular dystrophy etc.
Poor condition	Non-specified general disorders, e.g. age, ASA 4.

The high surgical risk group had significantly higher 30-day mortality (5.1%), more cardiac complications, and more procedure-related complications than group A, but similar endoleak and conversion rates. Results from multivariate analysis of pre-operative and operative variables and groups A, B and C are summarised in Table 2.

Late systemic complications occurred more frequently in groups B/C than A, but conversion and aneurysm rupture rates were the same. Two-year overall survival was less in group B (75.7%) and C (74.3%) than in group A (88.5%, p=0.0001), as were primary and secondary outcome rates. Classification into group B/C, pulmonary disorders, team experience <60 procedures and aneurysm diameter were factors found to be independently associated with late death on multivariate analysis.

A mathematical model was developed to enable comparison of patient survival between EVAR and conservative management of AAA >5cm, with an assumed annual rupture rate of 11% based on the literature. This concluded that, for up to one year, avoidance of operative mortality outweighs the benefit of reduced rupture rate, but thereafter, EVAR would afford an increasing survival advantage, with a two-year survival of 75% in the EVAR group compared to 63% where conservative management was allocated.

Table 2. Variables and groups associated with significantly higher 30-day mortality on multivariate analysis [16].

Factor	Odds ratio	p-value
Group B/C vs. A	1.8	0.039
ASA III or IV	1.9	0.03
Renal insufficiency	2.5	0.0003
Age >70 years	3.0	0.0004

The EVAR 2 trial [5]

The UK EVAR 2 trial ran in parallel with the EVAR 1 study and was designed to answer the question: would EVAR, in patients unfit for open repair, reduce the risk of aneurysm-related death from rupture and improve long-term survival and quality of life in comparison with no intervention?

The methodology was reported for both trials prior to the publication of results [13]. Inclusion criteria were any patients over 60 years of age with an AAA >5.5cm on CT, with anatomy suitable for EVAR. Decision for inclusion and device selection was self-governed by the individual centres. As previously discussed the exclusion criteria and selection for EVAR 2 was largely decided locally. Significant valvular disease, dysrythmias and congestive cardiac failure were considered exclusion criteria for EVAR 1, but not EVAR 2. Similarly, inability to ascend a flight of stairs without breathlessness, FEV1 <1.0L, pO_2 <8.0 kPa, and pCO_2 >6.5kPa constituted a relative indication for EVAR 2, as did a serum creatinine >200µmol/L. In addition, there was a recognition of 'fitness inflation', whereby a patient initially considered unfit for open repair or even any surgery may subsequently be deemed 'fit' in the light of increasing aneurysm size or symptoms.

In this trial, 338 patients were randomised to stenting (n=166) or no intervention (n=172) with comparable baseline characteristics. Cardiopulmonary status was noted to be worse than for patients enrolled in EVAR 1, and aspirin and statin use was low at 58% and 40% respectively. One hundred and fifty patients (90%) assigned EVAR received surgery within a median of 57 days, 144 of whom had successful endograft deployment. Forty-seven patients (27%) randomised for no intervention actually underwent AAA exclusion, 12 through open surgery. There were no patients lost to follow-up with a median time of 2.4 years. One hundred and forty-two patients across both groups died during follow-up with an overall four-year mortality of 64%, as estimated by Kaplan-Meier survival curves. Neither aneurysm-related nor all-cause mortality differed significantly between the EVAR and control groups. Nine patients (5%) in the EVAR group died from rupture before receiving elective treatment, with a median delay of 98 days between randomisation and rupture. In the same group, 14 patients (9%) were recorded as having procedure-related deaths. A total of

21 patients (12%) in the no intervention group died from aneurysm rupture, and only one of the 47 who crossed over and had repair died from the procedure (2%). *Post hoc* per-protocol analysis did not identify any significant difference in all-cause mortality between the two groups in the light of the 20% cross-over in treatment.

There were significant differences in postoperative complications and re-interventions between the two groups. At four years, 43% of EVAR patients had exhibited at least one complication with 26% requiring one or more re-interventions, compared to 18% and 4% (respectively) in the no-intervention group. Type 2 endoleak was the commonest graft-related complication in the EVAR group (10%), although only three required re-intervention, whereas Type 1 endoleaks occurred in ten patients (6%), of whom eight underwent surgery. Although the incidence of Type 1 endoleaks might initially suggest otherwise, the proportion of unsuccessful primary procedures and of re-interventions in EVAR 2 are very similar to those reported for EVAR 1. This may indicate that selection regarding anatomical suitability was consistent and not unduly influenced by considerations of fitness for open surgery.

Health-related quality of life was not significantly different between the two groups. Unsurprisingly, the mean estimated costs at four years were significantly higher for patients having undergone EVAR: £13,632 compared to £4983 in the no intervention group.

The results would appear to suggest that four years after EVAR in unfit patients, there is no benefit in terms of aneurysm-related or all-cause mortality, there are increased complication and re-intervention rates, greater hospital costs, and no improvement in quality of life compared with a conservative management policy. The results, however, are confounded by several factors, and firm conclusions should not necessarily be drawn. Firstly, considerable delay occurred between randomisation and intervention, resulting in rupture and death in 5%, somewhat high if one was to consider a surveillance group. Conversely, the rupture rate in the no intervention groups was low, only 12% after a median of 2.4 years, which may bias in favour of conservative treatment. Secondly, the Kaplan-Meier survival curves were noted to cross in favour of EVAR after two years, although, as only one third of patients in either group were alive at four years, it is unlikely that sufficient numbers would survive to realise this potential long-term benefit. Thirdly, considerable cross-over occurred, with more than one quarter of patients assigned conservative management undergoing EVAR. Although per-protocol analysis indicated that this alone did not confound mortality rates, when combined with the previously mentioned factors, one may consider the results of the trial less definitive.

Implications for current practice

The EVAR 2 trial results seem to indicate little potential benefit for the use of the endovascular devices in unfit patients. Based upon this evidence,

there is a danger of being dismissive of EVAR in all 'unfit' patients [17]. To do so would be to fail the patient, whose clinical picture may not quite equate to EVAR 2, but falls somewhere in between EVAR 1 and EVAR 2, thus highlighting the importance of decision-making on an individual basis. Since it is likely that prophylactic operations will not be effective on patients with short life expectancy [18], the focus should be on improving fitness rather than promoting early EVAR. In addition, accurate assessment of the anatomical suitability for EVAR remains an important part of the decision-making process, since the risk of complications in such patients are likely to increase with poor selection. Global pre-assessment is thus critical, but the clinician is still left with the original conundrum of balancing the operative risk against the risk of rupture.

Summary

◆   The level II evidence shows potential benefit for EVAR in unfit patients surviving more than 12 months, but indicates that age is an independent risk factor for morbidity and mortality.

◆   The EVAR 2 trial suggests that unfit patients should not be offered endovascular repair.

◆   It may be justified to offer EVAR to unfit patients with a high degree of anatomical suitability, after extensive pre-assessment and individualised attention to medical problems.

References

1.   Zarins CK, White RA, Schwarten D, et al. Aneurex stent graft versus open surgical repair of abdominal aortic aneurysms: multicenter prospective clinical trial. J Vasc Surg 1999; 29: 292-308.

2.   Pearson S, Hassen T, Spark JI, et al. Endovascular repair of abdominal aortic aneurysm reduces intraoperative cortisol and perioperative morbidity. J Vasc Surg 2005; 41(6): 919-25.

3.   Brady AR, Thompson SG, Fowkes FG, et al. UK Small Aneurysm Trial Participants. Abdominal aortic aneurysm expansion: risk factors and time intervals for surveillance. Circulation 2004; 110(1): 16-21.

4.   Buth J, Laheij RJF. Early complications and endoleaks after endovascular abdominal aortic aneurysm repair: report of a multicenter study. J Vasc Surg 2000; 31: 134-46.

5.   EVAR trial participants. Endovascular aneurysm repair and outcome in patients unfit for open repair of abdominal aortic aneurysm (EVAR trial 2): randomised controlled trial. Lancet 2005; 365(9478): 2187-92.

6.   Older P, Smith R, Courtney P, et al. Preoperative evaluation of cardiac failure and ischaemia in elderly patients by cardiopulmonary exercise testing. Chest 1993; 104: 701-4.

7.   Compton CN, Dillavou ED, Sheehan MK, et al. Is abdominal aortic aneurysm repair appropriate in oxygen-dependent chronic obstructive pulmonary disease patients? J Vasc Surg 2005; 42(4): 650-3.

8.   O'Hara PJ, Hetzer NR, Krajewski LP, et al. Ten-year experience with abdominal aortic aneurysm repair in octogenarians: early results and late outcomes. J Vasc Surg 1995; 21: 830-8.

9.   Minor ME, Ellozy S, Carroccio A, et al. Endovascular aortic aneurysm repair in the octogenarian: is it worthwhile? Arch Surg 2004; 139(3): 308-14.

10. Lange C, Leurs LJ., Buth J, *et al.* EUOROSTAR collaborators. Endovascular repair of abdominal aortic aneurysm in octogenarians: an analysis based on EUROSTAR data. *J Vasc Surg* 2005; 42(4): 624-30.

11. Owens B, Felts J, Spitznagel E. ASA physical status classification: a study of consistency rating. *Anaesthesiology* 1978; 49: 239-43.

12. Rutherford R, Flanigan D, Gupta S, *et al.* Suggested standards for reports dealing with lower limb ischaemia. *J Vasc Surg* 1986; 4: 80-94.

13. Brown LC, Epstein D, Manca A, *et al.* The UK EndoVascular Aneurysm Repair (EVAR) trials: design, methodology and progress. *Eur J Vasc Endovasc Surg* 2004; 27: 372-81.

14. Biancari F, Hobo R, Juvonen T. Glasgow Aneurysm Score predicts survival after endovascular stenting of abdominal aortic aneurysm in patients from the EUROSTAR registry. *Br J Surg* 2006. Epub 93(2): 191-4.

15. Sbarigia E, Speziale F, Ducasse E, *et al.* What is the best management for abdominal aortic aneurysm in patients at high surgical risk? A single-center review. *Interventional Angiology* 2005; 24(1): 70-4.

16. Buth J, van Marrewijk CJ., Harris PL, *et al.* Outcome of abdominal aortic aneurysm repair in patients with conditions considered unfit for an open procedure: a report on the EUROSTAR experience. *J Vasc Surg* 2002; 35(2): 211-20.

17. Takagi H, Umemoto T, Buskins E, *et al.* Endovascular repair of abdominal aortic aneurysm/authors' reply. *Lancet* 2005; 366(9489): 890-2.

18. Cronenwett JL. Endovascular aneurysm repair: important mid-term results. *Lancet* 2005; 365(9478): 2156-8.

Chapter 6

The role of medical therapy and endovascular repair in the management of small abdominal aortic aneurysms

Janet T Powell MD PhD FRCPath, Professor, Section of Vascular Surgery

Imperial College at Charing Cross, London, UK

Introduction

The diagnosis of small abdominal aortic aneurysm (AAA) takes with it a heightened risk of cardiovascular death [1, 2]. Although commonly, small AAAs are not associated with symptoms, the presence of an aneurysm should be considered as manifest cardiovascular disease and all such patients should receive medical therapy, including statins and antiplatelet drugs, to prevent secondary complications. This message has not yet reached all vascular surgeons, the primary referral point for patients with small AAA. Therefore, the first goal in the management of small AAA is to ensure that patients receive proper secondary prevention for cardiovascular disease. This is likely to confer additional benefits, such as a reduced growth rate of small AAAs [3].

Some 10-15 years ago there was considerable debate as to whether surgical intervention was required for small AAAs. This area of debate and the scientific approach of vascular surgeons led to the formulation of two multicentre randomised trials, both designed to show that early open repair of small AAA would save lives [4, 5]. These trials took place in the era before endovascular aneurysm repair was developed technologically and available widely. Both trials were supported by not-for-profit organisations and were fully powered, with the enrolment of more than 1000 patients in each. Neither trial managed to provide evidence for the hypothesis that early surgical repair of small AAAs was associated with improved patient survival. Surveillance was safe and not associated with an impaired quality of life. The costs of a policy of surveillance were considerably less than a policy of early surgery, particularly since about one third of patients died before their aneurysms reached the threshold aneurysm size for surgery. Delaying surgery until the aneurysm diameter exceeded 5.5cm was not associated with an increased surgical mortality. Nevertheless, the elective 30-day mortality for open surgical repair in these trials was significant and much higher than the rates currently being reported for endovascular repair. This has led to company-sponsored trials of surveillance versus endovascular repair for small aneurysms, but limited finance may mean that these trials are not fully powered [6].

These skeleton facts provide the framework for discussion concerning the management of patients with small AAA.

Medical therapy for small abdominal aortic aneurysms

There has been one reasonably sized trial based on the hypothesis that beta-blockers would slow small aneurysm growth rates [7]. Propranolol was the drug used, following the finding that this drug slowed the rate of aortic root dilatation in Marfan's syndrome. However, the small aneurysm trial failed to show any benefit for propranolol therapy and this treatment was associated with a high prevalence of side effects, leading to patient withdrawal. A smaller trial showed similar results, so that propranolol cannot be considered a suitable therapy to retard aneurysm growth. The only other published trials have used antibiotics, based on the hypotheses that these drugs would slow aneurysm growth through mechanisms of either metalloprotease inhibition or elimination of *Chlamydia pneumoniae*. These trials have been small, essentially phase II trials and hence very underpowered. Although a fully powered trial of doxycycline therapy in the USA has been proposed, funding such a trial has posed numerous problems. None of these trials have included best medical therapy (statins and antiplatelet drugs) as baseline conditions. In other areas of cardiovascular disease, any benefits of antibiotic therapy are short-lived (six months) and longer follow-up, to two years, suggests that antibiotic therapy may be associated with a worse prognosis [8].

There is a body of evidence accumulating to show that statins improve survival in patients with AAA, particularly those undergoing open surgical repair [9-11]. Most recently, evidence has been presented to suggest that statin therapy is associated with an almost 50% reduction in AAA growth rates, patients on statin therapy having growth rates of only 2.0mm/year compared to 3.6mm/year in the remainder [3]. These data come from a reasonably sized retrospective study. Although this publication calls for randomised trials of statin therapy to slow AAA growth, 'the horse has bolted' and there now are compelling reasons as to why such trials, for patients with small AAA are unethical. Together these studies only re-emphasise the need for statin therapy in all aneurysm patients. Statins have pleiotropic effects, stabilising atherosclerotic plaques, reducing inflammation and decreasing the expression of some matrix metalloproteinases in addition to reducing circulating cholesterol and LDL-cholesterol concentrations. Therefore, any effects of statins on aneurysm growth may occur through several plausible, synergistic mechanisms apart from the direct reduction of circulating cholesterol (which probably would not influence aneurysm growth rates [12]).

There are two further medical therapies that might be applied to contain the growth rate of small AAA, to reduce the likelihood of surgery ever being needed. First those patients who are current smokers should be given all available treatments to stop smoking, since this is likely to be associated with a 20-25% reduction in annual growth rates [12]. Many patients with small AAA have a history of hypertension and recent randomised trials have emphasised the role of angiotensin blockade, either alone or in combination therapy, for treatment of hypertension in those with cardiovascular disease [13]. The effect of optimal treatment of hypertension, including therapy with ACE inhibitors, on aneurysm growth is unclear, but it is very unlikely to be detrimental. There is some circumstantial evidence to indicate that ACE inhibitors could have an important effect to slow AAA growth [14].

So, for a patient with a small AAA, step one should be consultation with a cardiologist, angiologist or vascular physician to institute optimal medical therapy. It is probable that such therapy will reduce mean aneurysm growth rates by more than 50%. This could mean that, on average, a 4cm diameter AAA would take ten years or more to reach the threshold of 5.5cm and those with aneurysms smaller than 4cm in diameter might never reach the critical threshold within their lifetime.

Consensus and criticisms arising from the small aneurysm trials

The two trials [4, 5] included patients with aortic diameters 4.0-5.5cm, but the US trial was almost exclusively male, whilst the UK trial included women. Subsequent to these trials, the MASS aneurysm screening trial has shown that a policy of surveillance for aneurysms up to 6cm in men also was safe, rupture below this threshold diameter being very rare in men [15]. Elective surgical mortality was very different in the two intervention trials; 5.6% in the UK trial and 2.7% in the US trial, but despite these differences, early surgery did not improve long-term survival in either trial. By now, all patients from the UK trial have been followed-up for ten years and preliminary data indicate that even at ten years there is no survival benefit associated with a policy of early elective surgery. The mean annual growth rate of aneurysms 4.0-5.5cm in diameter is about 3mm/year. If this could be reduced to a target of 1mm/year many patients with small aneurysms would never attain an aneurysm diameter where rupture was a threat, so that no surgery would ever be needed. These trials were conducted before the widespread availability of statins, taken by only 2% of patients in the UK trial. If statins had been used in all these trial patients would the outcome have favoured surveillance even more strikingly?

Should endovascular repair be considered for small aneurysms?

The protagonists for intervention would prefer to suggest that the surgical mortality was too high in the small aneurysm trials and that the very low 30-day mortality associated with endovascular repair of small aneurysms in EUROSTAR and single centre studies would ensure that endovascular repair was better than surveillance for small aneurysms [16]. The case that is often made compares mortality from single centre experiences in the USA with results, now a decade old, from the UK Small Aneurysm Trial; since this trial had a higher operative mortality than the US trial, this is scientific trickery [17]. The interventionalists add the further argument that endovascular repair of small aneurysms is safer than endovascular repair of large aneurysms [16]. The rapid advances in medical technology and therapeutics are changing the face of medicine. Whilst in private healthcare systems expensive prophylaxis may be condoned, in public funded healthcare systems it is not. Therefore, the place of endovascular repair of small aneurysms is very much in doubt. The Belgian authorities already have come to the decision that endovascular repair is not cost-effective for large AAA and the focus should shift to improving survival following AAA repair [18]. In addition, since the technology is not fully stabilised, in

Belgium endovascular repair must be funded from research budgets, with ongoing rigorous evaluation of its performance, particularly for complications and secondary interventions.

The medical device companies have made considerable investment in endovascular technologies. Competition exists and every company seeks new markets and new clinical situations in which to use its already approved devices. Despite the Belgian position, with current evidence it seems reasonable to support the use of endovascular repair in large aneurysms, because aneurysm-related mortality and early survival is much better than after open repair. However, there is no level I evidence at all for the role of endovascular grafting of small aneurysms. The companies have offered to breach this gap in evidence by supporting two trials, one in the USA and one in Europe. However, the level of funding support offered will not permit a fully powered randomised trial. Can the conduct of underpowered clinical trials be considered ethical? Further, company-sponsored trials are recognised to overestimate treatment effects by about 30% [19]. Therefore, the community of vascular surgery should not anticipate that the results of these company-sponsored trials will be decisive. If a trial addresses an important clinical question and is well designed, not-for-profit agencies will offer support.

The results of these two company-sponsored trials of endovascular repair versus surveillance also are likely to depend on the anatomical stringency of 'suitable for endovascular repair' and the number of women included, since both these factors influence aneurysm rupture rates. Recent studies have suggested that if the aneurysm morphology is suitable for endovascular repair, the risk of rupture is considerably reduced [20, 21]. Other evidence has reported a much increased rate of AAA rupture when the renal artery is involved in the dilated segment of aorta [22]. Therefore, the rupture risk of small aneurysms in these two new trials could be much lower than the 1% observed in the small aneurysm trials [4, 5]. Several studies have suggested that the rupture rate of AAA in women is higher than men and aneurysms in women rupture at smaller diameters than aneurysms in men. The inclusion of a large proportion of women, therefore, might partially offset the reduced rupture rate likely in those with AAA anatomically suitable for endovascular repair. Whether newer devices with suprarenal fixation will influence outcomes also is uncertain and the trials would not have sufficient power to analyse such a subgroup of patients.

Disadvantages associated with early endovascular repair of small aneurysms

Another disadvantage of proposing endovascular repair in younger, fitter patients with small AAA, is the uncertainty concerning the durability of endovascular repair and the extent of radiation exposure associated with repeated CT surveillance scans. The recent endovascular repair trials have shown that the complications of endografting and secondary procedures are considerable and are not limited to the first year after aneurysm exclusion [23, 24]. In the EVAR 1 trial [24], 81/517 (15%) patients needed a secondary intervention, including two fatalities following rupture. The highest rates of intervention were in the first six months after intervention, but complications and interventions occurred steadily thereafter, with even a hint that the rate of re-interventions accelerated again after 2-3 years. With such a history, we cannot think of reducing surveillance to improve cost-effectiveness and quality of life, which continuing surveillance is likely to erode, for those with endovascular grafts.

Endovascular grafts are subject to a continuous cycle of quality improvement and it is possible that in the future, grafts will be more durable and surveillance protocols less intense. The patient with a small aneurysm might be better waiting until these improved grafts are available, even if by then their aneurysm is a little larger in diameter.

Cost-effectiveness arguments also are likely to weigh against early endovascular intervention. Endovascular repair is more expensive than open repair, with the additional costs of ongoing surveillance for endoleaks, endotension and graft migration.

Summary

♦   Secondary prevention of cardiovascular disease with statins and antiplatelet drugs must be offered, in addition to treatment of hypertension with ACE inhibitors. These treatments may also reduce aneurysm growth rate by more than 50%.

♦   There is no evidence to indicate that lower intervention-associated mortality would alter the conclusions of the small aneurysm trials, in favour of surveillance.

♦   Endovascular technology has not yet stabilised and durability remains in question, so that for small AAAs, watchful waiting remains the best policy for management.

♦   The current trials of endovascular repair versus surveillance for small aneurysms are company-sponsored and may not lead to robust results.

References

1. Brady AR, Thompson SG, Fowkes FGR, Powell JT. Aortic aneurysm diameter and risk of cardiovascular mortality. *Arterioscler Thromb Vasc Biol* 2001; 21: 1203-7.

2. Norman P, Le M, Pearce C, Jamrozik K. Infrarenal aortic diameter predicts all-cause mortality. *Arterioscler Thromb Vasc Biol* 2004; 24: 1278-82.

3. Schouten O, Van Laanen J, Boersma E, *et al*. Statins are associated with a reduced infrarenal abdominal aortic aneurysm growth. *Eur J Vasc Endovasc Surg* 2006: in press.

4. The UK Small Aneurysm Trial Participants. Mortality results for randomised controlled trial of early elective surgery or ultrasonographic surveillance for small abdominal aortic aneurysms. *Lancet* 1998; 352: 1649-55.

5. Lederle FA, Wilson SE, Johnson GR, *et al* for Aneurysm Detection and Management Veterans Affairs Cooperative Study Group. Immediate repair compared with surveillance of small abdominal aortic aneurysms. *N Engl J Med* 2002; 346: 1437-44.

6. Cao P for CAESAR trial collaborators. Comparison of surveillance vs Aortic Endografting for Small Aneurysm Repair (CAESAR) trial: study design and progress. *Eur J Vasc Endovasc Surg* 2005; 30: 245-51.

7. Propranolol trial investigators. Propranolol for small abdominal aortic aneurysms: results of a randomized trial. *J Vasc Surg* 2002; 35: 72-9.

8. CLARICOR trial group. Randomised placebo controlled multicentre trial to assess short term clarithromycin for patients with stable coronary heart disease: CLARICOR trial. *Br Med J* 2006; 332: 22-4.

9. Kertai MD, Boersma E, Westerhout CM, *et al*. A combination of statins and beta-blockers is independently associated with reduction in the incidence of perioperative mortality and nonfatal myocardial infarction in patients undergoing abdominal aortic aneurysm surgery. *Eur J Vasc Endovasc Surg* 2004; 28: 343-52.

10. Kertai MD, Boersma E, Westerhout CM, *et al*. Association between long-term statin use and mortality after successful abdominal aortic aneurysm surgery. *Am J Med* 2004; 116: 96-103.

11. Durazzo AE, Machado FS, Ikeoka DT, *et al*. Reduction in cardiovascular events after vascular surgery with atorvastatin: a randomised trial. *J Vasc Surg* 2004; 39: 967-75.

12. Brady AR, Thompson SG, Fowkes FGR, Greenhalgh RM, Powell JT. Abdominal aortic aneurysm expansion: risk factors and time intervals for surveillance. *Circulation* 2004; 110: 16-21.

13. Opie LH, Commerford PJ, Gersh BJ. Controversies in stable coronary artery disease. *Lancet* 2006; 367: 69-78.

14. Moran CS, McCann M, Karan M, *et al*. Association of osteoprotegerin with human abdominal aortic aneurysm progression. *Circulation* 2005; 111: 3119-25.

15. Ashton HA, Buxton MJ, Day NE, *et al* for Multicentre Aneurysm Screening Study Group. The Multicentre Aneurysm Screening Study (MASS) into the effect of abdominal aortic aneurysm screening on mortality in men: a randomised controlled trial. *Lancet* 2002; 360: 1531-9.

16. Harris PL, Vallabhaneni SR, Desgranges P, *et al*. Incidence and risk factors of late rupture, conversion and death after endovascular repair of infrarenal aortic aneurysms: The EUROSTAR experience. *J Vasc Surg* 2004; 32: 739-49.

17. Zarins CK, Crabtree T, Arko FR, *et al*. Endovascular repair or surveillance of patients with small AAA. *Eur J Vasc Endovasc Surg* 2005; 29: 496-503.

18. Bonneux L, Cleemput I, Vrijens F, *et al*. HTA De electieve endovasculaire behandeling van het abdominale aorta aneurysma (AAA). KCE Reports 2005; 23A (http// :kenniscentrum.fgov.be/documents/D20051027332.pdf).

19. Djulbegovic B, Lacevic M, Cantor A, *et al*. The uncertainty principle and industry-sponsored research. *Lancet* 2000; 356: 635-8.

20. Lederle FA, Johnson GR, Wilson SE, Ballard DJ, *et al*. Rupture rate of large abdominal aortic aneurysms in patients refusing or unfit for elective repair. *JAMA* 2002; 287: 2968-72.

21. Hinchcliffe RJ, Alric P, Rose D, *et al*. Comparison of morphological features of intact and ruptured aneurysms of infrarenal abdominal aorta. *J Vasc Surg* 2003; 38: 88-92.

22. Hatakeyama T, Shigematsu H, Muto T. Risk factors for rupture of abdominal aortic aneurysm based on three-dimensional study. *J Vasc Surg* 2001; 33: 453-61.

23. Blankensteijn JD, de Jong S, Prinssen M, *et al*. Two-year outcomes after conventional or endovascular repair of abdominal aortic aneurysms. *N Engl J Med* 2005; 352: 2398-405.

24. EVAR Trial Participants. Endovascular aneurysm repair versus open repair in patients with abdominal aortic aneurysm (EVAR trial 1): randomised controlled trial. *Lancet* 2005; 365: 2187-92.

Chapter 7

Failed EVAR: tricks of the trade

Geoffrey Gilling-Smith MS FRCS, Consultant Vascular Surgeon
Richard G McWilliams FRCS FRCR, Consultant Interventional Radiologist
Royal Liverpool University Hospital, Liverpool, UK

Introduction

Endovascular repair relies on a covered stent graft to isolate an aneurysm from the circulation and thus prevent rupture of the aneurysm, haemorrhage and death. The repair has unquestionably failed if the aneurysm subsequently ruptures and the patient suffers a fatal haemorrhage. The repair may also be considered to have failed if the patient remains, or is again, at risk of death from aneurysm rupture. In the opinion of the authors, the repair should also be considered a failure if it results in interruption of blood flow to the kidneys and/or the lower limbs.

The risk of aneurysm rupture depends on the tensile strength of the aneurysm wall and on the force applied against the wall from within the aneurysm. This in turn depends on the pressure within the aneurysm sac and failure to isolate the aneurysm from systemic arterial pressure leaves the aneurysm susceptible to rupture. Should rupture occur, the risk of fatal haemorrhage depends on the presence or absence of blood flow within the aneurysm sac.

Failure to isolate the aneurysm from both systemic arterial pressure and blood flow leaves the patient at risk of rupture, haemorrhage and death. Failure to isolate the aneurysm from either pressure or flow, but not both, may not however, constitute failure of the repair. Pressurisation of the aneurysm in the absence of flow may result in rupture, but this is likely to be a benign event. Indeed, fenestration of the aneurysm has been proposed as a treatment for aneurysm sac hygroma [1]. Conversely, the presence of blood flow within the aneurysm may not matter if the aneurysm is not at systemic pressure, since haemorrhage cannot occur unless the aneurysm ruptures.

Endovascular repair may fail primarily at the time of stent graft implantation, or secondarily after a period of successful isolation of the aneurysm.

Primary failure

This may occur if the stent graft cannot be deployed as intended, either because it is not possible to access the aorta, or because of failure of stent graft deployment. A more common problem is failure to isolate the aneurysm from the circulation, despite successful graft deployment. This may occur if the procedure has not been planned correctly and the stent graft is too small (i.e. undersized relative to the diameters of the aortic and iliac anastomotic seal zones), or too short (resulting in inadequate engagement of the iliac arteries). This may also occur if a shelf of calcified aortic, or possibly iliac, arterial wall protrudes into the lumen and prevents the graft from apposing against the full length of the intended seal zone.

Access problems

Stent graft delivery systems have an outer diameter of between 20 and 24 French. Access may, therefore, be difficult if the external iliac arteries are small, or if there is stenotic disease of either external or common iliac arteries.

Measurement of the external iliac diameter is an essential part of planning for endovascular repair. If the external iliac artery has a diameter of less than 8mm, attempts to pass a large stent graft delivery system may result in extensive intimal injury and/or rupture of the vessel. Consideration should be given to alternative approaches. The maximum external diameter of the graft delivery system varies with the type of commercial endograft, and it may be possible to select a system with a smaller profile. Alternatively, the endograft may be delivered via an iliac conduit [2]. This involves exposure of the common iliac artery through a retroperitoneal incision in the iliac fossa. A short length of 10mm diameter prosthetic graft is then anastomosed to the front of the common iliac artery. The conduit is ligated distally and then punctured with a needle in the normal way to allow introduction of a sheath, passage of wires and catheters and finally passage of the endograft delivery system. In the authors' experience, this technique is often less than satisfactory. It can be difficult to control bleeding from around the delivery system once this is introduced into the conduit and the technique inevitably reduces significantly the length of common iliac artery available for fixation and seal. There is also an increased risk of inadvertent irradiation of the operator's hands. Open surgical repair remains a reasonable option in a fit patient.

Stenotic disease of the iliac arteries can present a problem, particularly if there is extensive calcification. If localised, a lesion can be dilated by balloon angioplasty prior to passage of the delivery system, but there is a risk of subsequent disruption of the intima and dissection once flow is restored. Some, therefore, advocate stenting of iliac lesions prior to introduction of the delivery system, but the authors do not recommend this. Subsequent passage of the stent graft delivery system can result in proximal displacement of the stent, which is not ideal.

Access may also be difficult if there is marked tortuosity of the iliac arteries, particularly if these are calcified. Although modern delivery systems have some flexibility, they will not advance easily through tortuous arteries and every effort must be made to straighten the arteries prior to advancement of the delivery system. In most cases, the iliac arteries can be straightened by employing a stiffer wire. This will result in corrugation of the iliac intima, which may be injured by passage of the delivery system (Figure 1). Perhaps a more important problem is the tendency for the iliac arteries to resume their tortuosity once the stiff wire is withdrawn at the end of the procedure. This can result in kinking of the graft and it may sometimes be necessary to smooth out the kinks by deploying an additional stent such as a Wallstent (Figure 2).

If the iliac arteries cannot readily be straightened by introduction of a stiffer wire, it may be possible to straighten the arteries by dividing the circumflex iliac arteries at the level of the inguinal ligament and pulling a loop of redundant external iliac artery down into the groin incision. A short segment of artery can subsequently be resected if necessary.

Occasionally the delivery system will advance easily through the iliac arteries but then impact on the side of an angulated aneurysm. It is usually possible to resolve this problem by advancing the system while manually straightening the aneurysm. The operator stands on the same side of the patient as the delivery system and places a hand across the anterior abdominal wall. The fingers are then curled in gently to define the side of the aneurysm. Finally, the operator pulls the aneurysm towards him or herself, whilst advancing the delivery system with the other hand. The manoeuvre requires a certain amount of faith since it must be performed blind (i.e. without fluoroscopy).

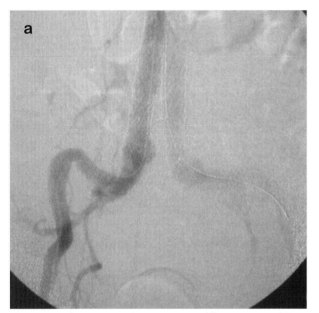
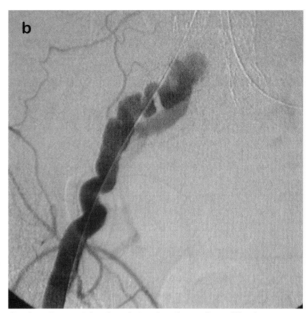

Figure 1. a) Tortuous right external iliac artery with a soft wire in place. b) After introduction of a stiff wire. Note the corrugation of the intima.

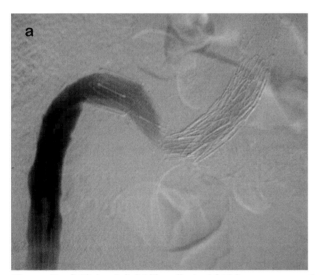
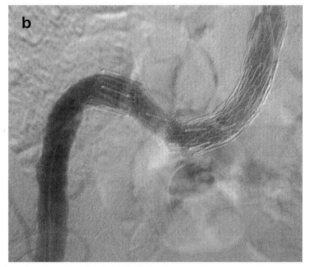

Figure 2. a) Kinked right iliac limb. b) This was corrected by deployment of a Wallstent.

Problems with graft deployment

Occasionally the delivery system will malfunction and fail to allow deployment of the graft. If it is not possible to initiate deployment, the delivery system can be withdrawn and endovascular repair attempted with another device if one is available, or on another occasion if it is not. A more challenging situation arises if the system allows partial deployment of the endograft, but then will not release the top stent or contralateral limb. A variety of endovascular manoeuvres have been described to deal with such a situation, but it may occasionally be necessary to resort to open repair to rescue the situation.

Partial or complete coverage of one or both renal artery ostia is a serious problem, which fortunately occurs only rarely. It may occur if the anatomy of the juxtarenal aorta is not defined clearly on angiography prior to graft deployment. This is more likely if the renal arteries arise more anteriorly or posteriorly than usual and it is important during planning to note carefully the positions of the renal ostia on CT. If these are anterior or posterior, the C-arm must be rotated to obtain left or right anterior oblique views so that angiography is performed with the C-arm at 90° to the longitudinal axis of the lowermost renal artery. Inadvertent coverage of one or both renal ostia may also occur if the graft has been partially deployed in the suprarenal aorta, but cannot then be drawn down into an infrarenal position. Some interventionists apparently favour this technique when employing endografts that have neither barbs nor hooks. The top of the endograft is allowed to flare within the supra-renal aorta and then drawn down into position. The problem with this technique is that the flared portion of the endograft may catch on a calcified plaque in the suprarenal aorta or on the origin of the uppermost renal artery. Even if the graft is initially deployed in the correct position, one or more renal artery origins may be covered if the endograft is subsequently pushed proximally during introduction of the contralateral limb.

As soon as the problem is recognised, every attempt must be made to draw the endograft distally so as to restore renal blood flow. It may be possible to pull the endograft caudally by inflating a large angioplasty balloon within the body of the endograft (i.e. immediately above the flow divider) and pulling this towards the groin. An alternative is to introduce a Sos-Omni catheter via the ipsilateral limb. The catheter is reformed within the body of the endograft and drawn caudally to engage the contralateral limb. A soft wire is then passed via the catheter into the contralateral limb, snared within the contralateral iliac artery and exteriorised through a sheath in the contralateral groin. Traction on both ends of the femoro-femoral wire (with the Sos-Omni still in place over the bifurcation of the endograft) may be sufficient to pull the endograft down into the desired position. It should be noted, however, that if the endograft has hooks or barbs, excessive traction in a caudal direction might result in tearing of the aorta.

If repeat angiography following such manoeuvres reveals persistent shuttering of one or both renal artery origins, the authors advise stenting of the affected renal artery or arteries. If angiography reveals absence of flow into one or more renal arteries, consideration should be given to immediate conversion, removal of the endograft and possibly bypass on the renal artery or arteries. In some patients it may be preferable to accept the loss of one kidney.

Endoleak

Completion angiography may reveal proximal or distal endoleak. In general, every attempt should be made to deal with such endoleaks during the primary procedure, since there is a risk of early rupture of the aneurysm if they persist [3].

Proximal endoleak may be due to undersizing of the graft relative to the aorta, to a shelf of calcified plaque preventing apposition of the endograft against the aortic neck or to maldeployment of the graft within a short, conical or diseased aortic neck.

In many cases, a proximal endoleak can be 'sealed' by gentle balloon dilatation of the endograft within the aneurysm neck. If this fails, alternative strategies include deployment of a large Palmaz stent or stent graft cuff within the aneurysm neck. Whichever is employed, it is important to measure carefully the distance from the lowermost renal artery origin to the endograft flow-divider, so as to ensure that the stent or cuff can be deployed proximal to the flow-divider. If the cuff is too long, it may deploy within one or other stent graft limb and compromise flow to the other limb.

If these techniques fail to resolve the problem, or if the endoleak is attributed to an inadequate length of good quality aortic neck, one may either elect to convert to open repair at the time or plan for deployment of a fenestrated cuff at a later date.

Distal endoleak may also be resolved by gentle dilatation of a moulding balloon within the iliac limb. If this fails, it may be necessary to employ an additional graft limb to extend the repair into the external iliac artery.

Completion angiography may also reveal evidence of side-branch reperfusion. In the authors' opinion, such endoleaks can safely be left. Most will seal spontaneously. Embolisation or laparoscopic clipping can be performed at a later date, if the endoleak persists and is thought to present a risk to the patient.

Planning errors

Many of the aforementioned problems can be avoided by meticulous attention to detail during planning of the endovascular repair and by rejection of cases of borderline anatomic suitability. Obsessive attention to detail, anticipation of problems and consideration of strategies to be employed should difficulties arise will in most cases ensure that the repair is straightforward and successful.

Secondary failure

Following successful endograft deployment and isolation of the aneurysm from blood flow (as determined by completion angiography and/or predischarge CT scanning), the aneurysm may again be at risk of rupture if the seal between the endograft and the aorta or iliac arteries becomes deficient, if a modular endograft separates into its component parts, or if there is a tear in the graft fabric.

Migration

The most important cause of late failure is migration of the stent graft and loss of seal at the proximal anastomotic zone [3]. Stent grafts are subject to significant haemodynamic forces [4]. These tend to displace the proximal part of the graft in a caudal direction. If the aneurysm is capacious, these forces may also result in displacement of the centre of the endograft towards the side of the aneurysm and disengagement of one or both iliac limbs from the iliac arteries - the so-called firehose effect. If a modular graft is employed, these forces may also result in disengagement of the iliac limb from the contralateral graft stump. A further consequence of migration is deformation of the graft, fracture of the graft stents and tear of the graft fabric.

Diagnosis of migration

Surveillance after endovascular repair should include serial abdominal radiography. Both PA and lateral views should be obtained according to a defined protocol, which ensures that the same film to focus distance and centering position are employed on every occasion. In this way, movement of the stent graft relative to the bony landmarks can be detected. It is important to note that the movements may be subtle. Films should always be compared with both the most recent and the first postoperative views. Plain radiography also outlines the shape of the endograft (Figure 3). Movement of the endograft will

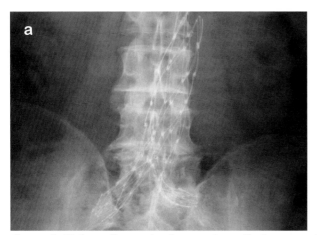 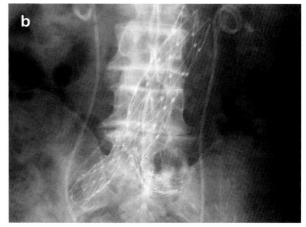

Figure 3. Plain radiograph of an endograft a) one and b) three years after the operation. Note the change in configuration.

usually be associated with a change in configuration, and any such change should prompt careful inspection of previous films to ascertain whether or not there has been any movement relative to the anastomotic seal zones. Plain radiography is also the method of choice to detect movement of a graft limb relative to the contralateral stump and/or fracture of stent graft wireforms.

If migration is suspected, the diagnosis can be confirmed by reference to the CT images. Review of these images will also permit an estimation of the magnitude of movement relative to the length of available aortic neck or iliac artery. Evidence of migration should, in general, prompt consideration of secondary intervention to prevent late graft-related endoleak. However, if there is less than 1cm of caudal displacement, and careful review of the images reveals that there is at least 1.5cm of aortic neck remaining available for seal, it may be judged safe to simply increase the frequency of radiographic examination and intervene only if there is evidence of further migration. In some patients the endograft migrates a short distance (perhaps to adopt a more 'comfortable' position within an angulated neck) and then migrates no further. As long as there remains a reasonable length of anastomotic seal, there is no need to intervene.

Management of migration

The length of proximal seal may be increased by deployment of a short cuff (Figure 4). However, this does not always resolve the problem. Although it may be possible to obtain secure fixation of the cuff to the aortic wall (the authors recommend a cuff with bare suprarenal stent and barbs), the endograft may continue to migrate caudally if the haemodynamic displacement force is greater than the radial force applied by the cuff against the fabric of the endograft. If the aneurysm is capacious, continued movement of the endograft will in due course result in disconnection and late endoleak.

An alternative strategy, therefore, is to reline the entire endograft (secondary endografting), employing either another bifurcated device or an aorto-uni-iliac device. The latter option is simpler, but mandates occlusion of the contralateral limb and restoration of

arterial continuity by means of a femoro-femoral cross-over graft. In some cases, it may be considered preferable to convert to open surgical repair.

Progressive disengagement of one or both iliac limbs or threatened dislocation of the contralateral limb from the endograft stump can usually be treated by deployment of an extension or interposition graft limb.

Graft-related endoleak

Evidence of late graft-related endoleak on follow-up CT or duplex ultrasound examination should, in general, prompt secondary intervention. Proximal endoleak may be treated by deployment of a cuff, secondary endografting or conversion to open surgical repair as described above. Distal endoleak or midgraft endoleak secondary to dislocation of the contralateral limb can usually be treated by deployment of an extension or interposition graft limb. Endoleak secondary to tear of the graft fabric will usually require secondary endografting or conversion to open surgical repair.

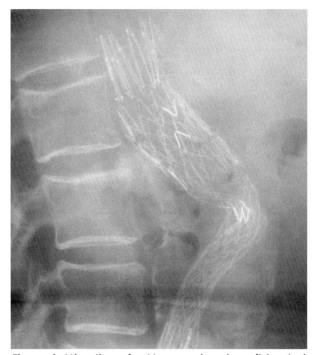

Figure 4. Migration of a Vanguard endograft treated by deployment of a Cook Zenith cuff. Note the deformation of the endograft, secondary to migration.

Side-branch endoleak

Side-branch endoleak is not in the opinion of the authors evidence of late failure, or an indication for secondary intervention, unless associated with expansion of the aneurysm and/or elevated intrasac pressure (see below). Options for intervention include embolisation, laparoscopic clipping, injection of a polymer such as Onyx within the aneurysm sac or laparotomy, incision of the aneurysm sac and under-running of the side-branch origins with a non-absorbable suture.

Expansion of the aneurysm

Continued expansion of the aneurysm after endovascular repair is considered by many to be evidence of failure of the repair. The authors do not agree with this view. Expansion is evidence only that the pressure within the aneurysm is greater than surrounding tissue pressure. It is not evidence that there is sufficient pressure to cause rupture. Furthermore, in the absence of endoleak, rupture is unlikely to result in fatal haemorrhage. Indeed, secondary intervention may not only be unnecessary, but in fact more hazardous than continued observation.

If follow-up imaging reveals continued or secondary expansion of the aneurysm, it is important to try and establish the probable cause and the likely risk of rupture, haemorrhage and death. Only then can one balance the risks of any proposed intervention against the risk of continued observation.

If there is evidence of graft-related endoleak on CT or duplex ultrasound, there is an appreciable risk of late rupture, haemorrhage and death. Urgent secondary intervention is indicated in most cases. If imaging reveals side-branch endoleak, it is rational to conclude that expansion is due to pressurisation of the aneurysm sac by the endoleak, and to proceed to treatment of the endoleak by one of the methods described above. In the authors' experience, however, intervention often fails to resolve the problem. The leak is abolished, but the aneurysm continues to expand and one must then consider alternative explanations.

Expansion may occasionally be due to low flow or intermittent endoleak and in all cases of expansion in which a cause is not apparent, it is important to perform further imaging. Triple-pass CT, contrast-enhanced duplex ultrasound or angiography may be necessary to visualise such leaks. If graft-related, the leak should in most cases be treated by secondary endografting. If not, a conservative approach is reasonable.

Careful review of plain radiographs taken throughout follow-up may reveal evidence of migration, impending dislocation of a modular graft limb or impending disengagement of graft limbs from the iliac arteries. It has been postulated that in such cases, reduction in the length of the anastomotic seal between the endograft and native aorta or iliac artery may allow transmission of systemic pressure to the sac so that expansion is the first sign of threatened graft-related endoleak. In most cases, such abnormalities should prompt secondary intervention. Options include deployment of a cuff or limb extension, secondary endografting and/or conversion to open surgical repair (see above).

Other causes of expansion include accumulation of extracellular material within the aneurysm sac (sac hygroma) and transmission of pressure through thrombus sealing a porous graft. Pressure may also be transmitted through thrombus sealing a previously demonstrated endoleak.

Where the cause of expansion remains unclear, it may help to measure intrasac pressure directly by translumbar puncture under fluoroscopic control. If the pressure is high, and the aneurysm is large, secondary endografting may be considered. If, however, the pressure is relatively low and/or the aneurysm is small, it is difficult to justify secondary intervention. Continued observation is, however, important since expansion of the aneurysm may lead to expansion of the aneurysm neck, migration and late proximal endoleak.

Summary

◆ Endovascular repair has failed if the patient remains or is again at risk of death from aneurysm rupture.

◆ It is better to prevent failure than to try and treat it. Careful selection and planning are the keys to success.

◆ Stent graft migration is the most important cause of late failure after endovascular repair.

◆ Graft-related endoleak should in general be treated by secondary intervention.

◆ Side-branch endoleak can often be safely observed.

◆ Expansion of the aneurysm after endovascular repair does not necessarily indicate failure of treatment.

References

1. Risberg B, Delle M, Lonn L, *et al.* Management of aneurysm sac hygroma. *J Endovasc Ther* 2004; 11: 191-5.
2. Lee WA, Berceli SA, Huber TS, *et al.* Morbidity with retroperitoneal procedures during endovascular abdominal aortic aneurysm repair. *J Vasc Surg* 2003; 38: 459-63.
3. Harris PL, Vallabhaneni SR, Desgranges P, *et al.* Incidence and risk factors of late rupture, conversion, and death after endovascular repair of infrarenal aortic aneurysms: the EUROSTAR experience. European collaborators on stent-graft techniques for aortic aneurysm repair. *J Vasc Surg* 2000; 32: 739-49.
4. Mohan IV, Harris PL, Van Marrewijk CJ, *et al.* Factors and forces influencing stent-graft migration after endovascular aortic aneurysm repair. *J Endovasc Ther* 2002; 6: 748-55.
5. Dias NV, Ivancev K, Malina M, *et al.* Intra-aneurysm sac pressure measurements after endovascular aneurysm repair: differences between shrinking, unchanged, and expanding aneurysms with and without endoleaks. *J Vasc Surg* 2004; 39: 1229-35.

Chapter 8

Thoracic stent grafts: current pitfalls and future developments

Graham Munneke MRCP FRCR, Clinical Fellow, Interventional Radiology

Matt Thompson MD FRCS, Professor of Vascular Surgery

Robert Morgan MRCP FRCR, Consultant Radiologist

St. George's Vascular Institute, St. George's Hospital, London, UK

Introduction

It is 15 years since the first reports in the literature by Parodi [1] and Volodos [2] of the endovascular exclusion of aneurysms of the abdominal and thoracic aorta respectively. Current indications for thoracic aortic stent grafts include descending thoracic aneurysms, complicated Type B dissection, traumatic aortic transection, aortobronchial fistula, penetrating ulcers and false aneurysms [3, 4]. Promising medium-term results have substantially increased referrals from cardiothoracic surgeons to their endovascular colleagues. A recent review of the literature [5] found published reports on the treatment of 1518 patients, with a variety of descending aortic pathologies between 1994 and 2004. Overall, there was a 97% primary technical success and a 30-day mortality of 5.5%. The total endoleak rate was 7.7% and less than 2% of patients suffered neurological complications. These results compare very favourably with the best surgical results [6], but doubts remain over the long-term durability of endovascular repair. Early devices were custom made from surgical graft material with Gianturco-Z stents attached at the proximal and distal ends of the graft to provide fixation. The body of the device was not supported by stents and if fixation failed or the device migrated it was prone to collapse into the aneurysm sac. The first generation commercial endografts were superior to custom-made devices in two ways. Firstly, they consisted of graft material supported along the entire length by nitinol stents leading to far superior column strength. Secondly, the devices were mounted in sophisticated delivery sheaths which aided the smooth passage of the stent to the landing zone and its accurate deployment thereafter. The most commonly used first generation devices were the Gore Excluder and the Medtronic Talent stent graft. Both had longitudinal support struts. In some patients, the longitudinal struts were shown to fatigue and fracture over time. Although there were no documented clinical sequelae, fracture of the longitudinal struts might have the potential for tearing of the graft material or erosion by the fractured struts through the aortic wall [7]. As a result of this possibility, the Gore device was withdrawn temporarily from the market and modified. The four devices currently available for use in Europe are described in detail below (Figure 1). They represent a significant advancement over what has been available previously, but are still not perfect. Notable common shortcomings are the need for large calibre delivery systems which may give rise to difficulties in accessing the thoracic aorta and injuries to the iliac arteries. Moreover, the large calibre delivery systems mean that the days of percutaneous thoracic intervention are still some way off. Finally, none of the devices are available in the small sizes necessary for

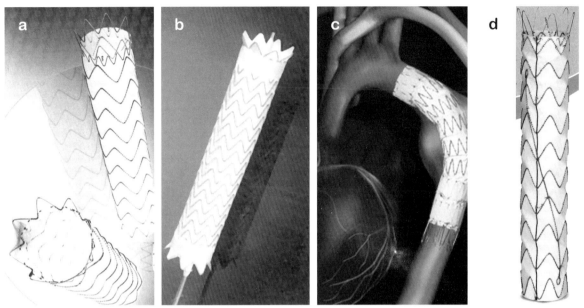

Figure 1. Current thoracic devices. a) Medtronic Valiant. b) Gore TAG. c) Cook TX2. d) Bolton Relay.

treating young patients suffering traumatic aortic injury.

Commercially available devices

Valiant (Medtronic, Santa Rosa, CA, USA)(Figure 2)

The Valiant thoracic stent graft is the successor of the Talent thoracic device, more than 16,000 of which have been implanted worldwide. The Valiant device, like Talent, is constructed of an external skeleton of nitinol stents sewn to thin-walled polyester graft material by non-absorbable sutures. The principal problem with the Talent device was that friction generated within the delivery sheath meant that an inordinate amount of force was required to unsheath the stent when deploying it around the aortic arch. This frictional force also limited the length of device it was possible to produce. The longest available Talent device was only 13cm. Valiant utilises the Xcelerant delivery system, used in the same company's abdominal aortic stent graft. This has a screw mechanism to withdraw the sheath, eliminating the effort required to deploy the device and allowing for the production of longer lengths. Valiant no longer has a longitudinal supporting strut. This makes it more

flexible and should allow it to conform better to tortuous aortic arches. It also eliminates the possibility of longitudinal strut fracture, a potential of the previous design [7].

The device was originally launched in 2005 in two configurations. One configuration is available with a proximal uncovered ('FreeFlo') stent, and the second without a proximal uncovered stent (closed web design). The closed web design is available as a straight or tapered device. The closed web was designed specifically for dissections where a bare stent may traumatise the flap. However, the closed web design has been known to angulate and droop on exiting the delivery sheath making accurate deployment difficult. As a result of this, the device has been withdrawn by Medtronic for use as a proximal stent, limiting its use to that of an extension after initial deployment of a free-flow stent graft.

Additional stent grafts may be deployed in a modular fashion, if additional coverage is required. Proximal 8 markers and distal 0 markers identify the extent of the graft material. A middle 8 marker on the extensions demonstrates the minimum overlap permissible (approximately three stent lengths). Devices with a proximal bare stent may not be used as extensions.

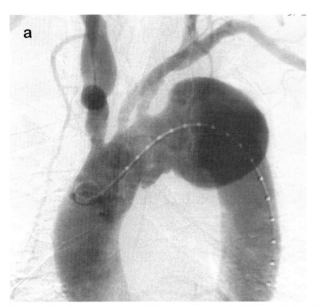 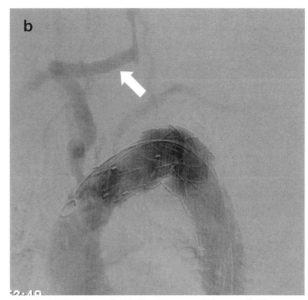

Figure 2. a) Aneurysm of the aortic arch. b) Exclusion by a Valiant stent graft. Note the carotid-carotid bypass graft (white arrow).

An advantage of the system is that it is now available in a good range of lengths and wide diameters. Sizes range from 24-46mm in 2mm intervals and three lengths between 110mm and 215mm (covered length). The delivery system varies from 22-25 French, depending on the diameter of stent graft used. The recommended oversizing is 10-20% for aneurysms and up to 10% for dissections. A minimum 15mm proximal and distal landing zone is suggested.

As mentioned previously, the stent graft is mounted in the Xcelerant delivery system. Deployment of the self-expanding stent may be achieved in two ways. For accurate deployment, rotation of the handle around a screw gear produces controlled withdrawal of the covering sheath. If more rapid deployment is required, a quick release trigger disengages the screw gear allowing deployment by pulling back the handle. When using the former method, the torque within the system has a tendency for the stent to move proximally by a few millimeters. Gentle traction on the delivery system is required to counteract this and hold the stent position stationary. Pharmacologically-induced hypotension should be employed (to a mean arterial pressure of 80-100mmHg), to avoid the wind sock effect. The first two springs should be released with the device slightly proximal of the desired

position. The device is then withdrawn to the desired location after check angiography and the rest of the stent graft is released.

In summary, the system represents a significant step forward with good controlled delivery and a useful range of diameters and lengths. The delivery system is very flexible and is a major advance on the previous Talent device. A range of smaller sizes for younger patients is desirable and the production of smaller delivery systems would be beneficial for all devices.

TAG thoracic endoprosthesis (W.L. Gore, Flagstaff, AZ, USA) (Figure 3)

The Gore TAG device replaced the Excluder thoracic device that had been withdrawn in 2002, following reports of strut fracture in some patients [7]. The new stent retains Gore's unique SIM-PULL deployment system, but has had a number of improvements. Notably, the longitudinal support strut has been removed and the graft material has been changed to non-porous expanded polytetrafluoro-ethylene (PTFE), as in the revised abdominal Excluder.

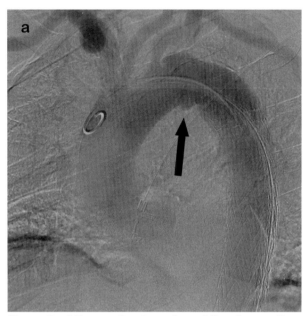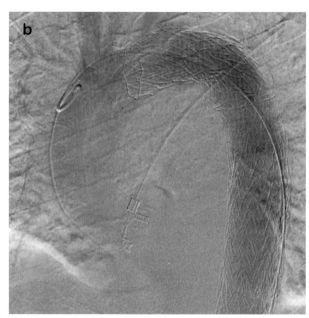

Figure 3. a) Traumatic dissection of the descending aorta (black arrow). b) Appearance post-deployment of two Gore TAG stent grafts.

The expanded PTFE graft is heat sealed to a nitinol stent exoskeleton. This avoids the use of sutures and the possibility of graft leaks through suture holes. Sealing cuffs are positioned at both ends. The ends of the stent are crenulated. There are radiopaque gold markers at the bases of the crenulations, 1cm from the ends of the endoprosthesis. The stent is mounted on the end of a delivery catheter constrained within an expanded PTFE sleeve. The catheter is inserted through a 30cm introducer sheath (20-24 French, depending on stent diameter). The catheter itself is low profile and is easily trackable around the aortic arch. Once in position, the stent is released by traction on a cord which unzips the restraining sleeve. The stent graft deploys from its centre outwards in less than one second. This reduces the possibility of the cardiac output causing stent malposition during deployment.

The TAG device is available in diameters of 26-40mm, enabling the treatment of patients with un-diseased aortic dimensions of 23-37mm. Lengths between 10-20cm are available and several overlapping grafts may be deployed to treat longer lesions.

The stent is extremely easy to position and deploy. Its ease of use and rapid delivery definitely have advantages in situations such as aortic rupture, when speed of deployment and exclusion of the aortic tear is paramount. However, the 'all or nothing' nature of the delivery system is also its major disadvantage. If the stent jumps forward or back during release there is no way to reposition it, except by attempting to drag it back with a balloon. For this reason, we don't use the device if accurate positioning is essential. Therefore, the device is used for lesions when the landing zones are not close to essential vessels, such as the left common carotid or coeliac arteries. One other important drawback of the system is the requirement for introduction into the vascular system through a sheath. Although the device itself is quite small, the sheaths are relatively large. Moreover, the sheath diameters quoted by the manufacturers refer to the inner rather than the outer diameters. For example, the 24 French sheath required by the 37 and 40mm diameter grafts, actually has an outer diameter of 9.1mm corresponding to a sheath size of 27 French. The large sheath sizes for the Gore device should be taken into consideration when the iliac arteries are of borderline calibre.

Zenith TX2 endograft (William Cook Europe, Bjaeverskov, Denmark)

The new Cook thoracic stent graft is similar in construction and delivery to their existing abdominal stent graft. It is available in both a one-piece design and two-piece modular configurations to treat varying lengths of aortic pathology. The stent graft is constructed of stainless steel Z stents sutured to polyester fabric graft. In both configurations, fixation is enhanced by 5mm long caudally orientated barbs which protrude through the fabric at the proximal end. At the distal end an uncovered stent with cranially orientated barbs is present. The TX2 proximal and distal components fit into each other with a two stent overlap.

The stent graft is mounted on a central core within a braided sheath. The sheath has a hydrophilic coating to facilitate introduction. Trigger wires hold the device in position even when the sheath has been retracted. The proximal stent is pinched-in toward the central core allowing blood to pass around the stent and making proximal repositioning a possibility. Once a satisfactory position has been achieved, two trigger wires release the proximal and distal stent attachments and allow the delivery system to be withdrawn.

The TX2 endoprosthesis is available as a single piece or a two-piece device. The one-piece design is rather short (81-85mm long) and is suited to patients with short lesions, such as aortic transections. The two piece device is the more versatile of the two configurations, and is available in a wider range of sizes. The two-piece endoprosthesis is available in 28-42mm diameters and in both straight and 4mm tapered proximal components. Both the straight and tapered components are available in at least two lengths for each diameter ranging from 108-216mm. Proximal and distal extensions are available. Cook recommend oversizing by 10-25% and at least a 3cm landing zone.

The delivery system will be familiar to those who have used the Zenith abdominal graft. It allows accurate positioning and keeps the graft stable during deployment. The device has the lowest profile sheath, only 20 French for diameters of up to 34mm, and 22 French for the larger sizes. This makes the endoprosthesis attractive for patients with narrow access vessels. On the negative side, although the proximal fixation barbs prevent migration, they make the device less suitable for patients with thoracic dissection because of the potential for trauma to the fragile intima, producing further dissection. However, this has not as yet been seen in clinical practice.

Relay (Bolton Medical, Sunrise, FL, USA)

This is a relatively new endoprosthesis with only a small number of implants worldwide. The stent graft comprises nitinol stents stitched to surgical graft material with an uncovered proximal bare stent. The proximal fixation and sealing zone has an independent 'freeflex' articulation with the body of the stent graft that is said to make it very conformable around the aortic arch. Middle markers denote a spiral support strut that must be aligned with the outermost curvature of the arch.

The stent is mounted on a dual sheath Transport™ delivery system. A rigid outer sheath facilitates device insertion into the abdominal aorta. The stent graft is advanced to the thoracic aorta inside the inner sheath. Deployment is achieved by withdrawing the inner sheath. The proximal bare stent is held closed within an apex grip allowing forward and backward repositioning in the semi-deployed situation.

The Relay device is available in diameters of 22-46mm and the larger sizes may be specified with a 4mm taper. The covered lengths are between 9-20cm and 10cm extension grafts are offered.

As yet, little is known about this graft; however, the presence of a longitudinal support strut raises some concerns. As mentioned above, when present on other devices, such struts have been prone to fracture. Although in this device it is placed in a spiral position, the possibility of future strut failure remains.

Future directions

Percutaneous access

As has been mentioned above, the large diameter delivery sheaths for thoracic devices may cause iliac artery rupture, most notably in female patients. Advances in technology and materials should see their profile reduce with time. The smallest calibre thoracic device is currently 20 French and wholly percutaneous thoracic stent grafting has been performed with large calibre percutaneous closure devices [8]. Future generations of low profile stent grafts may enable routine percutaneous treatment with the aid of suture-mediated arterial closure devices.

Expanding the indications for thoracic endografting

In general, proximal and distal landing zones of adequate (15-20cm) normal calibre aorta are required for adequate graft fixation. In cases such as arch aneurysms, Type A dissection and thoraco-abdominal aneurysms, these are available. It is known that the left subclavian artery may be covered, usually without clinical sequelae [9]. The same is of course not true for the other supra-aortic branches. Strategies to extend the length of aorta available include surgical bypass of the carotid and subclavian arteries, branched stent grafts or a combination of the two.

Bypass grafting

Depending on how proximal the landing zone must be, the left common carotid and innominate arteries may be covered following extra-anatomic bypass (Figure 4). Combinations of carotid-subclavian, carotid-carotid and ascending aorta to innominate and left carotid grafts may be employed [10-12]. The latter may be performed with the use of aortic side clamping, obviating the need for extracorporal circulation or deep hypothermic circulatory arrest and their attendant risks. Others have even proposed complete arch coverage combined with supra-aortic bypass and a femoro-axillary bypass graft to provide inflow [13]. This technique has not been widely practised, as thrombosis of the graft would be catastrophic.

Several small series have shown that extra-anatomic bypass of the arch vessels may be achieved with low procedural mortality and excellent long-term patency of the grafts [14-16].

Branched grafts

The development of stent grafts with side branches is a more elegant, but technically demanding method of complete arch reconstruction. Thus far, the majority of work on this subject has been performed by teams led by Timothy Chuter in the USA and Kanji Inoue in Japan. The Japanese device has between one and three side branches and is inserted femorally. Traction wires attached to the side branches are snared from brachial and carotid access, allowing the stents to be drawn into position in their target vessels. The main stent and its side branches are then balloon expanded into position. The majority of their experience is with the single branched (left subclavian) variant of the device [17]. As it is debatable as to the need to preserve left subclavian perfusion, the added complexity of the procedure does not seem justified. However, they have successfully treated an arch aneurysm with a triple-branched graft [18]. The procedure took eight hours and required 573ml of contrast media.

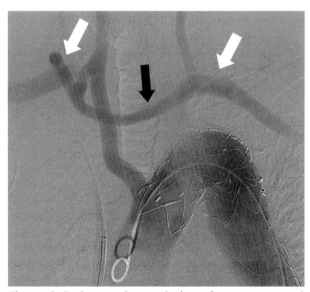

Figure 4. Endovascular exclusion of an aneurysmal aberrant right subclavian artery. All the supra-aortic vessels are supplied by the right carotid artery via carotid-carotid (black arrow) and carotid-subclavian bypass grafts (white arrows).

Chuter *et al* first bench-tested prototype branched stent grafts on a saline perfused rubber model of the thoracic aorta [19]. The first three devices were triple-branched designs and the fourth had a single side branch for the innominate artery. He concluded that only the single-branch design was easy enough to insert, orientate and deploy to merit its use in patients. He further concluded that multi-branch devices, such as the Inoue graft required a level of technical expertise that was unlikely to be widely available. The team went on to use the single-branch modular graft to treat a patient with a pseudo-aneurysm of the aortic arch [20]. Carotid-carotid and carotid-left subclavian bypasses were first performed. The device was a two-piece modular design. The proximal bifurcated segment had a long narrow innominate limb and a wide short aortic limb. It was inserted via the right carotid artery below the bypass graft. It was deployed in the ascending aorta leaving the long limb in the innominate artery and the short limb in the arch. The bypass graft maintained perfusion of the right carotid circulation during its occlusion by the delivery sheath. The short limb was then cannulated from femoral access and a tube extension graft deployed down to the descending thoracic aorta to exclude the aneurysm.

These cases show what is feasible with branched technology, but as yet there are no commercially available devices to allow more widespread application.

Fenestrated grafts

Although the development of branched graft technology is very challenging, it should be slightly easier to develop and implant devices with fenestrations at the proximal end for the left subclavian and common carotid arteries and at the distal end of one or more of the visceral arteries [8]. It is likely that fenestrated graft technology will advance quicker than branched graft designs.

Conclusions

Much progress has been made since the early days of homemade custom devices. The second generation commercial devices represent a large step forward, but there is still room for refinement and improvement. Time will tell whether they suffer from design-related problems like their predecessors. The indications and results of thoracic endografting are still to be fully evaluated and validated by randomised trials. In particular, there are little data on their efficacy in chronic aneurysmal dissections and their role in uncomplicated dissection is unknown. Advances on the horizon should lead to the possibility of the procedure becoming totally percutaneous, and branched or fenestrated grafts may open up the whole aorta to treatment.

Summary

- Much progress has been made since the early days of homemade custom devices.

- The second generation commercial devices represent a large step forward, but there is still room for refinement and improvement.

- The indications and results of thoracic endografting are still to be fully evaluated and validated by randomised trials.

- There are little data on their efficacy in chronic aneurysmal dissections and their role in uncomplicated dissection is unknown.

- Advances on the horizon should lead to the possibility of the procedure becoming totally percutaneous.

- Branched or fenestrated grafts may open up the whole aorta to treatment.

References

1. Parodi JC, Palmaz JC, Barone HD. Transfemoral intraluminal graft implantation for abdominal aortic aneurysms. *Ann Vasc Surg* 1991; 5: 491-9.

2. Volodos NL, Karpovich IP, Troyan VI, *et al*. Clinical experience of the use of self-fixing synthetic prostheses for remote endoprosthetics of the thoracic and the abdominal aorta and iliac arteries through the femoral artery and as intraoperative endoprosthesis for aorta reconstruction. *Vasa Suppl* 1991; 33: 93-5.

3. Matravers P, Morgan R, Belli A. The use of stent grafts for the treatment of aneurysms and dissections of the thoracic aorta: a single centre experience. *Eur J Vasc Endovasc Surg* 2003; 26(6): 587-95.

4. Munneke G, Loosemore T, Smith J, Thompson M, Morgan R, Belli AM. Pseudoaneurysm after aortic coarctation repair presenting with an aortobronchial fistula successfully treated with an aortic stent graft. *Clin Radiol* 2006; 61(1): 104-8.

5. Sayed S, Thompson MM. Endovascular repair of the descending thoracic aorta: evidence for the change in clinical practice. *Vascular* 2005; 13(3): 148-57.

6. Brandt M, Hussel K, Walluscheck KP, *et al*. Early and long-term results of replacement of the descending aorta. *Eur J Vasc Endovasc Surg* 2005; 30(4): 365-9.

7. Ellozy SH, Carroccio A, Minor M, *et al*. Challenges of endovascular tube graft repair of thoracic aortic aneurysm: midterm follow-up and lessons learned. *J Vasc Surg* 2003; 38(4): 676-83.

8. Anderson JL, Adam DJ, Berce M, *et al*. Repair of thoracoabdominal aortic aneurysms with fenestrated and branched endovascular stent grafts. *J Vasc Surg* 2005; 42(4): 600-7.

9. Hausegger KA, Oberwalder P, Tiesenhausen K, *et al*. Intentional left subclavian artery occlusion by thoracic aortic stent-grafts without surgical transposition. *J Endovasc Ther* 2001; 8(5): 472-6.

10. Kato N, Shimono T, Hirano T, *et al*. Aortic arch aneurysms: treatment with extraanatomical bypass and endovascular stent-grafting. *Cardiovasc Intervent Radiol* 2002; 25(5): 419-22.

11. Munneke GJ, Loosemore TM, Belli AM, *et al*. Aneurysm of an aberrant right subclavian artery successfully excluded by a thoracic aortic stent graft with supra-aortic bypass of three arch vessels. *Cardiovasc Intervent Radiol* 2005; 28(5): 653-5.

12. Dambrin C, Marcheix B, Hollington L, *et al*. Surgical treatment of an aortic arch aneurysm without cardio-pulmonary bypass: endovascular stent-grafting after extra-anatomic bypass of supra-aortic vessels. *Eur J Cardiothorac Surg* 2005; 27(1): 159-61.

13. Criado FJ, Barnatan MF, Rizk Y, *et al*. Technical strategies to expand stent-graft applicability in the aortic arch and proximal descending thoracic aorta. *J Endovasc Ther* 2002; 9 Suppl 2: II32-8.

14. Czerny M, Zimpfer D, Fleck T, *et al*. Initial results after combined repair of aortic arch aneurysms by sequential transposition of the supra-aortic branches and consecutive endovascular stent-graft placement. *Ann Thorac Surg* 2004; 78(4): 1256-60.

15. Carrel TP, Do DD, Triller J, *et al*. A less invasive approach to completely repair the aortic arch. *Ann Thorac Surg* 2005; 80(4): 1475-8.

16. Schumacher H, Bockler D, Bardenheuer H, *et al*. Endovascular aortic arch reconstruction with supra-aortic transposition for symptomatic contained rupture and dissection: early experience in 8 high-risk patients. *J Endovasc Ther* 2003; 10(6): 1066-74.

17. Saito N, Kimura T, Odashiro K, *et al*. Feasibility of the Inoue single-branched stent-graft implantation for thoracic aortic aneurysm or dissection involving the left subclavian artery: short- to medium-term results in 17 patients. *J Vasc Surg* 2005; 41(2): 206-12.

18. Saito N, Kimura T, Toma M, *et al*. Images in cardiovascular medicine. Endovascular treatment of a giant aortic arch aneurysm with a triple-branched stent graft. *Circulation* 2005; 112(12): e151-2.

19. Chuter TA, Buck DG, Schneider DB, *et al*. Development of a branched stent-graft for endovascular repair of aortic arch aneurysms. *J Endovasc Ther* 2003; 10(5): 940-5.

20. Chuter TA, Schneider DB, Reilly LM, *et al*. Modular branched stent graft for endovascular repair of aortic arch aneurysm and dissection. *J Vasc Surg* 2003; 38(4): 859-63.

Chapter 9

EVAR for thoracic aneurysms: selection criteria and adjuvant procedures

Keith G Jones MS FRCS, Consultant Vascular Surgeon

King's College Hospital, London, UK

Introduction

The concept and development of endovascular stent grafting for the treatment of thoracic aortic disease has generally focused upon cases deemed unfit or unsuitable for open surgery [1]. Although the early practice by Dake and colleagues [2] was described in four patients, all deemed surgical candidates, subsequent patients were those considered not fit for open repair. The favourable early outcomes of thoracic endografting were, therefore, in an unfavourably selected group, with the prerequisites to success being vascular access and anatomical suitability [3]. Indeed, Mitchell *et al* describe suitability as entailing a relatively straight segment of aorta and the absence of nearby important side branches [3]. Nevertheless, they also describe the need for operative correction of the subclavian artery in order to obtain an adequate proximal neck. This was an early example of how the use of adjuvant procedures could increase the endovascular suitability of patients.

The diminished risk of mortality and morbidity has often resulted in endovascular stenting being considered as the treatment of choice for patients with thoracic aortic disease (Figure 1). This is not surprising when a review of endovascular repair of the thoracic aorta has reported a 97% success rate in 1518 cases (of which 810 were aneurysms), with a 30-day mortality of 5.5% [4].

Although referral patterns may be dependent upon local unit policies and specialist interest, the utilisation of thoracic aortic endografting continues to increase. Whilst the primary selection criteria continue to be based upon anatomical suitability, the development of adjuvant procedures to create suitable landing zones will continue to increase numbers of patients suitable for treatment using thoracic stent grafts. This chapter examines the current selection criteria for thoracic stent grafting and describes those adjuvant procedures, which have been developed to increase its applicability.

Selection criteria

Need for intervention

Thoracic aneurysmal disease is known to be increasing, with an incidence of approximately 10 per 100,000 patient years [5], of which 40% affects the descending thoracic aorta. For large aneurysms, if left untreated, the two-year mortality rate may be in excess of 70%, with the major cause of death being rupture. There is, therefore, a need for prophylactic

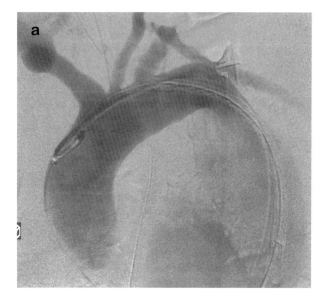

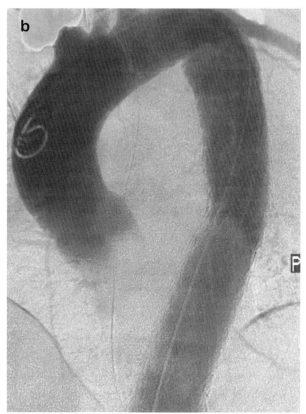

Figure 1. a) Intra-operative angiogram showing the endovascular treatment of an aneurysm of the descending thoracic aorta. The stent is shown in position pre-deployment, with a good proximal landing zone. b) Intra-operative angiogram showing successful deployment of two endografts. The proximal bare stents are at the origin of the left subclavian artery, giving complete exclusion of the aneurysm. *Courtesy of St. George's Hospital, London.*

intervention, and this must be balanced against procedural risks.

The recommended aneurysm size for open intervention in asymptomatic patients, based on expected rate of complications, is 55mm for the ascending and 65mm for the descending aorta, respectively. Both of these are lowered in patients with Marfan's syndrome, because of the increased risk of rupture associated with this condition. Nevertheless, these recommendations need to be balanced against comorbidity, and because of the lower risks associated with endovascular thoracic repair, there may be an argument for intervention at a smaller size, maybe 55mm. Indeed, some authors even describe intervention at an aneurysmal size of 50mm [6].

Aetiology

The majority of thoracic aneurysms are either secondary to medial degeneration or chronic dissection, and are entirely suitable for endovascular repair, provided they have a suitable landing zone, or one can be created. The remaining aneurysms are due to connective tissue disease, non-infectious aortitis, bacterial and fungal infections, or are false aneurysms, due to previous surgery or trauma. Endovascular repair has been performed for all of these aneurysm types, although the endovascular treatment of mycotic aneurysms may be regarded as palliative. Nevertheless, there are several series, with good medium-term follow-up, which would suggest endovascular repair to be curative, especially those for primary mycotic aneurysms arising in previously normal areas of aorta [7]. The best graft material to use for mycotic aneurysm stent graft procedures remains unclear; however, if a stent graft is inserted into a potentially infected bed, the recommendation would be for continuation of lifelong antibiotics [7-8].

Open versus endovascular

There is no evidence to favour either endovascular or open repair in comparable patients with thoracic aortic aneurysm. The case against open repair has been the higher associated morbidity and mortality, whereas for endovascular repair the downside is related to the unknown durability of devices, and the need for secondary intervention. However, medium-term results from single centres [6, 9] and registry reports [10] would favour an endovascular approach, especially since the majority of secondary interventions would be endovascular in nature. Ultimately, however, it may be the development of hybrid (combined open and endovascular) procedures, which are shown to produce the best outcomes and increase the number and range of treatable thoraco-abdominal aneurysms.

Risk of paraplegia

The risk of paraplegia is much less for endovascular (1-5%) than for open (5-10%) procedures, although why extensive coverage of the descending thoracic aorta is not associated with an increased paraplegia rate is not known. For a combined abdominal and thoracic aortic repair or, if the patient has had a previous AAA repair, consideration needs to be given to an increased risk of about 10%. For these patients, a prophylactic lumbar drain should be inserted.

Suitable access

The determining factor for suitability of access is the passage of the 24 French delivery system. This may be restricted either by vessel size or tortuosity. The small series of mycotic aneurysms described by Sayed et al is indicative of the possible difficulties female patients may present, with the three thoracic endografts being delivered by femoral, iliac and aortic punctures respectively [8].

Pre-procedural imaging is extremely important in the selection of suitable access vessels prior to thoracic stent graft insertion. It is important that the CT angiogram, duplex scan or conventional angiogram includes the vessels of the pelvis and the groins, and that the tortuosity of the iliac arteries is fully appreciated. It may be necessary to overcome tortuosity using a guidewire passed retrogradely from the left brachial to the femoral artery, in an attempt to straighten the passage of the stent and assist deployment (body flossing). Retrograde guidewire cannulation of the brachial arteries can also be used to mark the origins of the left subclavian or innominate arteries (Figure 2a) in order to allow accurate placement of the proximal stent graft. In addition, Chuter et al have described a proximal insertion via the right carotid artery, with the benefits of a short introducer and increased ease of graft positioning. This approach should, however, be reserved for cases involving adjuvant procedures to the great vessels [11].

Landing zone anatomy

Proximal landing zone

The ideal length for the proximal landing zone is at least 2cm. If this length of normal aorta is present, even aneurysms arising in the proximal descending aorta can be treated without involvement of the branch vessels (Figure 1). However, early experience of thoracic stent grafting in the presence of proximal descending aortic disease was disappointing, primarily due to maldeployment and dissection [3]. In addition to the requirement for an adequate length of seal, the concavity of the arch results in lack of apposition of the stent graft, Type 1 endoleak and stent collapse due to extrinsic pressure. In an attempt to improve the number of aneurysms involving the distal arch, which were suitable for stent grafting, a number of adjuvant procedures have evolved. These include:

- covering the left subclavian origin +/- retrograde coiling;
- carotid-subclavian transposition or bypass;
- carotid-carotid bypass;
- innominate bypass;
- a combination with ascending and arch of aorta surgery;
- branched stent grafts.

These procedures have not only improved the degree of proximal fixation of devices, but, along with visceral and renal bypass procedures, have expanded the indications for endograft treatment to include Type Crawford I, II and III thoraco-abdominal aortic aneurysms.

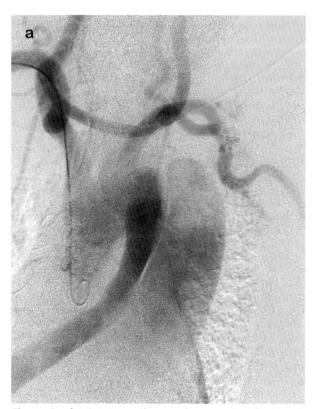
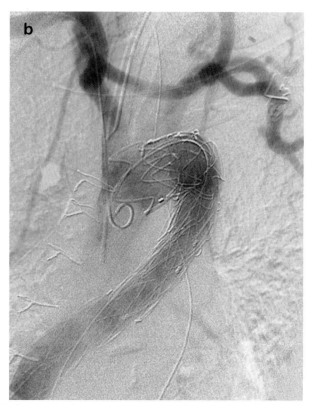

Figure 2. a) Intra-operative angiogram showing treatment of a thoracic aneurysm arising from a chronic Type B dissection. Note the functioning caroto-carotid cross-over graft and the graft from this to the left subclavian artery. The pigtail catheter is used to mark the innominate artery, as well as for intra-operative angiograms. b) Intra-operative angiogram post-stent graft deployment. Note the covered stent graft overlying the left common carotid and subclavian artery origins. A carotid cross-over graft maintains perfusion of the great vessels. *Courtesy of St. George's Hospital, London.*

Left subclavian artery

The EUROSTAR and UK thoracic stent graft registries show that placement of the stent over the origin of the left subclavian artery is required in up to 17% of cases, in order to obtain an adequate proximal landing zone [10]. Just over half of these patients had undergone pre-emptive subclavian artery revascularisation, either by transposition or bypass. In the other half, the subclavian artery was covered without a bypass procedure, relying on the adequacy of the collateral circulation to maintain left arm vascularisation. Bell *et al* showed the safety of this procedure in 2003. They describe covering the left subclavian artery origin in 17 of 67 stent procedures, without the need for revascularisation [9]. In addition, Rehders *et al* describe stenting over the left subclavian origin in 22 of 171 cases. At follow-up, only seven patients described mild symptoms of

subclavian steal syndrome [12]. It is, therefore, generally accepted that subclavian revascularisation is unnecessary, provided that the contralateral vertebral artery and the aortic branch from which it originates is patent. There are, however, several notable exceptions. These include:

- previous cardiac revascularisation using a left internal mammary graft;
- a left arm arteriovenous shunt for haemodialysis;
- right subclavian artery arising distal to the left (Lusoria artery);
- left-hand dominant professional patients [13].

Additionally, if the pre-operative risk of paraplegia is felt to be increased, due to planned extensive coverage of the descending thoracic aorta with a combined or previous abdominal aortic repair, then this risk may be diminished by prophylactic revascularisation [14].

Left common carotid artery

In some cases, the proximity of the aneurysm to the arch of the aorta requires deployment of the stent graft, not only over the left subclavian artery origin, but also over that of the left common carotid artery. This is not merely a factor of suitable length of apposition of the stent graft, but also relates to the ability of the proximal stent graft to fit snugly against the concavity of the arch. Without this apposition, not only is a Type 1 endoleak likely to occur, but also there is a risk that the extrinsic force of the blood will cause displacement, collapse or closure of the proximal stent. This problem would have occurred in the case represented in Figure 2a, where aneurysmal change had occurred in a chronic Type B dissection originating just distal to the left subclavian origin. The concavity of the aortic arch has a very acute angle and, in order to gain apposition, the stent would need to be placed within a landing zone beyond the apex of the arch and involving the origin of the left common carotid artery. Therefore, a carotid-carotid bypass has been performed, along with a carotid-left subclavian bypass, so allowing more proximal stent graft deployment (Figure 2b). As is the case with subclavian revascularisation, the carotid-carotid cross-over may be performed during the same procedure, immediately prior to stenting, or as an initial procedure at some time point prior to stenting.

Chuter et al describe the use of a cross-over graft in the treatment of a wide-necked aortic arch pseudoaneurysm. In this case, ligation of the proximal left common carotid artery was left until after the proximal endograft had been deployed via the right common carotid artery. In this instance, the 'temporary retrograde' cross-over graft flow diminished the risk of right cerebral hypoperfusion, whilst the delivery system was occluding the right common carotid.

There is good evidence for the durability of these hybrid procedures [6, 9, 15]; however, there is also a risk of stroke, presumably due to manipulation of the delivery system within the arch, resulting in the dislodgement of embolic material. In addition, with the use of prosthetic material to perform the extra-anatomical bypass, there is the inevitable risk of graft infection. For this reason, Czerny et al successfully describe surgical revascularisation of the left carotid artery, without the need for prosthetic graft insertion. This technique involves transposition of the left common carotid artery onto the innominate artery followed by transposition of the left subclavian artery into the former [16].

The innominate artery

For more proximal advancement of the stent graft, the origin of the innominate artery may be covered, but this requires a median sternotomy to allow prior grafting of the innominate artery. An inverted bifurcated graft is used, with a proximal anastomosis to a longitudinal arteriotomy in the ascending aorta and the distal anastomosis to the innominate and left common carotid arteries. Alternatively, one limb can be anastomosed onto the left subclavian artery, with the common carotid anastomosed end-to-side to the graft [17]. These cases require placement of the subsequent endograft over the arch of the aorta, which in turn requires flexibility of the sheath and the graft to allow both introduction and deployment of the device. Both Type 1 endoleak and neurological complications have been reported following this procedure [17-18].

Hybrid procedures of the proximal aortic arch

In those patients with aneurysm involving both the arch and the proximal descending aorta, the open management involves a two-stage procedure, with a proximal elephant trunk repair being followed by a distal repair of the descending aorta. The morbidity and mortality associated with this approach remain substantial, and there would appear to be a potential advantage for combining endovascular grafting with less invasive surgical techniques.

Greenberg et al describe 22 cases in which an elephant trunk repair of the proximal aorta was followed after a mean interval of seven months by retrograde insertion of an endograft into the elephant trunk [19]. Further adjuvant procedures included left subclavian revascularisation in five patients and mesenteric bypass in three patients. The mortality rate was 4.5% at one month, rising to 15.8% at 24 months.

A further variation is described by Karck et al [20]. They describe a single procedure utilising a hybrid prosthesis, with the stent component deployed antegradely into the descending aorta. The graft component is sutured to the wall of the distal arch, the great vessels are inserted onto a patch and the proximal anastomosis performed. The operation is performed via a median sternotomy and utilises hypothermic circulatory arrest and antegrade cerebral perfusion. The peri-operative mortality is reported as 4.5%, which is comparable to the two-stage hybrid procedure.

To date, there are no objective data to compare these procedures and long-term durability results, in combination with accurate morbidity data, are required before the optimal hybrid can be determined.

Branched stent grafts

The expected development of branched stent grafts for the treatment of thoracic aortic disease has not occurred, and is well behind that which is allowing the fenestrated/branched graft treatment of peri and suprarenal aortic aneurysms [11]. Further progress in this field is awaited.

Distal landing zone

A 2cm landing zone is also required to effect a seal in the distal neck of the aneurysm. This can often involve coverage of the visceral and renal vessels, with the potential risk of visceral and renal ischaemia. To counter this, several adjuvant procedures have been developed. These include:

- scallops or fenestrations of the distal stent to allow overstenting of the coeliac axis without occlusion;
- branched grafts to the visceral vessels;
- extra-anatomical surgical revascularisation prior to stenting.

Fenestrated or branched stent grafts

In 2001, Stanley et al described a case in which a fenestration was cut in a Cook Zenith stent graft (William A. Cook Australia Pty. Ltd, Brisbane, Australia), in order to accommodate a coeliac trunk situated 0.5cm below the distal extent of a thoracic aneurysm [21]. Inoue et al had previously (1997) described the use of a single branched graft in order to perfuse the coeliac trunk [22].

There was little development of these techniques until recently. In 2005, Anderson et al demonstrated the feasibility of using fenestrated and branched stent grafts to treat thoraco-abdominal aneurysms [23]. In three of the four initially reported cases, previous abdominal surgery would have made a hybrid approach high risk, and in one of these, the whole graft procedure was performed percutaneously. However, these cases require high quality imaging both pre-operatively, to allow for complex graft customisation and design, and intra-operatively to facilitate the difficult catheter manipulations. For this reason, fenestration and branch grafting with respect to the mesenteric vessels involved in thoraco-abdominal aneurysms can only be viewed as experimental and is limited to highly specialised centres.

Visceral/renal revascularisation

The recent advancement of endovascular treatment to include Type II, III and IV thoraco-abdominal aneurysms has occurred due to the development of hybrid procedures designed to retrogradely revascularise the visceral and renal vessels.

In 2002, Ballard et al described a technique for visceral perfusion during open repair of Type III aneurysms. This utilised a trifurcated graft, arising from the aorta distal to the aneurysm, and anastomosed to the visceral vessels, so allowing perfusion during the aneurysm repair [24]. This concept has been utilised in combination with endovascular stenting, with surgical grafts being taken from the distal infrarenal aorta or the common iliac arteries to revascularise the coeliac trunk via the hepatic artery, the superior mesenteric artery and both renal arteries. The origin of the grafts, or an additional side conduit,

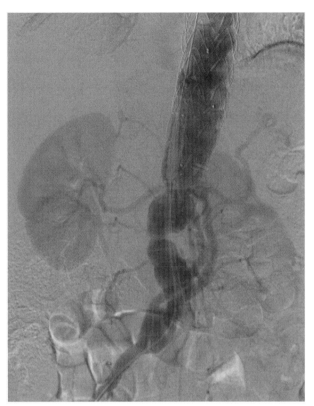

Figure 3. Intra-operative angiogram showing a hybrid repair of a thoraco-abdominal aneurysm. The distal aspect of the stent is covering the origins of the visceral vessels. Visceral revascularisation is from the right common iliac artery. *Courtesy of St. George's Hospital, London.*

can then be used for insertion of the stent graft delivery system (Figure 3).

In 1999, Quinones-Baldrich *et al* described a Type IV thoraco-abdominal aneurysm with associated visceral artery aneurysms, where a combined surgical approach of retrograde perfusion of the visceral

vessels and endovascular grafting allowed successful occlusion with minimal mesenteric ischaemia [25]. This case would have been very high risk for surgery alone because of previous aortic surgery.

Rimmer *et al* described a similar hybrid procedure in a high risk patient with a Type III thoraco-abdominal aneurysm, in whom previous thoracic and abdominal surgery had been performed [26]. An inverted bifurcated graft was anastomosed to each iliac artery and the four limbs anastomosed to the hepatic artery, superior mesenteric artery and both renal arteries respectively. The origins of the visceral and renal vessels were ligated and a thoracic endograft deployed across them. The subsequent series of 29 patients treated by this technique, involved patients who were deemed to have an excessively high risk of morbidity and mortality if offered open surgery. Nevertheless, the favourable results associated with this technique, resulting in the complete exclusion of the aneurysm and the absence of paraplegia, has led to the hybrid approach now being preferred to open surgery, for the treatment of Crawford Type I, II and III thoraco-abdominal aneurysms [27]. The benefits include, avoidance of a thoracotomy and its associated respiratory morbidity, the absence of thoracic aortic clamping, diminished mesenteric ischaemia and the reduced risk of paraplegia.

Clearly, as with all endovascular aneurysm procedures, longer-term durability data are required, but it is difficult to see how open surgery alone will have any advantages over this hybrid approach. Additionally, it remains to be seen if branch graft technology will develop to allow complete endovascular procedures, which can compare favourably with the hybrid approach.

Summary

◆ Endovascular stent grafting should be the preferred treatment of aneurysms of the descending thoracic aorta.

◆ The utilisation of branch vessel revascularisation procedures facilitates endovascular repair of thoraco-abdominal aneurysms.

◆ Evolution of fenestrated/branched grafts may allow complete endovascular treatment.

◆ The risks of paraplegia and the need for CSF drainage should always be considered.

◆ It is safe to cover the left subclavian artery origin, in the majority of cases.

◆ Passage of the stent graft often requires more proximal access than the common femoral artery.

References

1. Volodos NL, Karpovich IP, Troyan VI, *et al*. Clinical experience of the use of self-fixing synthetic prosthesis for remote endoprosthetics of the thoracic and the abdominal aorta and iliac arteries through the femoral artery and as endoprosthesis for aorta reconstruction. *Vasa* 1991; 33: 93-5.

2. Dake MD, Miller DC, Semba RS, *et al*. Transluminal placement of endovascular stent-grafts for the treatment of descending thoracic aortic aneurysms. *N Engl J Med* 1994; 331: 1729-34.

3. Mitchell RS, Dake MD, Semba CP, *et al*. Endovascular stent-graft repair of thoracic aortic aneurysms. *J Thorac Cardiovasc Surg* 1996; 111: 1054-62.

4. Sayed S, Thompson MM. Endovascular repair of the descending thoracic aorta: evidence for the change in clinical practice. *Vascular* 2005; 13(3): 148-57.

5. Elefteriades JA. Natural history of thoracic aneurysms: indications for surgery, and surgical versus nonsurgical risks. *Ann Thorac Surg* 2002: 74(5): 1204-9.

6. Criado FJ, Abul-Khoudoud OR, Domer GS, *et al*. Endovascular repair of the thoracic aorta: lessons learned. *Ann Thorac Surgery* 2005; 80 (3): 857-63.

7. Jones KG, Bell RE, Sabharwal T, *et al*. Treatment of mycotic aortic aneurysms with endoluminal grafts. *Eur J Vasc Endovasc Surg* 2005; 29(2): 139-44.

8. Sayed S, Choke E, Helme S, *et al*. Endovascular stent graft repair of mycotic aneurysms of the thoracic aorta. *J Cardiovasc Surg (Torino)* 2005; 46(2): 155-61.

9. Bell RE, Taylor PR, Aukett M, *et al*. Mid-term results for second-generation thoracic stent grafts. *Br J Surg* 2003: 90: 811-7.

10. Lears LJ, Bell R, Degrieck Y, *et al*. Endovascular treatment of thoracic aortic diseases: combined experience from the EUROSTAR and UNITED KINGDOM Thoracic Endograft registries. *J Vasc Surg* 2004; 40: 670-80.

11. Chuter TA, Schneider DB, Reilly, *et al*. Modular branched stent graft for endovascular repair of aortic arch aneurysm and dissection. *J Vasc Surg* 2003; 38(4): 859-63.

12. Rehders TC, Petzsch M, Ince H, *et al*. Intentional occlusion of the left subclavian artery during stent-graft implantation in the thoracic aorta: risk and relevance. *J Endovasc Ther* 2004; 11(6): 659-66.

13. Riambau V, Caserta G, Garcia-Madrid C, *et al*. When to revascularise the subclavian artery in aortic thoracic stenting? In: *Hybrid vascular procedures.* Brancherau A, Jacobs C, Eds. Armonk, NY: Edition Futura Publishing, 2004: 85-90.

14. Tiesenhausen K, Hausegger KA, Oberwalder P, *et al*. Left subclavian artery management in endovascular repair of thoracic aortic aneurysms and aortic dissections. *J Card Surg* 2003; 18: 429-35.

15. Ozsvath KJ, Roddy SP, Clement Darling III R, *et al*. Carotid-carotid crossover bypass: is it a durable procedure? *J Vasc Surg* 2003; 37(3): 582-5.

16. Czerny M, Zimpfer D, Fleck T, *et al*. Initial results after combining repair of the aortic arch aneurysms by sequential transposition of the supra-aortic branches and consecutive endovascular stent-graft placement. *Ann Thorac Surg* 2004; 78(4): 1256-60.

17. Gottardi R, Lammer J, Grimm M, *et al*. Entire rerouting of the supraaortic branches for endovascular stent-graft placement of an aortic arch aneurysm. *Eur J Cardiothorac Surg* 2006; 29(2): 258-60.

18. Melissano G, Civilini E, Bertoglio L, *et al*. Endovascular treatment of aortic arch aneurysms. *Eur J Vasc Endovasc Surg* 2005: 29(2): 131-8.

19. Greenberg RK, Haddad F, Svensson L, *et al.* Hybrid approaches to thoracic aortic aneurysms. The role of endovascular elephant trunk completion. *Circulation* 2005; 112: 2619-26.

20. Karck M, Chavan A, Charlady N, *et al.* The frozen elephant trunk technique for treatment of extensive thoracic aortic aneurysms, operative results and follow-up. *Eur J Cardiothorac Surg* 2005; 28(2): 286-90.

21. Stanley BM, Semmens JB, Lawrence-Brown MM, *et al* Fenestration in endovascular grafts for aortic aneurysm repair: new horizons for preserving blood flow in branch vessels. *J Endovasc Ther* 2001; 8: 16-24.

22. Inoue K, Iwase T, Sato M, *et al.* Transluminal endovascular branched graft placement for a pseudoaneurysm reconstruction of the descending thoracic aorta including the celiac axis. *J Thorac Cardiovasc Surg* 1997; 114: 859-61.

23. Anderson JL, Adam DJ, Berce M, *et al.* Repair of thoraco-abdominal aortic aneurysms with fenestrated and branched endovascular stent grafts. *J Vasc Surg* 2005; 42(4): 600-7.

24. Ballard JL, Abou-Zamzam Jr AM, Teruya TH. Type III and IV thoraco-abdominal aortic aneurysm repair: results of a trifurcated / two graft technique. *J Vasc Surg* 2002; 36: 211-6.

25. Quinones-Baldrich WJ, Panetta TF, Vescera CL, *et al.* Repair of type IV thoraco-abdominal aneurysm with a combined endovascular and surgical approach. *J Vasc Surg* 1999; 30: 555-60.

26. Rimmer J, Wolfe JHN. Type III thoraco-abdominal aortic aneurysm repair: a combined surgical and endovascular approach. *Eur J Vasc Endovasc Surg* 2003: 26(6): 677-9

27. Black SA, Wolfe JHN, Clark M, *et al.* Complex thoraco-abdominal aortic aneurysms: endovascular exclusion with visceral revascularisation. *J Vasc Surg* 2006: in press.

Chapter 10

EVAR for acute and chronic thoracic dissections: evidence and recommendations

Marcus Brooks MA MD FRCS (Gen Surg), Specialist Registrar

Robert Morgan MRCP FRCR, Consultant Radiologist

Matt Thompson MD FRCS, Professor of Vascular Surgery

St. George's Vascular Institute, St. George's Hospital, London, UK

Introduction

A review of the contemporary management of thoracic aortic dissection using endovascular techniques is important as commercial thoracic endografts are increasingly available and the understanding of aortic wall pathology is rapidly evolving. Pre-morbid diagnosis using CT and MRI has led to the diagnosis of associated aortic syndromes, penetrating aortic ulcer (PAU) and intramural haematoma (IMH). In both acute and chronic dissection, patency of primary or secondary entry tears may lead to aortic expansion and rupture. In animal models, covered stents achieved closure of the primary entry tear and false lumen thrombosis [1]. Dake at Stanford reported deployment of an endovascular stent in the thoracic aorta in 1994 and Palma, in 1997, reported EVAR for thoracic dissection [2, 3].

Incidence

Hospital admissions data in the UK (ICD10:I71.0) for the years 1999-2003 code a median of 851 admissions annually with acute aortic dissection. This provides an approximate UK incidence estimate of 6:100,000 person-years. This figure is consistent with UK and USA population-based studies of 2.6-3.5:100,000 person-years.

Definitions

In an aortic dissection, an intimal tear (primary intimal tear) allows blood to flow into the aortic media or adventitia creating a 'false' lumen [4]. The native or 'true' lumen becomes compressed (Figure 1). The false lumen may be a blind ending, but frequently re-entry occurs at natural fenestrations, including the visceral and renal side-branch origins. Secondary tears develop in chronic dissections.

Intramural haematoma (IMH) is a radiological diagnosis of blood within the aortic wall without communication with the aortic lumen. Most (50-85%) develop within the descending aorta and are associated with hypertension [5]. IMH may account for 5-20% of cases diagnosed clinically as acute dissection [6, 7]. Progression of IMH to acute dissection (16-47%) or aortic rupture (20-45%) has been observed [8, 9].

Penetrating aortic ulcers (PAUs) develop at the edge of atherosclerotic aortic plaques. PAU can stabilise, rupture or dissect [10, 11]. It appears that painful deep ulcers with adjacent haematoma are more prone to rupture [11].

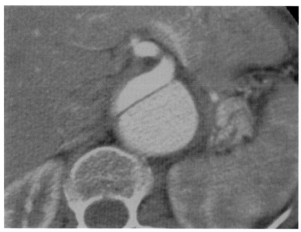

Figure 1. Contrast-enhanced CT scan showing compression of the true lumen (shown here supplying the coeliac axis) by the expanding false lumen in a Type B aortic dissection.

Classification

Thoracic dissections can be classified by either the site of the primary intimal tear (Stanford classification) or by their direction of propagation and extent (De Bakey classification, Table 1) [13]. Acute dissection is defined as within two weeks of the onset of symptoms.

Natural history

In order to understand the role for EVAR in the management of thoracic aortic dissection, the natural history must be understood. Firstly, it must be appreciated that in a patient who has suffered a non-

Table 1. Stanford and De Bakey classifications of thoracic aortic dissection.

Stanford	
Type A	All dissections involving the ascending aorta
Type B	All dissections not involving the ascending aorta
De Bakey	
Type I	Origin in ascending aorta, propagates distally into arch
Type II	Origin in ascending aorta, confined to ascending aorta
Type III	Origin in descending aorta, extends distally only

Pathophysiology

Classically, aortic dissection is associated with cystic medial necrosis. Microscopically, changes are observed in the intima (thickening, fibrosis, calcification and extracellular fatty acid deposition) and extracellular matrix (apoptosis, elastosis and cellular disruption) [12]. Inherited (Marfan's syndrome, Ehlers-Danlos syndrome [Type IV], annulo-aortic ectasia, bicuspid aortic valve, coarctation of the aorta and familial aortic dissection) or acquired (cocaine abuse, syphilis, Takayasu's arteritis, Bechet's disease) conditions pre-dispose to dissection. The aortic intima can also be disrupted by trauma or surgery.

traumatic aortic dissection, the entire aorta and its main side branches are at risk of future dissection, rupture or aneurysm formation.

Acute Stanford Type A dissection

Thoracic aortic dissection, originating from an intimal tear in the ascending aorta, has a mortality of 24% by 24 hours, 29% by 48 hours and 49% by two weeks [14]. Death results from aortic rupture, stroke, pericardial tamponade, visceral ischaemia, coronary ischaemia or aortic valve disruption.

Acute Stanford Type B dissection

Dissection originating in the descending aorta is less lethal; with medical intervention alone, 90% of patients will survive one month, 60-80% survive five years, and 40-45% survive ten years [15, 16]. Increasing age, aortic rupture and side-branch malperfusion are predictors for early deaths [17, 18]. However, this condition is not benign. Patients who develop acute complications (side-branch ischaemia or rupture) have a mortality approaching that of Type A dissections, up to 25% by 48 hours, despite surgical intervention [19, 20].

Chronic thoracic aortic dissection

The incidence of late false lumen aneurysms may be as high as 20%. The actuarial freedom from aortic enlargement in patients with an aortic diameter greater than 40mm following acute dissection is less than 30% at five years [21]. In an observational study of 110 patients managed medically in the acute phase, false lumen flow was an independent risk factor for late dissection-related death (Hazard ratio 5.6, 95% CI 1.1-28), but did not influence overall survival [22]. Persistence of flow within the false lumen increases the risk of late complications in most [19, 23], but not all studies [24, 25]. What is clear is that spontaneous thrombosis of the false lumen is rare (<4%) [14].

Intramural haematoma (IMH)

Studies in Caucasian patients with ascending aortic IMH report 30-day mortality of 21% [9]. Comparable studies in Asian patients suggest that IMH is relatively benign [26]. It appears that the risk of rupture is greatest when IMH affects the ascending aorta.

Definitive treatment

Patients with thoracic aortic dissection require rapid diagnosis and evaluation for evolving complications using CT and ECHO. Patients managed conservatively should be in an HDU/ITU setting with invasive blood pressure monitoring, beta-blockade and arterial vasodilators to achieve a systolic blood pressure of less than 140mmHg and pulse rate less than 60bpm. Pain relief will reduce catecholamine release and its effect on blood pressure.

Stanford Type A dissection

The majority of Type A thoracic aortic dissections are unsuitable for endovascular intervention because the coronary ostia or arch side branches are involved in the dissection. However, a few patients may be suitable when the primary entry tear is in the descending aorta. Kato and Shimono, from Japan, report experience of 28 patients with Type A dissections managed with EVAR [27, 28]. In ten patients, the primary entry tear was in the descending aorta and covering this resulted in successful thrombosis of the arch dissection. Open ascending aortic replacement frequently leaves a distal dissection flap. Erbel et al observed that high flow in the distal false lumen on transoesophageal ECHO was associated with significant late mortality (43%) [23]. Palma reports combining open aortic repair with EVAR for the distal dissection [3].

Type B dissection

The International Register of Aortic Dissections (IRAD) includes 46 patients treated with EVAR for Type B aortic dissections, with in-hospital mortality of 6.5% [17]. In 2004, EUROSTAR reported the outcome of 131 patients (43% symptomatic) undergoing EVAR for thoracic dissections [29]. Technical success was achieved in 89%, with low rates of paraplegia (0.8%) and mortality (6.5% elective and 12% emergency). Short-term follow-up was encouraging; at a median of 12 months, 90% of patients were alive with no significant increase in median aortic diameter. In both registries, and many published case series, there is a failure to differentiate between intervention for acute complications, intervention for chronic complications, and 'prophylactic' intervention in asymptomatic patients.

Nienaber has published the only case-control studies of EVAR for thoracic aortic dissection. In

Table 2. Published case series of EVAR for acute and chronic thoracic dissection.

Author	Country	Year	N	Indication	Technical success (%)	30-day mortality (%)	Follow-up (months)	Late survival (%)
Nienaber et al [31]	Germany	2003	11	Impending rupture	100	0	15	100.0
Dake, Kato et al [32]	USA	1999	19	Malperfusion	100	16	13	84.2
Doss et al [33]	Germany	2003	9	Impending rupture	100	0	N/A	N/A
Nienaber et al [30]	Germany/ Italy	1999	12	Chronic	100	0	3	100.0
Hausegger et al [34]	Austria	2001	5	Chronic	100	0	N/A	N/A
Won et al [35]	Korea	2001	12	Chronic	91	0	12	91.0
Bortone et al [36]	Italy	2002	12	Acute & Chronic	71	8	10	91.7
Shimono et al [37]	Japan	2002	37	Acute & Chronic	94	3	24	97.3
Buffolo et al [38]	Brasil	2002	181	Acute & Chronic	91	2	2	87.4
Lopera et al [39]	USA/ Columbia	2003	10	Acute & Chronic	90	0	30	80.0
Lambrechts et al [40]	Belgium	2003	11	Acute & Chronic	100	0	6	81.8
Lonn et al [41]	Sweden	2003	20	Acute & Chronic	100	15	13	85.0
Bortone et al [42]	Italy	2004	43	Acute & Chronic	96	7	20	83.7
Dialetto et al [43]	Italy	2005	28	Acute & Chronic	100	11	18	89.3
Eggebrecht et al [44]	Germany	2005	38	Acute & Chronic	100	3	18	73.7
			448		94	4	15	87.5 (n=434)

1999, 12 patients undergoing EVAR for chronic (greater than one month) Type B aortic dissections were compared to historical matched controls undergoing open repair [30]. EVAR was associated with zero morbidity or mortality as compared to four deaths and five serious adverse events following open repair. In 2003, 11 patients managed acutely with EVAR for complications were compared with 11 historical controls [31]. In the EVAR group, exclusion of the proximal tear was achieved in all patients, there were no procedure-related complications, and at a mean follow-up of 15 months, no patient had died. In the historical controls, three patients died within nine hours of admission to ITU and one late death occurred due to aortic rupture.

Table 2 summarises the main uncontrolled case series reporting EVAR for Type B aortic dissection (n=448, median age 60 years). The large number of patients in Buffolo's series is the result of EVAR being performed routinely in otherwise uncomplicated aortic dissections [38]. In all the other series, EVAR was reserved for acute complications, impending rupture or malperfusion, or chronic false lumen patency or dilatation. No series was consecutive, and exclusions were common due to unfavourable anatomy (e.g. entry site too close to the left subclavian artery, small or dissected iliac arteries, complex anatomy, multiple re-entry tears, small true lumen) or a preference for open surgery.

A single stent (median length 10cm) achieved technical success in closing the primary entry tear in

87% of patients (50-100%). In only one series was primary entry tear exclusion achieved in less than 90% of patients [36]. In that series, 8 of 14 patients had chronic dissections with multiple entry and re-entry points and compression of the true lumen. In the same authors' later experience, technical success had improved to 96%, perhaps reflecting the importance of patient selection and experience in EVAR for complex chronic dissections [45]. The false lumen was successfully thrombosed at the level of the stent in 83% of patients (60%-100%). The distal false lumen thrombosed less frequently (0-80%) [32, 34, 35, 46].

EVAR in the acute phase was also effective at correcting side-branch hypoperfusion for both dynamic and combined dynamic/static obstruction [32]. The most frequently performed additional procedure was left subclavian-carotid bypass (10%-80%). Other additional procedures confounding interpretation of these studies included coronary artery bypass grafting, percutaneous coronary angioplasty, aorto-innominate bypass and renal artery stenting. In only one series was a procedure converted to open repair (0.24% total). Reported 30-day mortality was 4.2% (0%-16%). Paraplegia developed in just one patient (0.24% total) and five patients suffered strokes (1.2% total). Late follow-up ranged from six to 30 months (median 15 months). Survival at the end of follow-up was 87.5% (74%-100%).

Highest mortality was observed when intervention was performed in the acute setting. In Eggebrecht's study, no mortality was observed in patients undergoing EVAR for chronic dissection, as compared to 40% mortality for acute complications (p=0.001) [44]. High acute mortality was observed by Kato who hypothesised that it was due to the fragility of the acutely dissected aorta, particularly when rigid first generation stents were deployed [47]. Two authors associate severe atherosclerosis of the aortic arch with an increased risk of stroke and rupture [41, 43].

Summary and recommendations

EVAR has found a role in the management of both acute and chronic thoracic aortic dissection. The EUROSTAR commentators note that short-term outcome for thoracic dissections are better than thoracic aneurysms [29]. Favourable outcomes has fuelled enthusiasm for EVAR for thoracic dissections and led to exploration of EVAR as a means of altering the natural history of this condition, to prevent late complications and dissection-related deaths.

Acute thoracic dissection

Acute thoracic dissection is defined as occurring within two weeks of symptom onset. Current recommendations are that EVAR should only be performed in this time period for the management of 'uncomplicated' Type A aortic dissections with the entry tear in the descending aorta and acute complications of Type B dissections, specifically:

- absolute indications:
  - rupture;
  - branch vessel malperfusion;

- relative indications:
  - persisting pain;
  - poorly controlled hypertension;
  - false lumen expansion.

Iliac artery access problems can usually be overcome by deployment via the abdominal aorta or supra-aortic arch arteries. Covering the subclavian artery, which in our experience rarely needs revascularisation, or carotid-carotid bypass and covering the left carotid origin can achieve proximal fixation. The dilated aortic arch (>38mm) remains a challenge and is a relative contraindication to EVAR with current stent grafts. We recommend coverage of the majority of the descending thoracic aorta, as in our early experience short stent grafts were associated with a high rate of late aortic dilatation. This approach does not appear to significantly increase the paraplegia rate.

EVAR should also be considered in patients with expanding IMH (Figure 2) or complicated PAU, as both conditions are potentially fatal and easily managed by stent graft exclusion of the affected aortic segment. EVAR may find a role as a 'hybrid' procedure to manage the distal dissection in conjunction with an open ascending or arch repair in Type A dissection.

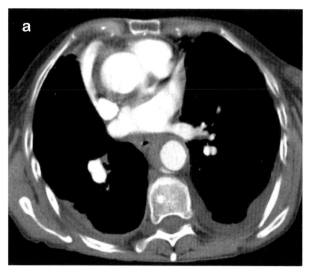
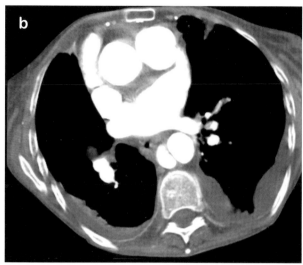

Figure 2. a) Contrast-enhanced CT scan showing progression of intramural haematoma. b) This progresses into a Type B aortic dissection in a 67-year-old lady who presented with spinal cord infarction.

There will never be a randomised trial of EVAR in the acute setting, as mortality with conservative measures and open surgery (>85%) is higher than that reported for EVAR (<20%) [48-50]. It is, therefore, vital that data from these patients are entered into registries, in order to better define indications for intervention and record long-term outcome.

'Early' chronic thoracic dissection

The uncontrolled studies already presented suggest that morbidity and mortality are highest when stenting is performed in the acute setting, even in patients without complications [44, 46]. Uncontrolled studies also support the hypothesis that early intervention, within the first six months to one year, is associated with aortic remodelling and might be the optimal time for intervention in patients who avoid early complications [51]. Patients with persistent false lumen flow and early dilatation (>4cm) are at significantly increased risk of late complications. The INSTEAD multicentre European randomised trial has been performed to investigate the role of EVAR in such patients [52]. In 2006, INSTEAD will report two-year outcomes comparing best medical therapy with and without EVAR in patients in a clinically stable condition with patent false lumens 14 days after acute dissection.

'Late' chronic thoracic dissection

Regardless of the early intervention performed, all patients must be on life-long treatment for hypertension. Beta blockers are the treatment of choice with a treatment goal of blood pressure less than 120/80mmHg. Calcium channel blockers are an alternative in patients who are beta-blocker intolerant. Regular follow-up and re-assessment of aortic size is recommended for life because of the high incidence of late complications, including aortic dilatation and further dissection [14]. Current consensus is that intervention is indicated in the chronic phase only if the aortic diameter exceeds 6cm, false lumen expansion exceeds 1cm/year or recurrent pain is experienced.

Abdominal fenestrations and re-entry points are of particular concern for the future, even after technically successful thoracic EVAR [39]. These arise from the 'natural' fenestrations at the origins of the visceral and renal side branches (Figure 3). Despite successful thrombosis of the thoracic false lumen, the aortic false lumen frequently remains patent and may continue to enlarge. A covered stent can only be deployed at this level if a branched stent is used or the visceral and renal arteries are first revascularised and ligated. EVAR has shown favourable outcome in the treatment of thoracic and thoraco-abdominal

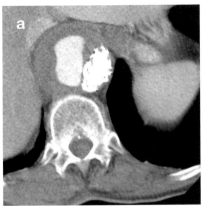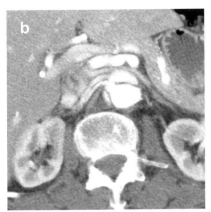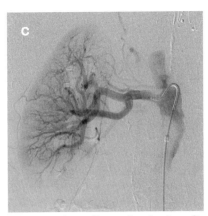

Figure 3. a) False lumen filling despite successful exclusion of the primary entry tear by a thoracic stent graft. b) The natural fenestrations at the level of the right renal artery are demonstrated on CT and c) angiogram. A right renal artery stent has subsequently significantly reduced false lumen flow.

aortic aneurysms associated with chronic aortic dissection (Chapter 9).

Conclusions

Lower rates of morbidity (including paraplegia) and mortality are reported in uncontrolled studies of EVAR for both acute and chronic thoracic aortic dissection, when compared to open surgery. EVAR achieves technical success in the exclusion of both primary and secondary entry tears and partial or complete false lumen thrombosis in most patients. Even if only partial false lumen thrombosis is achieved, false lumen wall stress is reduced and late dilatation and rupture may be prevented.

Since 2001, EVAR has been recommended by the European Society for Cardiology Task Force to seal entry into the false lumen for the management of acute complications [14]. The consensus that patients with acute Type B aortic dissection should be managed medically, except in the presence of life-threatening complications, has not changed. However, this consensus was agreed when it became clear that open surgery failed to improve outcome. The same

might not be true for EVAR, which appears to have lower procedure-related morbidity and mortality. EVAR, with off-the-shelf availability of thoracic devices (Chapter 8), will allow intervention in a proportion of the patients who develop side-branch malperfusion, retrograde dissection, or aortic rupture, who currently die with medical management.

Registry data and randomised controlled trials will help answer the question as to whether early intervention alters the natural history of aortic dissection, and, if so, in which patients prophylactic EVAR is indicated. EVAR performed in the late phase for aneurysmal dilatation is technically difficult and may require a combined or hybrid open surgical approach. Intervention for chronic dissections should be confined to specialist settings with a large endovascular experience and facilities for open thoracic aortic surgery.

Finally, if as anticipated, the indications for EVAR are broadened for thoracic dissection, technical success must not be mistaken for clinical success. Many of these patients are elderly with significant comorbidities and it is their general health status not their aortic disease that usually determines their long-term outcome.

Summary

◆ Open surgery (or EVAR) should be performed early for Type A dissection or IMH in the ascending aorta. (C)*.

◆ EVAR is the treatment of choice for acute complicated Type B aortic dissection (impending rupture, retrograde dissection and side-branch malperfusion) (C).

◆ Patients who survive an acute dissection require optimal medical management and close long-term surveillance (B).

◆ EVAR in the acute or 'early' chronic phase may prevent late false lumen dilatation and prevent dissection-related deaths (C). The results of the INSTEAD trial (A) are awaited.

◆ EVAR will become the treatment of choice for the management of chronic complications of thoracic aortic dissections (D).

* Grade of evidence, Oxford centre for evidence-based medicine.

References

1. Kato N, Hirano T, Takeda K, *et al*. Treatment of aortic dissections with a percutaneous intravascular endoprosthesis: comparison of covered and bare stents. *J Vasc Interv Radiol* 1994; 5(6): 805-12.

2. Dake MD, Miller DC, Semba CP, *et al*. Transluminal placement of endovascular stent-grafts for the treatment of descending thoracic aortic aneurysms. *N Engl J Med* 1994; 331(26): 1729-34.

3. Palma JH, Almeida DR, Carvalho AC, *et al*. Surgical treatment of acute type B aortic dissection using an endoprosthesis (elephant trunk). *Ann Thorac Surg* 1997; 63(4): 1081-4.

4. Larson EW, Edwards WD. Risk factors for aortic dissection: a necropsy study of 161 cases. *Am J Cardiol* 1984; 53: 849-55.

5. Maraj R, Rerkpattanapipat P, Jacobs LE, *et al*. Meta-analysis of 143 reported cases of aortic intramural hematoma. *Am J Cardiol* 2000; 86(6): 664-8.

6. Mohr-Kahaly S, Erbel R, Kearney P, *et al*. Aortic intramural hematoma visualized by transesophageal echocardiography: findings and prognostic implications. *J Am Coll Cardiol* 1994; 23: 658-64.

7. Nienabe, CA, von Kodolitsch Y, Petersen B, *et al*. Intramural hemorrhage of the thoracic aorta: diagnostic and therapeutic implications. *Circulation* 1995; 92: 1465-72.

8. Nienaber CA, Eagle KA. Aortic dissection: new frontiers in diagnosis and management: part I: from etiology to diagnostic strategies. *Circulation* 2003; 108(5): 628-35.

9. Evangelista A, Mukherjee D, Mehta RH, *et al*. Acute intramural hematoma of the aorta: a mystery in evolution. *Circulation* 2005; 111(8): 1063-70.

10. Ganaha F, Miller DC, Sugimoto K, *et al*. The prognosis of aortic intramural hematoma with and without penetrating atherosclerose ulcer: a clinical and radiological analysis. *Circulation* 2002; 106: 342-8.

11. von Kodolitsch Y, Nienaber CA. Penetrating ulcer of the thoracic aorta: natural history, diagnostic and prognostic profiles. *Z Kardiol* 1998; 87: 917-27.

12. von Kodolitsch Y, Aydin MA, Koschyk DH, *et al*. Predictors of aneurysm formation after surgical correction of aortic co-arctation. *J Am Coll Cardiol* 2002; 39: 617-24.

13. Daily PO, Trueblood HW, Stinson EB, *et al*. Management of acute aortic dissection. *Am Thorac Surg* 1970; 10: 237-47.

14. Erbel R, Alfonso F, Boileau C, *et al*. Diagnosis and management of aortic dissections. *Eur Heart J* 2001; 22: 1642-81.

15. Bernard Y, Zimmermann H, Chocron S, *et al*. False lumen patency as a predictor of late outcome in aortic dissection. *Am J Cardiol* 2001; 87(12): 1378-82.

16. Umana JP, Lai DT, Mitchell RS, *et al*. Is medical therapy still the optimal treatment strategy for patients with acute type B aortic dissections? *J Thorac Cardiovasc Surg* 2002; 124(5): 896-910.

17. Suzuki T, Mehta RH, Ince H, *et al*. Clinical profiles and outcomes of acute type B aortic dissection in the current era: lessons from the International Registry of Aortic Dissection (IRAD). *Circulation* 2003; 108 Suppl 1: II312-7.

18. Tsai TT, Bossone E, Isselbacher EM, *et al*. Clinical characteristics of hypotension in patients with acute aortic dissection. *Am J Cardiol* 2005; 95(1): 48-52.

19. Bogaert J, Meyns B, Rademakers FE, *et al.* Follow-up of aortic dissection: contribution of MR angiography for evaluation of the abdominal aorta and its branches. *Eur Radiol* 1997; 7(5): 695-702.

20. Meszaros I, Morocz J, Szlavi J, *et al.* Epidemiology and clinicopathology of aortic dissection. *Chest* 2000; 117(5): 1271-8.

21. Kato M, Bai H, Sato K, *et al.* Determining surgical indications for acute type B dissection based on enlargement of aortic diameter during the chronic phase. *Circulation* 1995; 92(9 Suppl): II107-12.

22. Akutsu K, Nejima J, Kiuchi K, *et al.* Effects of the patent false lumen on the long-term outcome of type B acute aortic dissection. *Eur J Cardiothorac Surg* 2004; 26(2): 359-66.

23. Erbel R, Oelert H, Meyer J, *et al.* Effect of medical and surgical therapy on aortic dissection evaluated by transesophageal echocardiography: implication for prognosis and therapy (The European Cooperative Study Group on Echocardiography). *Circulation* 1993; 83: 1604-15.

24. Kozai Y, Watanabe S, Yonezawa M, *et al.* Long-term prognosis of acute aortic dissection with medical treatment: a survey of 263 unoperated patients. *Jpn Circ J* 2001; 65(5): 359-63.

25. Juvonen T, Ergin MA, Galla JD, *et al.* Risk factors for rupture of chronic type B dissections. *J Thorac Cardiovasc Surg* 1999; 117(4): 776-86.

26. Kaji S, Akasaka T, Horibata Y, *et al.* Long-term prognosis of patients with type A aortic intramural hematoma. *Circulation* 2002; 106 (suppl I): I-248-I-252.

27. Kato N, Shimono T, Hirano T, *et al.* Transluminal placement of endovascular stent-grafts for the treatment of type A aortic dissection with an entry tear in the descending thoracic aorta. *J Vasc Surg* 2001; 34(6): 1023-8.

28. Shimono T, Kato N, Tokui T, *et al.* Endovascular stent-graft repair for acute type A aortic dissection with an intimal tear in the descending aorta. *J Thorac Cardiovasc Surg* 1998; 116(1): 171-3.

29. Leurs LJ, Bell R, Degrieck Y, *et al.* Endovascular treatment of thoracic aortic diseases: combined experience from the EUROSTAR and United Kingdom Thoracic Endograft registries. *J Vasc Surg* 2004; 40(4): 670-9; discussion 679-80.

30. Nienaber CA, Fattori R, Lund G, *et al.* Nonsurgical reconstruction of thoracic aortic dissection by stent-graft placement. *N Engl J Med* 1999; 340(20): 1539-45.

31. Nienaber CA, Ince H, Weber F, *et al.* Emergency stent-graft placement in thoracic aortic dissection and evolving rupture. *J Card Surg* 2003; 18(5): 464-70.

32. Dake MD, Kato N, Mitchell RS, *et al.* Endovascular stent-graft placement for the treatment of acute aortic dissection. *N Engl J Med* 1999; 340(20): 1546-52.

33. Doss M, Balzer J, Martens S, *et al.* Surgical versus endovascular treatment of acute thoracic aortic rupture: a single-center experience. *Ann Thorac Surg* 2003; 76(5): 1465-9; discussion 1469-70.

34. Hausegger KA, Tiesenhausen K, Schedlbauer P, *et al.* Treatment of acute aortic type B dissection with stent-grafts. *Cardiovasc Intervent Radiol* 2001; 24(5): 306-12.

35. Won JY, Lee DY, Shim WH, *et al.* Elective endovascular treatment of descending thoracic aortic aneurysms and chronic dissections with stent-grafts. *J Vasc Interv Radiol* 2001; 12(5): 575-82.

36. Bortone AS, Schena S, D'Agostino D, *et al.* Immediate versus delayed endovascular treatment of post-traumatic aortic pseudoaneurysms and type B dissections: retrospective analysis and premises to the upcoming European trial. *Circulation* 2002; 106(12 Suppl 1): I234-40.

37. Shimono T, Kato N, Yasuda F, *et al.* Transluminal stent-graft placements for the treatments of acute onset and chronic aortic dissections. *Circulation* 2002; 106(12 Suppl 1): I241-7.

38. Buffolo E, da Fonseca JH, de Souza JA, *et al.* Revolutionary treatment of aneurysms and dissections of descending aorta: the endovascular approach. *Ann Thorac Surg* 2002; 74(5): S1815-7; discussion S1825-32.

39. Lopera J, Patino JH, Urbina C, *et al.* Endovascular treatment of complicated type-B aortic dissection with stent-grafts: midterm results. *J Vasc Interv Radiol* 2003; 14(2 Pt 1): 195-203.

40. Lambrechts D, Casselman F, Schroeyers P, *et al.* Endovascular treatment of the descending thoracic aorta. *Eur J Vasc Endovasc Surg* 2003; 26(4): 437-44.

41. Lonn L, Delle M, Falkenberg M, *et al.* Endovascular treatment of type B thoracic aortic dissections. *J Card Surg* 2003; 18(6): 539-44.

42. Bortone AS, De Cillis E, D'Agostino D, *et al.* Stent graft treatment of thoracic aortic disease. *Surg Technol Int* 2004; 12: 189-93.

43. Dialetto G, Covino FE, Scognamiglio G, *et al.* Treatment of type B aortic dissection: endoluminal repair or conventional medical therapy? *Eur J Cardiothorac Surg* 2005; 27(5): 826-30.

44. Eggebrecht H, Schmermund A, Herold U, *et al.* Endovascular stent-graft placement for acute and contained rupture of the descending thoracic aorta. *Catheter Cardiovasc Interv* 2005; 66(4): 474-82.

45. Bortone AS, De Cillis E, D'Agostino D, *et al.* Endovascular treatment of thoracic aortic disease: four years of experience. *Circulation* 2004; 110(11 Suppl 1): II262-7.

46. Kato N, Hirano T, Shimono T, *et al.* Treatment of chronic aortic dissection by transluminal endovascular stent-graft placement: preliminary results. *J Vasc Interv Radiol* 2001; 12(7): 835-40.

47. Kato M, Kuratani T, Kaneko M, *et al.* The results of total arch graft implantation with open stent-graft placement for type A aortic dissection. *J Thorac Cardiovasc Surg* 2002; 124(3): 531-40.

48. Elefteriades JA, Hartleroad J, Gusberg RJ, *et al.* Long-term experience with descending aortic dissection: the complication-specific approach. *Ann Thorac Surg* 1992; 53(1): 11-20; discussion 20-1.

49. Walker PJ, Dake MD, Mitchell RS, *et al.* The use of endovascular techniques for the treatment of complications of aortic dissection. *J Vasc Surg* 1993; 18(6): 1042-51.

50. Miller DC, Mitchell RS, Oyer PE, *et al.* Independent determinants of operative mortality for patients with aortic dissections. *Circulation* 1984; 70(3 Pt 2): I153-64.

51. Kato M, Matsuda T, Kaneko M, *et al*. Outcomes of stent-graft treatment of false lumen in aortic dissection. *Circulation* 1998; 98(19 Suppl): II305-11; discussion II311-2.

52. Nienaber CA, Zannetti S, Barbieri B, *et al*. INvestigation of STEnt grafts in patients with type B Aortic Dissection: design of the INSTEAD trial - a prospective, multicenter, European randomized trial. *Am Heart J* 2005; 149(4): 592-9.

Chapter 11

Aortic arch branch vessel disease: the endovascular option

David Kessel MA MRCP FRCR, Consultant Vascular Radiologist

Leeds Teaching Hospitals NHS Trust, St. James's University Hospital, Leeds, UK

Introduction

Disease of the great vessels of the aortic arch is relatively uncommon compared to disease of the carotid bifurcation and there are a few conditions such as Takayasu's arteritis with a predilection for this area. The various presentations of arch vessel disease have been described previously [1]. They include, not only acute and chronic limb ischaemia, but also coronary and cerebral steal syndromes, TIA and stroke. This chapter will address recent advances in imaging assessment that help plan therapy, discuss some topics that are relatively problematic in the aortic arch vessels and outline the role of endovascular intervention in the supra-aortic vessels.

Imaging supra-aortic arterial disease

There are two aspects to the imaging of supra-aortic arterial disease: firstly, the origins of the great vessels themselves and secondly, the distal circulation in the upper limb and brain. In the context of this chapter, discussion will focus on the origins and the important distal sequelae in the arm.

Intra-arterial digital subtraction angiography (IADSA) has, until recently, been the mainstay of imaging of the aortic arch and its branches, but that is changing. This procedure is not without risk with a mortality of 0.1% and disabling stroke rate of about 1% in the NASCET trial. Clearly a non-invasive alternative which avoids this is desirable. Ultrasound is of limited used for imaging the arch and origins of the great vessels, as views are dependent on the patient's body habitus and the skill of the operator. As a consequence, it cannot reliably diagnose or exclude proximal disease. Conversely, ultrasound gives exquisite views of the vessels in the neck and arm.

Recent advances in contrast-enhanced magnetic resonance angiography (CEMRA) and computed tomography angiography (CTA) have added to the diagnostic armamentarium. Several studies comparing CEMRA and IADSA have shown that MRA has a high sensitivity with a tendency for detection of lesions offset by a tendency to overcall the degree of stenosis of the carotid and subclavian arteries [2, 3]. Unfortunately, CEMRA performs less well at aortic arch level; this is largely attributable to respiratory motion artefacts in patients who were unable to breath-hold for 30 seconds. Consequently, images may be degraded with diagnosis being uncertain in 15% and with 4% being uninterpretable. If the MRA appears normal, it is normal but artefact may simulate

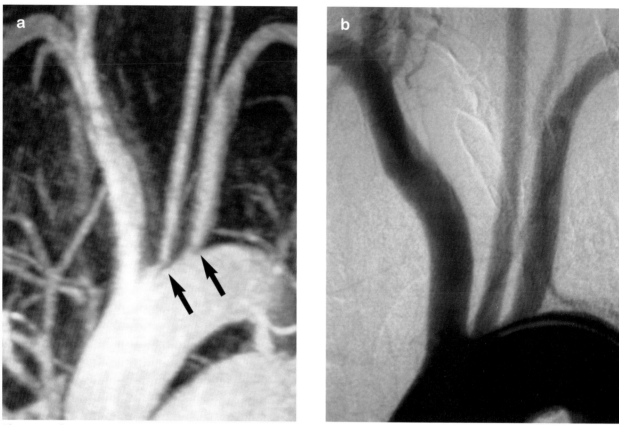

Figure 1. a) Pseudostenoses on MRA (black arrows) of the origins of the left common carotid and left subclavian arteries in a patient with left internal carotid artery stenosis. b) The IADSA is normal, allowing carotid artery stenting.

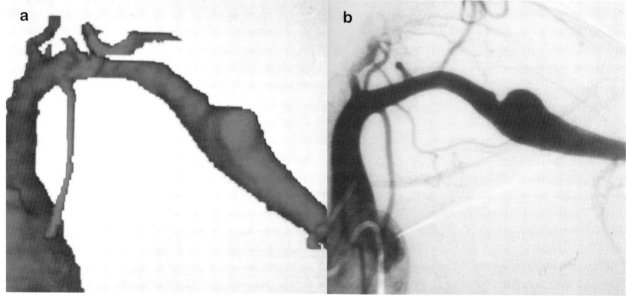

Figure 2. a) CT angiogram in a patient with thoracic outlet syndrome showing a subclavian artery aneurysm. b) Corresponding IADSA. The branches of the subclavian artery are clearly demonstrated.

stenosis (Figure 1). In reality it is not uncommon for DSA images to be degraded in the region of the arch due to cardiac and respiratory motion. CTA and MRA have the advantage of being able to assess the vessels from any perspective. In Wutke's study [2], three of the IADSA studies were found to have underestimated the degree of stenosis due to the angiographic projections not demonstrating the stenosis in true profile. In this respect, the ability to view CT and MRA reconstructions in multiple orientations may offset the inferior spatial resolution.

Recently, there have been great advances in CTA with the advent of multislice CT scanners. This has massively reduced image acquisition time largely eliminating concerns of respiratory motion. Imaging can be further improved by utilising cardiac gating to offset the effect of cardiac motion. CTA is threatening to replace diagnostic coronary angiography in the next few years. An area where CTA undoubtedly rules supreme is in the assessment of trauma and vascular injury [4]. Only CT can show the bones, soft tissues and blood vessels in such detail (Figure 2). Contemporary CTA is able to demonstrate the constellation of vascular injury from intimal tear through to false aneurysm and extravasation, and simultaneously assess the spine, lungs and airways. CT is unique in being able to demonstrate the track of penetrating injuries, such as knife and bullet wounds. CT may occasionally suffer from artefacts due to body habitus, metal fragments and metallic prostheses. In some cases other modalities may be needed to overcome this limitation, but it should be recognised that MRA will also suffer and in some cases even DSA is impossible.

As always, a pragmatic view should be taken to imaging, depending on the clinical questions to be answered. DSA will remain necessary for the time being when it is necessary to assess the small vessels in the hands and in some vascular malformations. CTA should be the investigation of choice for investigation of trauma to the aortic arch, thoracic inlet and neck. MRA is first choice for assessment of the arch and carotid arteries. Using this approach it will be rare to miss important vascular abnormalities and the risks of catheter angiography will be reduced, as only selected patients need be exposed to them.

Conditions affecting the supra-aortic vessels

Most aortic arch vessel disease is atheromatous in aetiology and shares the same risk factors as peripheral vascular disease elsewhere. There are, however, differences between upper and lower extremity arterial disease. Unlike vascular disease in the lower limbs, arch disease tends to be focal. Arko [5] reported an incidence of a proximal, ipsilateral atherosclerotic tandem lesion of an aortic arch vessel in only 1% of patients undergoing carotid endarterectomy. In patients with significant cervical carotid stenosis, only 17% had >30% innominate or subclavian artery stenosis [6]. Disease of the subclavian and innominate arteries is usually gradually progressive and frequently asymptomatic [7]. This is due to the presence of multiple collateral pathways. In contrast to the acute occlusion of an iliac artery, abrupt occlusion of the subclavian artery origin may be tolerated. Rehders [8] performed test balloon occlusion of the left subclavian artery (LSCA) prior to stent grafting to evaluate whether revascularisation would be necessary. None of the 22 patients tested developed symptomatic arm ischaemia during 30- minute balloon inflation. The reported incidence of symptomatic ischaemia following coverage of the LSCA during thoracic stent grafting ranges from 0-32% with under 3% of patients requiring late surgical revascularisation [8].

In addition to atheromatous disease there are other conditions that have a predilection for the great arteries of the aortic arch.

Takayasu's arteritis

Takayasu's arteritis is an inflammatory arteritis of unknown aetiology, commonest in Asians and typically affecting women aged between 20 and 40. Like many inflammatory conditions, the initial stage is difficult to diagnose, due to non-specific clinical features which may be ascribed to a viral illness. There is a subsequent stage of active vascular inflammation with thickening of the intima and media; during this phase the arteries may be tender. The late quiescent 'pulseless' stage is characterised by fibrosis of the media and adventitia, with the development of arterial stenoses and occlusions. Aneurysms may form when there is post-stenotic dilatation or if the media is destroyed. Diagnosis is based on clinical and radiological findings according to the modified Ishikawa criteria [9]: the presence of two major criteria, one major and two minor criteria or four minor criteria indicates a high probability of Takayasu's arteritis (Table 1).

Once the diagnosis has been established, various classifications have been proposed according to the distribution of the lesions [10]. Takayasu's arteritis frequently involves the supra-aortic circulation. Types I-III involve the aortic arch and its branches, Type IV the abdominal aorta, and Type V is generalised. Angiography used to be essential to the imaging diagnosis, but cross-sectional imaging gives far more information regarding the state of the vessel wall. Ultrasound gives exquisite images of superficial vessels such as the carotid artery. This may help establish the diagnosis, but treatment planning requires knowledge of the entire aorta and also the pulmonary arteries. In view of this, MRI scanning is an ideal modality, as it can cover large areas giving both angiographic and anatomic detail of the artery wall. Multislice CT scanners can give similar information, but with the disadvantage of using ionising radiation and iodinated contrast. Both CT and MRI can demonstrate not just mural thickening but also enhancement during the inflammatory phases of the disease. The optimal imaging techniques and characteristic findings can be seen in a pictorial review by Nastri et al [11].

Table 1. Criteria for diagnosis of Takayasu's arteritis.

	Arterial imaging	Clinical
Major	Arterial lesion	Symptoms >1 month
	Mid L subclavian artery	Intermittent claudication
	Mid R subclavian artery	Absent or asymmetric pulses
		Fever
		Neck pain
		Amaurosis or blurred vision
		Syncope
		Dyspnoea
		Palpitations
Minor	Arterial lesion	Signs
	Pulmonary artery	ESR >20mm/min
	L common carotid artery	Carotid artery tenderness
	Distal innominate artery	Hypertension
	Descending thoracic aorta	Aortic regurgitation
	Abdominal aorta	
	Coronary arteries	

The mainstay of treatment for the active phase of Takayasu's arteritis is corticosteroid, sometimes in combination with other immunosuppressive agents such as methotrexate. When there is ischaemia due to a focal lesion, angioplasty and stenting are indicated. Evidence regarding the efficacy of treatment is limited. The largest series to date reports treatment at 58 sites in 25 patients with active disease; the patients were on concomitant immunosuppressive therapy [12]. Twenty-three of the sites were supra-aortic. In keeping with other reports the initial technical success rate of angioplasty was 80-90%. Most authors have reported that the residual stenosis tends to be greater in patients with Takayasu's arteritis than in atheromatous disease. This may well reflect the degree of wall thickening caused by the inflammatory response. Min reported a restenosis rate of 25% in patients who had follow-up; this is in keeping with other authors' results. Giant cell arteritis can also affect the arch vessels, Both [13] treated cases of giant cell arteritis and Takayasu's arteritis in 33 lesions in 11 patients with similar rates of technical success and restenosis.

Radiotherapy

The arch vessels and carotid arteries are affected by radiotherapy for head and neck, breast and thoracic malignancies. Radiotherapy for breast cancer tends to affect the subclavian, axillary and innominate arteries, whilst therapy for head and neck tumours commonly involves the common carotid artery. Typically, long segments of artery are involved. External beam irradiation leads to arterial injury damaging the vessel wall and vasa vasorum. This results in intimal proliferation, medial necrosis and peri-advantitial fibrosis. Initial wall thickening leads to luminal reduction. This may be compounded by ischaemia due to damage to the vasa vasorum. Estimates based on ultrasound surveillance suggest that 12-22% of patients will develop significant carotid artery stenoses following cervical irradiation. Radiotherapy appears to increase the progress of atheromatous disease compared to controls. Despite this, there is usually a long interval between radiotherapy and onset of significant stenosis; this is typically in excess of five years.

In the presence of multiple vascular lesions or a 'hostile neck' with marked soft tissue scarring, endovascular therapy is an attractive option; this is particularly true in patients with a poor life expectancy. There is a suggestion that angioplasty and stenting for radiation-induced stenoses are less durable than in atheromatous disease. In a series of 16 patients with radiation-induced carotid artery stenosis, Ting [14] had a 94% success rate with 17% restenosis at a median follow-up of 30 months (Figure 3). This is not dissimilar to results in large series of carotid intervention. Hassen-Khodja [15] reported a retrospective review of 64 patients from 11 centres

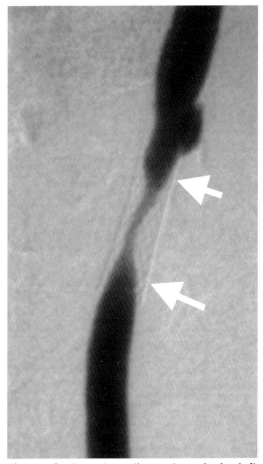

Figure 3. Symptomatic restenosis in left common carotid artery six months following carotid artery stenting for post-radiotherapy stricture. A second stent was placed and the artery has remained patent at two years follow-up.

treated by surgical bypass (79%), angioplasty and stenting (21%). Roughly one third of patients demonstrated involvement of multiple vessels, but only one third of these required revascularisation of more than a single trunk. There were five strokes in 30 patients undergoing carotid surgery and none in the 13 patients who were treated by stenting with a single restenosis. Interestingly, in this series there were no endovascular treatments for subclavian lesions, suggesting that a long segment of the vessel was involved.

Given the limited evidence available, it seems reasonable to treat radiotherapy-related supra-aortic occlusive disease in the same way as atherosclerotic stenosis.

Vertebral artery disease

The posterior circulation may be affected by arch disease in two distinct ways. Firstly, 'vertebral insufficiency' is most commonly due to vertebral artery flow reversal occurring distal to an occlusive lesion of the subclavian or innominate artery. Fortunately, the majority of these steals are asymptomatic. Symptomatic subclavian steal with vertigo and posterior fossa symptoms occurs when cerebral perfusion is significantly reduced during exercise of the upper limb or the heart in the presence of an internal mammary to coronary artery graft. True vertebral insufficiency is seen when there is flow-limiting stenosis in a dominant vertebral artery. These flow disturbances are usually readily rectified by endovascular or open repair. The second manifestation of vertebral artery stenosis is posterior circulation TIA or stroke.

Roughly one quarter of CVA occur in the posterior circulation territory and one fifth of these are associated with an extracranial vertebral artery stenosis [16,17]. Asymptomatic vertebral artery stenoses seem to have a relatively benign course with the risk of stroke relating to any associated carotid artery disease. The exception to this occurs when there is co-existing basilar artery disease. Intracranial vertebral artery stenosis is associated with an annual stroke rate of 7% [18]. There is comparatively little in the literature concerning the revascularisation of the vertebral artery. This probably reflects the fact that most vertebral artery disease has been managed medically. The vertebral artery arises from the postero-superior aspect of the subclavian artery, hence performing surgery on the vertebral artery origin is technically challenging and transposition may be a safer option, as with lesions of the aortic arch.

The proximal vertebral artery is often tortuous which makes it difficult to assess. MRA studies of the carotid arteries and aortic arch must be interpreted with caution. MIP images frequently suggest vertebral artery origin stenosis, so it is essential to review the source images on the MR workstation. Modern low profile angioplasty balloons and stent systems are ideally suited to treating small vessels like the vertebral artery. A small series reported 100% restenosis in four patients treated with angioplasty alone compared with only 10% in ten patients treated by stenting [17]. Chastain [19] reported 10% restenosis in a study of 49 patients treated with vertebral artery stenting and followed-up angiographically. Others have reported higher restenosis rates; Lin [20] treated 58 symptomatic patients with a 5% stroke rate and symptomatic relief was achieved in 97% of patients at a mean follow-up of 30 months. Symptoms recurred in only two patients. Angiography was performed in just under half of the patients and one quarter of these had recurrent stenosis. This suggests restenosis in 40-50% overall, but that the lesion characteristics had changed to make them asymptomatic. This is likely to be a reflection of the need to restore a smooth non-embologenic surface rather than maintain flow. Clearly, restenosis would be symptomatic in cases of vertebral insufficiency.

This limited evidence suggests that symptomatic vertebral artery stenoses can be treated by angioplasty and stenting with a stroke rate of around 5%, which is comparable to that for carotid stenosis. Stents probably provide a more durable angiographic result, but as restenosis may not be symptomatic the case for primary stenting is unproven.

Indications for endovascular therapy of the supra-aortic vessels

Given the relative rarity of disease of the supra-aortic arteries, both surgery and endovascular treatments of the great vessels of the aortic arch are uncommon. The therapeutic options are discussed elsewhere [1]. Hence, it is hardly surprising that there are no prospective randomised clinical trials to guide clinical practice. Such evidence as exists suggests that surgery provides a more durable result than endovascular therapy at the cost of an increased procedural morbidity [21].

As is always the case, endovascular and open surgical repair are complementary techniques. When deciding on the best treatment every patient should be considered on their own merits; management decisions will depend on several factors not least the local surgical and endovascular expertise. It is usually appropriate to try endovascular therapy for patients with arm claudication secondary to a proximal stenosis. The technical success rate will be close to 100% and immediate or late failure is unlikely to preclude surgery. The same cannot be said in the presence of complete occlusion of an arch artery as these are frequently difficult to traverse, especially if calcified (Figure 4). In most reports in occlusions, technical success rates vary from 14-40% [21]. Even with femoral and brachial access this is much lower than the success rates for traversing iliac artery occlusions. The brachial approach is analogous to the retrograde approach to an iliac occlusion from the ipsilateral femoral artery. The wire will generally either pass through with little difficulty or it will dissect; in this case it is unlikely to re-enter the aortic lumen. The femoral approach might be compared to retrograde recanalisation of an iliac occlusion from the contralateral femoral artery. This manoeuvre is often successful in the iliac artery, where it is possible to obtain a very stable catheter position with a reverse curve catheter; this is not the case in the aortic arch where the catheter will always be relatively unstable.

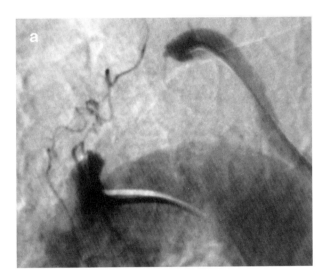

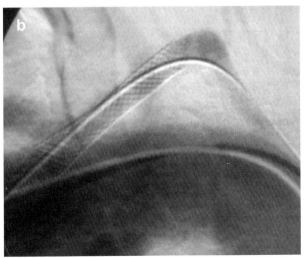

Figure 4. a) Left subclavian artery occlusion in a patient with severe arm claudication (note that the vertebral artery is occluded). The occlusion was traversed from the arm. b) Following placement of a stent the subclavian artery is widely patent.

It is not unreasonable to try to recanalise arch vessel occlusions, but attempts should not be prolonged or too vigorous as they are more likely to lead to complications. In these circumstances, extra-anatomical bypass grafting can be a simpler and more durable option, especially in young patients with claudication affecting their work. Extra-anatomical surgery relies on a suitable donor vessel and so is unsuitable in the presence of disease involving multiple arteries. In this instance a combined approach may be indicated with endovascular therapy to optimise arterial inflow to a surgical graft. The same applies to pre-operative inflow improvement when a left internal mammary artery (LIMA) to coronary graft is necessary distal to a stenosis of the LSCA. A 'coronary steal' syndrome due to development of a left SCA stenosis is also well described. A unique form of combined approach is employed when there are tandem lesions of the carotid artery. In this case, the inflow angioplasty/stent can be performed during carotid endarterectomy with the internal carotid artery clamped to prevent distal embolisation. The arterial sheath is inserted retrogradely and the working distance is very short with maximum stability. If the patient does not tolerate carotid artery occlusion much of the advantage of this approach is lost.

In acute limb ischaemia, surgery is required if there is significant tissue loss or compartment syndrome. This is not to say that angioplasty, stenting and thrombolysis do not have a role to play. Large emboli are usually managed surgically but any associated stenosis is most simply treated with primary stenting.

Summary

◆ Disease of the vessels of the aortic arch is relatively uncommon.

◆ Alternative causes such as Takayasu's arteritis and radiotherapy should be considered.

◆ Angiography and endovascular therapy are associated with a risk of stroke.

◆ The role of non-invasive imaging is increasing, with MRA the first choice for investigation of carotid artery disease and CTA for trauma.

◆ Vertebral artery disease should only be treated if symptomatic.

◆ Surgery probably produces more durable results, but will rarely be precluded by an attempt at endovascular therapy.

References

1. Kessel D. Supra-aortic intervention. *Endovascular Intervention: Current Controversies.* Wyatt MG, Watkinson AF, Eds. Shrewsbury, UK: tfm publishing, 2004.

2. Wutke R, Lang W, Fellner C, *et al.* High resolution, contrast-enhanced magnetic resonance angiography with elliptical centric k-space ordering of supra-aortic arteries compared with selective X-ray angiography. *Stroke* 2002; 23: 1522-9.

3. Willinek WA, von Falkenhausen M, Born M, *et al.* Noninvasive detection of steno-occlusive disease of the supra-aortic arteries with three-dimensional contrast-enhanced magnetic resonance angiography. A prospective, intra-individual comparative analysis with digital subtraction angiography. *Stroke* 2005; 36: 38-43.

4. Nunez DB, Torres-Leon M, Munera F. Vascular injuries of the neck and thoracic inlet: helical CT-angiographic correlation. *RadioGraphics* 2004; 24: 1087-100.

5. Arko FR, Buckely CJ, Lee SD, *et al.* J combined carotid endarterectomy with transluminal angioplasty and primary stenting of the supra-aortic vessels. *Cardiovasc Surg* 2000; 41: 737-42.

6. Fields WS, Lemak NA. Joint study of extra-cranial arterial occlusion: VII subclavian steal - a review of 168 cases. *JAMA* 1972; 222: 1139-43.

7. Ackerman H, Diener HC, Seboldt H, *et al.* Ultrasonographic follow-up of subclavian stenosis and occlusion: natural history and surgical treatment. *Stroke* 1988; 19: 431-5.

8. Rehders TC, Petzshc M, Ince H, *et al.* Intentional occlusion of the left subclavian artery during stent-graft implantation in the thoracic aorta: risk and relevance. *J Endovasc Ther* 2004; 11: 659-66.

9. Sharma BK, Jain S, Suri S, *et al.* Diagnostic criteria for Takayasu arteritis. *Int J Cardiol* 1996; 54: S141-7.

10. Moriwaki R, Noda M, Yajima M, *et al.* Clinical manifestations of Takayasu arteritis in India and Japan: new classification of angiographic findings. *Angiology* 1997; 48: 369-79.

11. Nastri MV,. Baptista LPS,. Baroni RH, *et al*. Gadolinium-enhanced three-dimensional MR angiography of Takayasu arteritis. *RadioGraphics* 2004; 24: 773-86.

12. Min PK, Park S, Jung JH, *et al*. Endovascular therapy combined with immunosuppressive treatment for occlusive arterial disease in patients with Takayasu's arteritis. *J Endovasc Ther* 2005; 12: 28-34.

13. Both M, Jahnke T, Reinhold-Keller E, *et al*. Percutaneous management of occlusive arterial disease associated with vasculitis: a single center experience. *Cardiovasc Intervent Radiol* 2003; 26: 19-26.

14. Ting ACW, Cheng SWK, Yeung KA, *et al*. Carotid stenting for radiation-induced extracranial carotid artery occlusive disease: efficacy and midterm outcomes. *J Endovasc Ther* 2004; 11: 53-9.

15. Hassen-Khodja A, Kieffer. Radiotherapy-induced supra-aortic trunk disease: early and long-term results of surgical and endovascular reconstruction. *J Vasc Surg* 2004; 40: 254-61.

16. Wityk RJ, Chang HM, Rosengart A, *et al*. Proximal extracranial vertebral artery disease in the New England Medical Centre Posterior Circulation Registry. *Arch Neurol* 1998; 55: 470-8.

17. Cloud GC, Crawley F, Clifton A, *et al*. Vertebral artery origin angioplasty and primary stenting: safety and restenosis rates in a prospective series. *J of Neurol, Neurosurg and Psych* 2003; 74: 586-90.

18. Moufarrij NA, Little JR, Furlan AJ, *et al*. Vertebral artery stenosis: long-term follow-up. *Stroke* 1984; 15: 260-3.

19. Chastain HD Campbell MS, Iyer S, *et al*. Extracranial vertebral artery stent placement: in-hospital and follow-up results. *J Neurosurg* 1999; 91: 547-52.

20. Lin YH, Juang JM, Jeng JS, *et al*. Symptomatic ostial vertebral artery stenosis treated with tubular coronary stents: clinical results and restenosis analysis. *J Endovasc Ther* 2004; 11: 719-26.

21. Modarai B, Ali T, Dourado R, *et al*. Comparison of extra-anatomic bypass grafting with angioplasty for atherosclerotic disease of the supra-aortic trunks. *Br J Surg* 2004; 91: 1453-7.

Chapter 12

Evidence for the endovascular treatment of acute aortic syndrome

Mo Hamady MB ChB FRCR, Consultant, Interventional Radiology

St. Mary's Hospital, London, UK

Introduction

Acute aortic syndrome refers to a spectrum of acute aortic pathologies including aortic dissection (AD), intramural haematoma (IMH), penetrating aortic ulcer (PAU) and aortic transection.

The relatively new concept of acute aortic syndrome reflects recent advances in the management of thoracic aortic pathology and dramatic improvements in aortic imaging. Aortic pathology is frequently unsuitable for conservative medical treatment and many patients are also poor surgical candidates. For this reason, endovascular aortic repair using stent grafts (ESG) has been increasingly used as an alternative, minimally invasive intervention for the treatment of these patients. This chapter reviews the current evidence for endoluminal therapy in acute aortic syndrome.

Acute thoracic dissection

AD is a tear in the intima of the aorta, creating false and true lumens separated by an intimo-medial flap. The dissected aorta is at high risk of rupture, ischaemic complications and aneurysmal dilatation. The reported incidence of AD is about 3.5 cases per 100,000 population per year [1]. There is an expectedly higher incidence among males in their 5th and 6th

decade of life. AD is classified according to time and location. Acute AD is dissection within two weeks of the primary event. Stanford Type A AD involves the ascending aorta and/or the aortic arch, whereas Type B AD involves the descending thoracic aorta.

There is well established evidence that Type A AD is a highly lethal pathology and should be treated urgently with surgical replacement of the aorta. On the other hand, treatment of Type B AD remains a controversial issue. Medical treatment with blood pressure and heart rate control has been the gold standard, and achieves a 90% survival rate. However, a patent false lumen can lead to rupture or continuous dilatation of the aorta in 20-50% of cases within five years [2, 3]. The current indications for intervention in Type B AD include uncontrolled hypertension, relentless pain, visceral ischaemia and aneurysmal dilatation.

Surgery has been the traditional treatment modality for complicated Type B AD. However, it carries significant mortality and morbidity rates, which may exceed 50% in emergency situations [4]. Endovascular stent grafting (ESG) has recently emerged as an attractive alternative to the standard surgical treatment. It provides a minimally invasive approach, short procedural time, high technical success and significantly lower periprocedural complications. The principle of ESG in AD is to seal the primary entry tear site, thereby promoting the thrombosis of false lumen and redirecting the flow to the true lumen. Previous investigators have shown that false lumen thrombosis is associated with better long-term prognosis [5]. The safety and efficacy of ESG of the thoracic aneurysm has been established in several studies, and the reported technical success rate of stent deployment is high at around 98% [6, 7].

In a meta-analysis of 609 AD patients treated with ESG, the total in-hospital mortality was slightly over 5% and the two-year survival rate around 90%. This compares favourably with the standard medical treatment [8]. In the same meta-analysis, false lumen thrombosis was recorded in 75% of cases; however, the late re-intervention (surgical conversion or adjunctive endovascular stent) rate was relatively high at around 12%. This does not necessarily indicate failure of endovascular therapy, because aortic degenerative disease is a continuous process. This hypothesis is supported by data showing that further surgery was needed in 11-20% of medically treated patients and in 10-44% of patients initially treated surgically [4, 9]. Endovascular treatment may, in theory, play a significant role in the prevention of aortic growth, but as yet, there is no strong evidence from randomised trials or registries to support this hypothesis. There are data from the EUROSTAR and UK thoracic endograft registries. These were analysed in 2004 and show a 30-day mortality rate of 12% with a one-year cumulative survival rate of 90% for the use of ESG to treat patients with AD. Out of 131 patients with AD enrolled in these registries, false lumen thrombosis was achieved in 86% of cases [10].

One of the most devastating consequences of aortic intervention is neurological compromise. Nevertheless, the 1% reported incidence of paraplegia post-ESG is remarkably low compared to the 7-36% reported after surgical treatment [4]. Likewise, the incidence of stroke post-endovascular therapy is approximately 3% [10]. Surgical treatment for patients with AD complicated by peripheral ischaemia has a particularly high peri-operative mortality approaching 80% [11]. Consequently, interventional radiological techniques (percutaneous fenestration and/or stenting) have evolved in an attempt to reduce both morbidity and mortality following EVT. Slonim and colleagues reported their mid-term experience

with 40 patients treated percutaneously to relieve peripheral ischaemia [12]. They reported a 93% technical success rate and a 25% 30-day mortality rate. Procedure-related complications were recorded in nine patients (22%), with only three of them (7%) having significant clinical consequences. However, long-term data and larger patient numbers are needed to confirm the durability of this approach.

Intramural haematoma (IMH)

Although IMH was first described in 1920, recent development in imaging modalities and advancement in endovascular therapy has revived interest in this clinical entity. IMH is defined as haemorrhage into the aortic wall, with no radiological evidence of intimal tear. The prevalence of IMH in cases of acute aortic syndrome is about 6% [13]. Aortic IMH may progress in retrograde or antegrade fashion and spontaneous re-absorption has been reported in one third of cases [14]. In this same study involving follow-up on 50 patients with IMH, progression to frank AD was noted in 40% of cases.

The overall mortality associated with IMH is 21% [14]. The mortality associated with Type A IMH is even higher. Data from the IRAD registry have shown that, of 58 IMH patients, 23 were diagnosed with Type A IMH and that the mortality rate in this group was 39% [14]. By contrast, the 35 patients with Type B IMH had a mortality rate of 8%, suggesting a more benign course for Type B IMH. Other investigators have also noted the benign nature of Type B IMH. Von Kodolitsch and colleagues studied 66 patients with IMH and noted that the 17 patients with Type B IMH had a 10% in-hospital mortality, closely comparable to Type B AD [15]. Few predictors for IMH evolution have been well established. Several workers have suggested that location, maximum aortic diameter and the presence of an associated penetrating aortic ulcer were of prognostic value, but there is little evidence to support these suppositions [15, 16].

Although there has been a better understanding of the natural course of IMH, there is no strong evidence for a clear treatment strategy. Current management practice is centred mainly on the location of IMH according to Stanford classification. Patients with Type A IMH are treated primarily with open surgical repair, with the reported 30-day mortality varying between 10% and 37% [16-18]. Asymptomatic patients, or those with Type B IMH, are treated conservatively with frequent radiological imaging to assess disease progression. Harris *et al* studied 53 patients with Type B IMH. There was no significant difference in mortality rates between medical and surgical treatment (10% and 19% respectively) [18]. Similarly, the survival rate associated with medical treatment of 31 patients in the IRAD registry was 90% [14].

The presence of PAU in association with IMH may represent a different group of patients who need a more aggressive approach [19]. Although endovascular treatment (ESG) in isolated Type B IMH can potentially play a significant role in the management of this subset of patients, this management option has not been widely reported to date.

Penetrating aortic ulcer (PAU)

PAU is caused by ulceration of the intimal layer of the atherosclerotic plaque with haemorrhage into the medial layer of the aorta [19]. PAU usually involves the descending thoracic aorta with a clear predilection to the female sex. Characteristically, it affects elderly patients and is associated with severe and multiple comorbidities, and a high prevalence of aortic degenerative disease [20].

The natural history of this disease can result in significant complications. Ganaha *et al* studied 65 symptomatic patients with IMH, of which 31 had associated PAU; disease progression was noted in 48% of the patients in the PAU group. Likewise, in a retrospective review of 198 patients with AD, Coady *et al* reported a 40% risk of aortic rupture among patients with PUA at initial presentation [19]. Furthermore, Tittle *et al* have reported an incidence of late aortic rupture following initially successful medical treatment [21].

The current indications for intervention are symptomatic PAU with uncontrolled chest pain, an enlarging ulcer with IMH, and increasing haemothorax [1]. Surgical repair is considered the definitive treatment; however, it is associated with a significant risk of mortality and morbidity in those usually frail patients with several comorbidities. The Mayo Clinic group studied 105 patients with PAU of the descending thoracic aorta presenting over a 25-year period [22]. Over one third of these patients were treated surgically with an overall mortality of 30%. This compared with a 21% mortality rate for those patients treated medically.

Endovascular therapy, with its known minimally invasive technique, provides an attractive alternative and several studies have established the safety and efficacy of ESG in treatment of PAU, although absolute patient numbers remain small (Figure 1). Dake *et al*

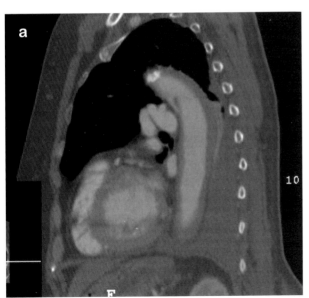
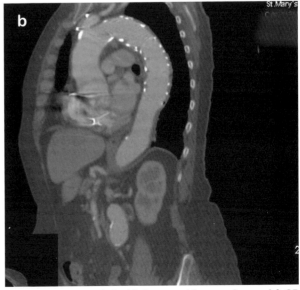

Figure 1. a) CT angiogram showing a penetrating aortic ulcer with an associated intramural haematoma. b) CT angiogram post-stent insertion demonstrates resolution of the aortic pathology.

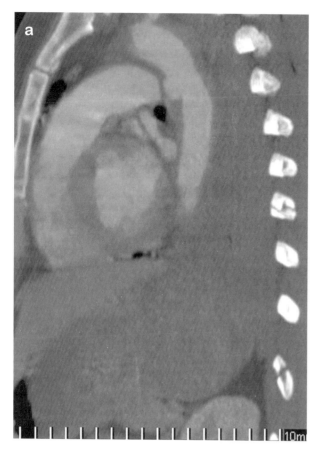

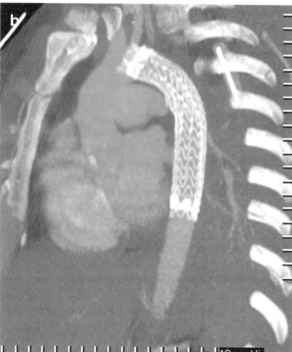

Figure 2. a) CT angiogram of the aortic arch showing an aortic transection. **b)** CT angiogram showing successful stent deployment for the treatment of an aortic dissection.

studied the midterm results of 26 patients with symptomatic PAU treated with ESG. They reported a 92% technical success rate, a peri-operative mortality rate of 15% and a five-year survival rate of 70%. Large aortic diameter and female sex were independent predictive factors for treatment failure [23]. Mitchell *et al* reported the treatment of ten PAU patients with first generation ESG. The early mortality was 8.7% with a 73% two-year survival [24]. Despite these encouraging short and mid-term results, more evidence is needed to establish the long-term efficacy of this treatment modality and to refine the criteria for patient selection.

Traumatic transection

Aortic transection is simply defined as disruption of the aortic wall. Complete disruption leads to aortic rupture, whereas partial disruption, with the blood flow precariously maintained within the vascular lumen by the adventitia and surrounding mediastinal tissues, causes contained transection compatible with initial survival.

Traumatic aortic rupture is a highly lethal condition with 90% of the victims perishing at the scene of the injury [25]. For those surviving the initial trauma, in-hospital mortality is 32% on the first day and 74% at two weeks respectively [25]. Furthermore, delayed aortic rupture is found in 30% of patients with a chronic traumatic aortic injury who survived the primary event [26]. Early intervention is, therefore, advocated for all patients who have suffered traumatic aortic transection.

Surgical replacement of the ascending aorta, including thoracotomy, single lung ventilation, aortic cross-clamping, anticoagulation and potentially extra-corporeal circulation has been the standard treatment modality for these patients. Unsurprisingly, these are highly unstable patients and the mortality and morbidity associated with surgical repair is significant. In a study of 263 patients with traumatic aortic rupture, Attar *et al* reported a 24% mortality rate and a 13% incidence of paraplegia [27].

ESG provides a minimally invasive technique for the treatment of these patients, obviating the need for aortic cross-clamping and full heparinisation in this patient group who have often suffered significant polytrauma (Figure 2). Melan *et al*, report the use of ESG to treat 15 patients with traumatic transection. The mortality and paraplegic rates in this study were 6.7% and 0% respectively, a significant improvement on the results of open surgery [28]. The EUROSTAR and UK stent graft registries contain data on 50 patients with traumatic aortic transection [10]. ESG treatment in this group resulted in a 96% primary technical success rate, a 6% early mortality rate and a one-year cumulative survival rate of 82%. In addition, neurological complications were only reported in 6% of these patients. Nevertheless, early ESG failure did occur, requiring secondary endovascular intervention [29]. The author has also experienced similar problems of graft failure in two patients who eventually required open surgical repair. The most likely explanation for the initial failure of ESG treatment is the disparity between the relative large size of thoracic aortic stents and the relatively small aortic size found in these often young, non-atherosclerotic individuals. Clearly, there is a need for the availability of smaller 'on the shelf' stent grafts to overcome this problem. To date, however, there are no randomised trials or large numbers of patients enrolled in international registries to draw clear evidence about the durability of endoluminal therapy in traumatic transection.

Summary

◆ Type A AD has a poor prognosis and should be treated surgically.

◆ Medical management remains the gold standard for the treatment of uncomplicated Type B AD.

◆ ESG is a safe and effective treatment for complicated AD, with good short and mid-term results.

◆ Type A IMH has a poor prognosis and should be treated surgically.

◆ ESG appears to be an appropriate treatment for PAU, although case numbers remain small.

◆ ESG can benefit patients with traumatic aortic transection.

◆ There are no long-term data regarding the use of ESG for the treatment of these conditions.

References

1. Meszaros I, Morocz J, Szlavi J, *et al*. Epidemiology and clinicopathology of aortic dissection. *Chest* 2000; 117: 1271-8.

2. Doroghazi RM, Slater EE, DeSanctis RW, *et al*. Long-term survival of patients with treated aortic dissection. *J Am Coll Cardiol* 1984; 3: 1026-34.

3. Wheat MW Jr. Acute dissection of the aorta. *Cardiovasc Clin* 1987; 17: 241-62.

4. Umana JP, Miller DC, Mitchell RS. What is the best treatment for patients with acute type B aortic dissections - medical, surgical, or endovascular stent-grafting? *Ann Thorac Surg* 2002; 74: S1840-3.

5. Erbel R, Oelert H, Meyer J, *et al*. Effect of medical and surgical therapy on aortic dissection evaluated by transesophageal echocardiography. Implications for prognosis and therapy. The European Cooperative Study Group on Echocardiography. *Circulation* 1993; 87: 1604-15.

6. Palma JH, de Souza JA, Rodrigues Alves CM, *et al*. Self-expandable aortic stent-grafts for treatment of descending aortic dissections. *Ann Thorac Surg* 2002; 73: 1138-41.

7. Dake MD, Kato N, Mitchell RS, *et al*. Endovascular stent-graft placement for the treatment of acute aortic dissection. *N Engl J Med* 1999; 340: 1546-52.

8. Eggebrecht H, Nienaber CA, Neuhauser M, *et al*. Endovascular stent-graft placement in aortic dissection: a meta-analysis. *Eur Heart J* 2006; 27: 489-98.

9. Bernard Y, Zimmermann H, Chocron S, *et al*. False lumen patency as a predictor of late outcome in aortic dissection. *Am J Cardiol* 2001; 87: 1378-82.

10. Leurs LJ, Bell R, Degrieck Y, Thomas S, *et al*. EUROSTAR; UK Thoracic Endograft Registry collaborators. Endovascular treatment of thoracic aortic diseases: combined experience from the EUROSTAR and United Kingdom Thoracic Endograft registries. *J Vasc Surg* 2004; 40: 670-9.

11. Fann JI, Sarris GE, Mitchell RS, Shumway NE, *et al*. Treatment of patients with aortic dissection presenting with peripheral vascular complications. *Ann Surg* 1990; 212: 705-13.

12. Slonim SM, Miller DC, Mitchell RS, *et al*. Percutaneous balloon fenestration and stenting for life-threatening ischemic complications in patients with acute aortic dissection. *J Thorac Cardiovasc Surg* 1999; 117: 1118-26.

13. Evangelista A, Mukherjee D, Mehta RH, *et al*. International Registry of Aortic Dissection (IRAD) Investigators. Acute intramural hematoma of the aorta: a mystery in evolution. *Circulation* 2005; 111: 1063-70.

14. Evangelista A, Dominguez R, *et al*. Prognostic value of clinical and morphologic findings in short-term evolution of aortic intramural haematoma. Therapeutic implications. *Eur Heart J* 2004; 25: 81-7.

15. von Kodolitsch Y, Csosz SK, Koschyk DH, *et al*. Intramural hematoma of the aorta: predictors of progression to dissection and rupture. *Circulation* 2003; 107: 1158-63.

16. Nienaber CA, von Kodolitsch Y, Petersen B, *et al*. Intramural hemorrhage of the thoracic aorta. Diagnostic and therapeutic implications. *Circulation* 1995; 92: 1465-72.

17. Robbins RC, McManus RP, Mitchell RS, *et al*. Management of patients with intramural hematoma of the thoracic aorta. *Circulation* 1993; 88(5 Pt 2): II1-10.

18. Harris KM, Braverman AC, Gutierrez FR, *et al*. Transesophageal echocardiographic and clinical features of aortic intramural hematoma. *J Thorac Cardiovasc Surg* 1997; 114: 619-26.

19. Coady MA, Rizzo JA, Hammond GL, Pierce JG, *et al*. Penetrating ulcer of the thoracic aorta: what is it? How do we recognize it? How do we manage it? *J Vasc Surg* 1998; 27: 1006-15.

20. Coady MA, Rizzo JA, Elefteriades JA. Pathologic variants of thoracic aortic dissections. Penetrating atherosclerotic ulcers and intramural hematomas. *Cardiol Clin* 1999; 17: 637-57.

21. Tittle SL, Lynch RJ, Cole PE, Singh HS, *et al*. Midterm follow-up of penetrating ulcer and intramural hematoma of the aorta. *J Thorac Cardiovasc Surg* 2002; 123: 1051-9.

22. Cho KR, Stanson AW, Potter DD, *et al*. Penetrating atherosclerotic ulcer of the descending thoracic aorta and arch. *J Thorac Cardiovasc Surg* 2004; 127: 1393-9.

23. Demers P, Miller DC, Mitchell RS, *et al*. Stent-graft repair of penetrating atherosclerotic ulcers in the descending thoracic aorta: mid-term results. *Ann Thorac Surg* 2004; 77: 81-6.

24. Mitchell RS, Miller DC, Dake MD, *et al*. Thoracic aortic aneurysm repair with an endovascular stent graft: the 'first generation'. *Ann Thorac Surg* 1999; 67: 1971-4.

25. Parmey LF, Mattingly TW, Manion WC, *et al*. Nonpenetrating traumatic injury of the aorta. *Circulation* 1958; 17: 1086-101.

26. Finkelmeier BA, Mentzer RM Jr, Kaiser DL, *et al*. Chronic traumatic thoracic aneurysm. Influence of operative treatment on natural history: an analysis of reported cases, 1950-1980. *J Thorac Cardiovasc Surg* 1982; 84: 257-66.

27. Attar S, Cardarelli MG, Downing SW, *et al*. Traumatic aortic rupture: recent outcome with regard to neurologic deficit. *Ann Thorac Surg* 1999; 67: 959-64.

28. Melnitchouk S, Pfammatter T, Kadner A, *et al*. Emergency stent-graft placement for hemorrhage control in acute thoracic aortic rupture. *Eur J Cardiothorac Surg* 2004; 25: 1032-8.

29. Idu MM, Reekers JA, Balm R, *et al*. Collapse of a stent-graft following treatment of a traumatic thoracic aortic rupture. *J Endovasc Ther* 2005; 12: 503-7.

Chapter 13

Carotid artery stenting: current evidence and review of current practice

Viktor Berczi MD PhD, Endovascular Fellow
Trevor J Cleveland FRCS FRCR, Consultant Vascular Radiologist
Sheffield Vascular Institute, The Northern General Hospital, Sheffield, UK

Introduction

In the UK, the incidence of stroke is 2/1000, i.e. approximately 120,000 patients will suffer their first stroke every year. Stroke patients use 10% of hospital bed-days and 5% of annual healthcare expenditure. Elderly patients are at higher risk; the incidence of TIA increases with age from 0.9 per 1000 (55-64 years of age) to 2.6 per 1000 (75-84 years of age). Other risk factors for stroke include: smoking, hypertension, heart disease, peripheral vascular disease, diabetes, previous TIA or stroke, elevated cholesterol, high plasma fibrinogen, male sex, African-American or Asian population, and family history [1].

About 80% of strokes are ischaemic and 20% haemorrhagic. Eighty percent of all ischaemic strokes occur in the carotid territory. Intracranial occlusive disease alone is rarely responsible and pure haemodynamic reasons are responsible in less than 2% of all strokes. The most important aetiology of carotid territory infarction is thrombo-embolism of the internal carotid/middle cerebral artery (50%), small vessel disease (25%), cardiogenic embolism (15%), haematological disease (5%) and non-atheromatous disease (kinking, coiling, fibromuscular dysplasia, arteritis, aneurysm) (5%) [2].

The clinical natural history of stroke secondary to carotid artery disease is mainly determined by carotid plaque progression and degeneration. For symptomatic patients, early trials (aspirin v no treatment) in the 1970s and 1980s demonstrated a significant reduction in the risk of stroke for patients on aspirin. In the placebo cohorts, the rate of stroke was 19-22% during the 24-36 months follow-up period. The stroke risk also depends substantially on the number of risk factors involved and the degree of carotid stenosis. Patients with zero to five risk factors, with six risk factors or over six risk factors have 17%, 23% and 39% stroke risk at two years. If the degree of carotid stenosis is 70-79%, 80-89%, or 90-99%, then the risk of stroke at two years is 12%, 18% or 26% [2]. The stroke rate is the greatest in the first year following presentation and declines over time.

Given the proven role of risk factor modification with drug therapy, there was still excessive risk of stroke, despite these, in patients with high-grade stenoses. This led to development of additional therapies for stroke prevention. Carotid endarterectomy (CEA) was developed and was subsequently shown to be beneficial for groups of patients with both symptomatic and asymptomatic stenoses (NASCET [3], ECST [4], ACST [5], ACAS [6]). In line with the continuing healthcare trend towards less invasive therapy, angioplasty, and subsequently stenting, has been introduced as an alternative, or additional, treatment option.

A short history of carotid stenting

Carotid angioplasty was first investigated in an animal model almost 30 years ago. Human carotid angioplasty was reported in 1980 as a combined surgical and endovascular procedure, where the proximal common carotid artery was angioplastied via carotid cut-down with concomitant carotid bifurcation endarterectomy. Initially, carotid angioplasty (without stenting - Figure 1) was indicated only when surgery was not possible, but the patient remained at an unacceptably high risk of stroke. At the time, angioplasty of the carotid territory was performed using equipment designed for peripheral vascular use.

Major developments during the last 25 years in endovascular carotid revascularisation include:

- primary stenting;
- dedicated devices (low profile balloons, stents and protection systems);
- use of guiding catheters and sheaths;
- effective antiplatelet regimes;
- closure devices.

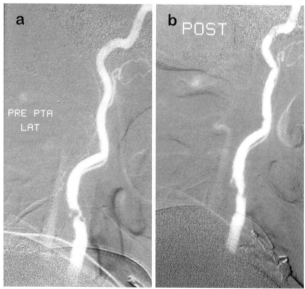

Figure 1. a) Carotid artery stenosis before angioplasty. b) The same stenosis as a) following balloon angioplasty.

The evidence for treating carotid lesions

All the early evidence was based on trials comparing CEA with best medical therapy of the time (BMT). Later, carotid artery angioplasty/stenting (CAS) was compared with CEA. No trials were done to directly compare the results of CAS with medical therapy alone. Some of the new trials (e.g. TACIT for asymptomatic patients) are aiming for direct comparison. In this chapter, trials including symptomatic patients are summarised; trials on asymptomatic patients are discussed in Chapter 16.

Randomised trials for symptomatic patients, CEA versus BMT

NASCET [3] and ECST [4]

ECST and NASCET included 6462 patients with ipsilateral carotid symptoms in the preceding six months. NASCET found no evidence that CEA benefited patients with a stenosis <50%. Patients with 50-69% stenoses showed small, but significant benefit. Gain in stroke-free survival was maximal in patients with 70-99% stenoses (surgical risk 8.9% at five years, medical risk 28.3% at five years; five CEA to prevent one ipsilateral stroke in three years). ECST demonstrated benefit only in patients with 70-99% carotid stenoses (surgical risk 10.5% at five years, medical risk 19.0% at five years; 12 CEA to prevent one ipsilateral stroke at five years).

Secondary analyses from NASCET suggest that patients over 75 years old benefit the most, especially those with the most severe disease (three CEAs to be performed to prevent one stroke at two years) [7]. Further secondary analysis demonstrated that women and men with >70% symptomatic stenosis had similar long-term benefit from CEA, although the peri-operative risks were higher for women. CEA was not beneficial for women with 50% to 69% stenosis without other risk factors for stroke [8].

Randomised trials for symptomatic patients, CEA vs. CAS

Leicester trial [9]

This was the first randomised trial to be published in 1998, albeit incomplete. It planned to randomise 300 symptomatic patients with an ipsilateral carotid stenosis >70% without preliminary diagnostic angiography. Stents were employed in all patients; protection devices were not available at the time. The Data Monitoring Committee suspended the trial after 17 patients had received their allocated treatment. The ten CEAs had no complications. However, five of the seven patients randomised to CAS suffered stroke (four periprocedural, one on day eight; three out of five disabling stroke at 30 days). It remains too small to influence clinical practice, but it reinforced the potential problem of treating a poorly selected population.

CAVATAS trial [10]

The Carotid and Vertebral Artery Transluminal Angioplasty Study (CAVATAS) is the largest, published study to date and shows equivalence between the two treatment modalities, in terms of prevention of disabling stroke/death up to three years. There were a total of 504 patients randomised with symptomatic >50% stenosis (majority had >70%) suitable for both CEA and CAS. Recruitment started in 1992, before routine use of dual antiplatelet therapy, primary stenting or cerebral protection devices. During the second half of the five-year recruitment period, stents - including Palmaz (Cordis), Strecker (Medi-Tech) and Wallstent (Schneider) - were increasingly used (in 26% overall).

The death/any stroke rate was 10.0% for the CAS group and 9.9% for the CEA patients. The death/disabling stroke rate was also not significantly different in the two groups (6.4% vs 5.9%). Delayed discharge due to wound haematoma was more likely in the surgical group (6.7% vs. 1.3%, p<0.0015). As a consequence of surgery, cranial nerve injury was documented in 8.7%. Significant (70-90%) restenosis was more likely to occur in the CAS group (14% vs. 6.7%, p<0.011). Cumulative freedom from death or disabling stroke at three years (including the 30-day risk) was 86% in both groups. No data were provided in this study for the three-year risk of death/any stroke rate.

The 10% risk of death/any stroke rate was higher than that observed in ECST (7.5%) and NASCET (5.8%), but there was an overlap between the confidence intervals. Explanations include: a high risk for the CAVATAS population compared to that of ECST or NASCET; primary stenting was performed in only 26% of patients; protection devices were not available; interventionalists had not received a standardised training in angioplasty. CAVATAS was a catalyst for a number of other randomised trials, including the ongoing ICSS, which is also referred to as CAVATAS 2.

The Wallstent study [11]

The third randomised trial of its kind has only been reported in abstract form. The commercially sponsored trial was abandoned after recruiting 219 symptomatic patients with an ipsilateral 60-99% carotid stenosis. Primary stenting with the Wallstent (Schneider, USA) without a protection device was performed. The 30-day risk of death/any stroke was 12.1% and 4.5% in the CAS and CEA group, respectively (p=0.049). In addition, 7% incidence of bradycardia and 4% incidence of groin haematoma was observed in the CAS patients. Comparable one-year data or restenosis rates were not published in the abstract.

The Lexington symptomatic study [12]

In a community hospital, 104 symptomatic patients with >70% ipsilateral carotid stenosis were randomised. CAS included primary stenting using the Wallstent (Boston Scientific) endoprosthesis without cerebral protection devices. By two years, no patient in either treatment arm had suffered a stroke. In the CAS group, one TIA and one leg amputation, and in the CEA group, one non-stroke death and four cranial nerve palsy were documented. The most unique finding of this study is the lack of stroke in either treatment arm during any part of the two-year follow-up period.

EVA 3S trial [13]

This is a multicentre, randomised trial in France, that was suspended after 80 patients had been randomised. An analysis of the patients included at that time led the investigators to conclude that the use of CAS without cerebral protection should not be continued. The trial was recommenced, and has recently been suspended again. The reasons for this and the conclusions are awaited.

In the first 80 symptomatic patients with >70% ipsilateral carotid stenosis, CAS was performed with primary stenting; cerebral protection devices were used at the discretion of the operator. In 7.5% of randomised patients, CAS could not be performed due to technical difficulties; these patients underwent CEA. In the remaining 73 patients, a cerebral protection device was used in 58 (80%). Overall, 30-day death/any stroke was 13.6%. Analysis of the subgroups showed that the risk of death/stroke for CAS without cerebral protection was 26.7% (4/15), compared to 10.3% (6/58). Based on these results the Data Monitoring Committee recommended stopping the unprotected CAS, despite the fact that the study was never powered to make this distinction, the observed differences were not statistically significant, and the lower limits of the confidence intervals were compatible with an absence of difference.

SAPPHIRE study [14]

In this trial, 334 patients, who were considered to be at high risk for open surgery, with symptomatic, >50% stenosis (1/3 of patients), and asymptomatic, >80% stenosis (2/3 of patients), were randomised for CEA or CAS. High risk for surgery was considered to be due to age >80 years, presence of congestive heart failure, severe COPD, previous endarterectomy with restenosis, previous radiation therapy or radical neck surgery, or lesions proximal or distal to the bulb or the proximal internal carotid artery. Primary stenting was performed with the Precise stent (Cordis) and the Angioguard (Cordis) protection system. The primary endpoint of the study was the cumulative incidence of a major cardiovascular event at one year, a composite of death, stroke, or myocardial infarction

within 30 days after the intervention or death or ipsilateral stroke between 31 days and one year. The trial was stopped prematurely because of slowing enrolment.

Patients randomised to CAS with cerebral protection were less likely to suffer death, stroke or MI (cumulative incidence for CAS and CEA was 12.2% and 20.1%, respectively, absolute difference, -7.9 percentage points; 95% CI -16.4 to 0.7%; p=0.004 for noninferiority, and p=0.053 for superiority).

It should be noted that more than half of patients considered for randomisation were excluded from the study, most of these patients being offered CAS and only a small fraction had CEA without randomisation. The complication rate of the asymptomatic patients was above what is now generally accepted as acceptable (above 4% in asymptomatic patients, there is no benefit in long-term stroke prevention [1]).

In summary, out of the six randomised trials above, two trials were abandoned and one was suspended, due to poor results in the unprotected CAS arm. The CAVATAS trial suggests equivalent results for CEA and CAS. The SAPPHIRE study indicated non-inferiority in terms of outcomes of CAS and CEA, but raised concerns in the asymptomatic patients.

Trials in progress, future trials

ICSS

An international, multicentre, randomised, controlled, open, prospective clinical trial, namely the International Carotid Stenting Study (ICSS), also known as CAVATAS 2, is recruiting. The objectives of the ICSS are to compare the risks, benefits and cost-effectiveness of a treatment policy of referral for carotid stenting, compared with referral for carotid endarterectomy. Symptomatic patients are included over the age of 40 years with atherosclerotic carotid stenosis, suitable for both stenting and surgery. The protocol recommends that a cerebral protection system should be used whenever the operator thinks one can be safely deployed. The combination of aspirin and clopidogrel is recommended to cover stenting procedures. All patients will receive best medical care. Neurologists will follow-up patients for five years. The primary outcome measure is the difference in the long-term rate of fatal or disabling stroke in any territory between patients randomised to stenting or surgery. The ICSS protocol incorporates a number of novel features to ensure patient safety, including the concept of probationary centres, proctoring of inexperienced investigators and monitoring of individual centre results on an ongoing basis. The protocol is also designed to mirror routine clinical practice.

CREST, SPACE

The multicentre Carotid Revascularization Endarterectomy vs. Stent Trial (CREST) in the USA for symptomatic (>50% stenosis) (30% of the participants) and asymptomatic (>70% stenosis) (70% of participants) patients compares the efficacy of carotid endarterectomy (CEA) and CAS in an ongoing clinical trial.

The Stent-Supported Percutaneous Angioplasty of the Carotid Artery versus Endarterectomy (SPACE) trial is investigating if both treatment modalities are equivalent in the treatment of severe symptomatic carotid stenoses in Germany, Austria and Switzerland (32 centres; the trial has recently closed and the early results are awaited). Patients with symptomatic (transient ischaemic attack or minor stroke) stenosis (<50%), eligible for both methods, were recruited into this trial. The primary endpoint is the incidence of an ipsilateral stroke or death between randomisation and day 30 after treatment.

Three of the ongoing trials, EVA-3S, SPACE and ICSS (CAVATAS 2), have prospectively agreed to combine individual patient data after completion of follow-up. This meta-analysis will provide results similar to a mega-trial and should also allow informative subgroup analyses. The results should determine whether CAS truly rivals CEA as the treatment of choice for carotid stenosis.

Recent non-randomised trials, reviews, registries

A recent, dual independent Cochrane Systematic Review, published in 2004, included all relevant papers up to June 2003. The objective of this review was to assess the benefits and risks of endovascular treatments compared with CEA or medical therapy. Meta-analysis of the data found no significant difference between the odds of death or any stroke at 30 days post-procedure (Odds Ratio [OR] endovascular: surgery 1.26, 95% CI 0.82 to 1.94). The odds of death or disabling stroke at 30 days were similar in the endovascular and surgical group (OR 1.22, CI 0.61 to 2.41). At one year following procedure, there was no significant difference between the two groups in preventing any stroke or death (OR 1.36, CI 0.87 to 2.13). Endovascular treatment significantly reduced the risk of cranial neuropathy (OR 0.12, CI 0.06 to 0.25). There was no significant difference between the two groups when the risk of death, any stroke or myocardial infarction was considered (OR 0.99, CI 0.66 to 1.48). There was substantial heterogeneity between the trials for four of the five outcomes. Data from randomised trials comparing endovascular treatment for carotid artery stenosis with CEA, suggest that the two treatments have similar early risks of death or stroke and similar long-term benefits. There is a strong case to continue recruitment in the current randomised trials comparing carotid stenting with endarterectomy[15].

Pooled data from ECST and NASCET (5893 patients with 33,000 patient-years of follow-up) showed that benefit from surgery was greatest in men, patients aged 75 years or older, and those randomised within two weeks after their last ischaemic event, and fell rapidly with increasing delay. For patients with 50% or higher stenosis, the number of patients needed to undergo surgery to prevent one ipsilateral stroke in five years was nine for men versus 36 for women, five for age 75 years or older versus 18 for younger than 65 years, and five for those randomised within two weeks after their last ischaemic event, versus 125 for patients randomised after more than 12 weeks. These results were consistent across the individual trials. Ideally, the procedure should be done within two weeks of the patient's last symptoms[16].

The aim of the Italian prospective registry (four centres, 416 patients; 63% symptomatic, 37% asymptomatic) was to evaluate the applicability and efficacy of the MoMa Device (Invatec, Roncadelle, Italy) for the prevention of cerebral embolisation during carotid artery stenting (CAS) in a real world population. No periprocedural strokes and deaths were observed. Complications during hospitalization included 16 minor strokes (3.84%), three transient ischaemic attacks (0.72%), two deaths (0.48%) and one major stroke (0.24%). The cumulative rate at discharge and 30 days was 4.56% for all strokes and deaths, and 0.72% for major strokes and deaths. All the patients underwent 30-day follow-up. These results match favourably with current available studies on carotid stenting with cerebral protection.

A contemporary meta-analysis (published in 2005) compared one-month composite rates of stroke or death, all stroke, disabling stroke, myocardial infarction, cranial nerve injury, and major bleeding and one-year rates of both minor and major ipsilateral stroke. The 30-day stroke and death rates associated with CAS and CEA were not significantly different. Lower rates of myocardial infarction and cranial nerve injury were observed with CAS compared with CEA [17].

Patient management

On the website of the Cardiovascular and Interventional Radiology Society of Europe (www.cirse.org), the "Quality assurance guidelines for the performance of carotid stenting" has been installed recently.

Radiological diagnosis

The goals of imaging are: to assess whether or not carotid disease is present; to assess the severity of carotid disease; to exclude or verify occlusion; to assess any unusual features or anatomy of the carotid bifurcation; and if stenting is planned, to assess the proximal and distal vessels. These goals should be achieved with minimal risk and be reliable.

Carotid duplex ultrasound (US) is non-invasive, cheap and widely available in comparison to other imaging modalities. For detection of occlusion it has excellent sensitivity (96%) and specificity (100%). However, sensitivity and specificity for diagnosing a stenosis of between 70-99% rarely reaches 90% in a review of 63 publications [18]. Duplex ultrasound is operator-dependent; it is poor at differentiating sub-occlusion from complete occlusion and detecting high carotid lesions; the origin of the arch branches or the circle of Willis cannot be directly assessed by ultrasound [18, 19]. Carotid plaque characteristics are known to have a correlation with the risk of neurological events; soft plaques denote higher risk than calcified plaques. The importance of carotid plaque morphology and its implication of success prediction will be addressed in Chapter 17.

Magnetic resonance angiography (MRA) avoids the risks of catheter-related embolic events, iodinated contrast nephrotoxicity, allergic reactions, and the use of ionising radiation. MRA does have its limitations with sensitivity and specificity values of 92-98% and 76-90% respectively, for diagnosing 70-99% carotid stenosis (Figure 2). There is also a tendency for MRA to overestimate stenoses in comparison to conventional digital subtraction angiography, although this may be partially explained by the greater number of projection images available at MRA [18]. In some centres, despite the limitations, MRA and ultrasound have replaced DSA to assess suitability for CEA in the majority of patients.

Computed tomography angiography (CTA), a new and minimally invasive method of visualising both intracranial and extracranial arteries, can be used alone or in combination with US in the diagnosis of ICA stenoses. Sensitivity and specificity when compared to DSA is between 85-100% and 63-100%, respectively. Recent studies have shown that 13-15.6% of the patients would have been offered CEA incorrectly if they were examined only by US and CTA. Multi-slice CTA, which promises to be better, has only recently become available routinely. The technique still requires ionising radiation and the use of a potentially nephrotoxic contrast medium, which limit its benefits over conventional angiography.

The limitations of these imaging techniques must be considered in light of the complication rates inherent in catheter angiography. The combined

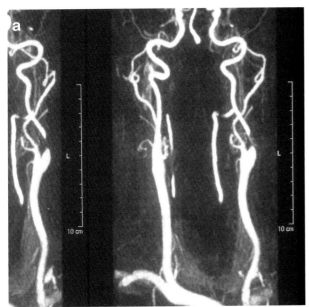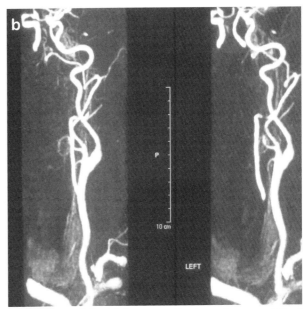

Figure 2. a) MR angiogram showing an apparent stenosis at the ICA origin. b) Same patient as a), except that all of the artery has been included in the reconstruction, showing that there is no stenosis.

transient/reversible and permanent neurological complication rate of selective cerebral angiography varies between 0.4-12.2% and 0-5.4%, respectively. The NASCET group suggest that the risk of major stroke or death due to angiography should be no more than 1%. The ACAS group calculated a 1.2% arteriogram risk. Recently, a study from Sheffield demonstrated that non-selective, arch aortography had no focal neurological complications in 311 patients (mean age 71.0 ± 9.2 years, 97% symptomatic, 3% awaited coronary bypass surgery). The lack of focal neurological complications demonstrated in this study may be attributed to this minimal manipulation and to the lack of dead space in the flushed catheters [19].

All symptomatic patients are referred for angiography following a routine duplex scan and neurological assessment in our centre. Arch angiography is performed to confirm the duplex findings and also to allow planning for any further intervention. Inappropriate stenting attempts on patients with diseased arch branch origins increase the risk of embolic complications from the stenting procedure. Patients with diseased origins are also likely to be at most risk from a selective diagnostic procedure and therefore using arch aortography in all

patients avoids this risk at the diagnostic stage. Non-selective, arch aortography that comprises minimal neurological risk is used as a gold standard modality in our centre for evaluating arch branches and carotid bifurcations until such time as MRA or CTA techniques become more reliable.

Pharmacological support

Optimisation of all risk factors, including best medical therapy, should be strictly observed in all patients. During the procedure, heparin is routinely administered to avoid thrombus forming on the catheters. The importance of administration of an anticholinergic prior to manipulation of the carotid bulb, in order to prevent sinus bradyarrythmias has been emphasised for more than 15 years. In Sheffield, 600 microgram glycopyrrolate is given; many other centres use atropine. Glycopyrrolate has a shorter duration of action than atropine and tachycardia is less pronounced.

Dual antiplatelet therapy inhibits platelet activation through two different pathways. Aspirin, a cyclo-oxygenase inhibitor, inhibits platelet thromboxane synthesis. In aspirin-intolerant patients, dipyridamole is generally used. Clopidogrel inhibits platelet adenosine diphosphate (ADP) receptors, thus preventing fibrinogen binding. It is now routine practice in most units to commence dual antiplatelet therapy prior to CAS.

A randomised trial showed significant benefit of aspirin plus clopidogrel versus aspirin plus 24-hour anticoagulation (heparin) [20]. Clopidogrel is recommended in addition to aspirin, and these drugs must both be fully active at the time of CAS. In order that this can be reasonably certain, a routine dose (75mg daily) must be given for at least three days before CAS, and longer is probably better. Dual antiplatelet therapy should be continued for at least four weeks following the intervention.

Cerebral protection devices

A growing body of data indicate that the use of cerebral protection devices may decrease the incidence of embolic neurological deficits associated with CAS. In Sheffield, current practice involves the use of cerebral protection devices in every case when it is technically possible. Chapter 14 will describe the types of and data on cerebral protection devices.

Follow-up and restenosis

The CAVATAS group published the rates of residual severe stenosis and restenosis, and their contribution to recurrent symptoms recently. In the analysed group, endovascular patients were treated by balloon angioplasty alone (88%) or stenting (22%). Patches were used in 63% of CEA patients. More patients had ≥70% stenosis of the ipsilateral carotid artery one year after endovascular treatment than after endarterectomy (18.5% versus 5.2%, p=0.0001). The results were significantly better after stenting compared with angioplasty alone at one month (p<0.001), but not at one year. Recurrent ipsilateral symptoms were more common in endovascular patients with severe stenosis (5/32 [15.6%]) compared with lesser degrees of stenosis at one year (11/141 [7.8%], p=0.02), but most were transient ischaemic attacks and none were disabling or fatal strokes. There were no recurrent symptoms in the nine CEA patients with >70% stenosis at one year. Further studies are required to determine whether newer carotid stenting techniques are associated with a lower risk of restenosis. The low rate of recurrent stroke in both endovascular and endarterectomy patients suggests that treatment of restenosis should be limited to patients with recurrent symptoms, very tight restenosis or progressive disease, but long-term follow-up data are required.

Summary

◆   Endovascular treatment for carotid stenosis has been performed for some years.

◆   There has been an improvement over this time in:
o   the equipment that is available;
o   understanding about which patients are at high risk of stroke;
o   imaging modalities to assess the carotid bifurcation;
o   drug therapy before, during and after CAS;
o   which patients are morphologically suitable for CAS and which are not.

◆   Data indicate that CAS can be performed with a similar safety profile to CEA.

◆   Further trials are being performed to clarify the situation further.

References

1. Naylor AR, Gaines PA. Carotid endarterectomy or stenting: an overview of the randomised trials. In: *Endovascular Intervention: Current Controversies.* Wyatt MG, Watkinson AF, Eds. Shrewsbury: tfm publishing Ltd, 2004: 127-33.

2. Mackey WC, Naylor AR. Carotid artery disease: natural history and diagnosis. In: *Comprehensive Vascular and Endovascular Surgery.* Hallet JW, Mills JL, Earnshaw JJ, Reekers JA, Eds. Edinburgh: Mosby, 2004: 521-31.

3. North American Symptomatic Carotid Endarterectomy Trial Collaborators. Beneficial effect of carotid endarterectomy in symptomatic patients with high-grade carotid stenosis. *N Engl J Med* 1991; 325(7): 445-53.

4. European Carotid Surgery Trialists' Collaborative Group. MRC European Carotid Surgery Trial: interim results for symptomatic patients with severe (70-99%) or with mild (0-29%) carotid stenosis. European Carotid Surgery Trialists' Collaborative Group. *Lancet* 1991; 337(8752): 1235-43.

5. Halliday A, Mansfield A, Marro J, Peto C, Peto R, Potter J, Thomas D. MRC Asymptomatic Carotid Surgery Trial (ACST) Collaborative Group. Prevention of disabling and fatal strokes by successful carotid endarterectomy in patients without recent neurological symptoms: randomised controlled trial. *Lancet* 2004; 363 (9420): 1492-1502.

6. Executive Committee for the Asymptomatic Carotid Atherosclerosis Study. Endarterectomy for asymptomatic carotid artery stenosis. *JAMA* 1995; 273: 1421-8.

7. Alamowitch S, Eliasziw M, Algra A, Meldrum H, Barnett HJ; North American Symptomatic Carotid Endarterectomy Trial (NASCET) Group. Risk, causes, and prevention of ischaemic stroke in elderly patients with symptomatic internal-carotid-artery stenosis. *Lancet* 2001; 357: 1154-60.

8. Alamowitch S, Eliasziw M, Barnett HJ; North American Symptomatic Carotid Endarterectomy Trial (NASCET); ASA Trial Group; Carotid Endarterectomy (ACE) Trial Group. The risk and benefit of endarterectomy in women with symptomatic internal carotid artery disease. *Stroke* 2005; 36: 27-31.

9. Naylor AR, Bolia A, Abbott RJ, Pye IF, Smith J, Lennard N, *et al.* Randomized study of carotid angioplasty and stenting versus carotid endarterectomy: a stopped trial. *J Vasc Surg* 1998; 28: 326-34.

10. CAVATAS investigators. Endovascular versus surgical treatment in patients with carotid stenosis in the Carotid and Vertebral Artery Transluminal Angioplasty Study (CAVATAS): a randomized trial. *Lancet* 2001; 357: 1729-37.

11. Alberts MJ. Results of a multicenter prospective randomized trial of carotid artery stenting versus carotid endarterectomy. *Stroke* 2001; 32: 325.

12. Brooks WH, McClure RR, Jones MR, Coleman TC, Breathitt L. Carotid angioplasty and stenting versus carotid endarterectomy: a randomized trial in a community hospital. *J Am Coll Cardiol* 2001; 38: 1589-995.

13. Mas JL, Chatellier G, Beyssen B; EVA-3S Investigators. Carotid angioplasty and stenting with and without cerebral protection: clinical alert from the Endarterectomy Versus Angioplasty in Patients With Symptomatic Severe Carotid Stenosis (EVA-3S) trial. *Stroke* 2004; 35(1): e18-20.

14. Yadav JS, Wholey MH, Kuntz RE, Fayad P, Katzen BT, Mishkel GJ, *et al*; Stenting and Angioplasty with Protection in Patients at High Risk for Endarterectomy Investigators. Protected carotid-artery stenting versus endarterectomy in high-risk patients. *New Engl J Med* 351: 1491-1501.

15. Coward LJ, Featherstone RL, Brown MM. Percutaneous transluminal angioplasty and stenting for carotid artery stenosis. *Cochrane Database Syst Rev* 2004; Issue 2: CD000515.

16. Rothwell PM, Eliasziw M, Gutnikov SA, Warlow CP, Barnett HJ; Carotid Endarterectomy Trialists Collaboration. Endarterectomy for symptomatic carotid stenosis in relation to clinical subgroups and timing of surgery. *Lancet* 2004; 363(9413): 915-24.

17. Qureshi AI, Kirmani JF, Divani AA, Hobson RW II. Carotid angioplasty with or without stent placement versus carotid endarterectomy for treatment of carotid stenosis: a meta-analysis. *Neurosurgery* 2005; 56: 1171-81.

18. Nederkoorn PJ, van der Graaf Y, Hunink MG. Duplex ultrasound and magnetic resonance angiography compared with digital subtraction angiography in carotid artery stenosis: a systematic review. *Stroke* 2003; 34: 1324-32.

19. Berczi V, Randall M, Balamurugan R, Shaw D, Venables GS, Cleveland TJ, Gaines PA. Safety of arch aortography for assessment of carotid arteries. *Eur Vasc Endovasc Surg* 2006; 31(1): 3-7.

20. McKevitt FM, Randall MS, Cleveland TJ, Gaines PA, Tan KT, Venables GS. The benefits of combined anti-platelet treatment in carotid artery stenting. *Eur J Vasc Endovasc Surg* 2005; 29(5): 522-7.

Chapter 14

Carotid filters: evidence, availability and the future

Sumaira Macdonald MB ChB (Comm.) MRCP FRCR PhD

Consultant Vascular Radiologist & Honorary Clinical Senior Lecturer

Freeman Hospital, Newcastle upon Tyne, UK

Introduction

Endovascular management of significant carotid stenosis has evolved significantly from its inception in the 1980s, when it comprised a rudimentary angioplasty technique. The current state of the art involves protected primary carotid stenting with dedicated low-profile rapid-exchange equipment and effective procedural pharmacological support. The development and integration of protection devices has been an important step in the quest to reduce the periprocedural stroke risk.

Carotid stenting (CAS), as the endovascular option is now known, has some potential advantages over carotid endarterectomy (CEA). These include avoidance of a neck incision and, therefore, of cranial nerve injury and neck haematoma, and avoidance of carotid cross-clamping. This latter presumptive benefit, however, clearly has the potential to constitute a drawback. Endovascular manipulation of atherosclerotic plaque which, in symptomatic patients has by definition become unstable and produced symptoms by cerebral embolisation, is hazardous without control of the distal internal carotid artery (ICA). The use of a cerebral protection filter presents perhaps the ideal solution in that it promises distal control without the need for flow arrest. For the dual reasons of widespread availability and intuitive philosophy, filters are the most commonly used protection device, used in 90% of CAS treatment episodes at the current time. Alternative strategies 'protect' the brain at the expense of constant procedural cerebral perfusion i.e. by flow arrest (distal or proximal balloon occlusion) or by flow reversal.

Availability

It is perhaps apposite to discuss availability before evidence base. Just as in any rapidly evolving technical arena, innovative procedures are trialled by pioneers and early positive reports fuel uptake and availability before any real evidence is accrued. Social theorists describe an s-curve portraying the diffusion of innovations. The five stages involved in this 'diffusion' are the launch by innovators, followed in successive stages by early adopters, the early majority, the late majority and finally, the laggards. The speed of diffusion accelerates to a peak (the 'tipping point'), which occurs on average at 20% adoption [1]. This tipping point happened relatively early in the time-line of the development and availability of filters.

The first protection device that was commercially available was the distal balloon occlusion device, the PercuSurge GuardWire™ (Medtronic, Santa Rosa, USA), which was based on Theron's original concept [2]. Filters released to trialling centres became available towards the end of 1999-2000. These prototype devices were wire-mounted on long 300cm wires. Their crossing profiles have gradually diminished and their delivery and retrieval systems have become 'monorail' or 'rapid-exchange'-compatible, like every other step of the CAS procedure. Two filters currently allow the operator to first cross the lesion with a high-quality 0.014" guidewire with subsequent filter placement (EmboShield™, Abbott Vascular, Abbott Park, Illinois, USA and SpideRX™, Ev3 Europe, 75008 Paris, France). The advantages of this technical refinement include improved one-to-one torque and responsiveness, and the ability to cross extremely tight tortuous lesions without resorting to 'buddy wiring' (the prior placement of a separate 0.014" wire) or pre-filter placement predilatation.

The uptake in the use of cerebral protection is elegantly displayed in Figure 1. Between 1997 to 2003, there was a steep increase in use of protection devices as they became available within the German Cardiology Carotid Stenting Registry (ALKK) [3]. Seventy-one percent of these devices were filters.

Devices used within the International Carotid Stenting Study (ICSS) must have a CE Mark (Conformité Européenne) and have satisfied the Steering Committee. Steering Committee approval rests on availability of peer-reviewed published safety and/or efficacy data, in addition to CE marking.

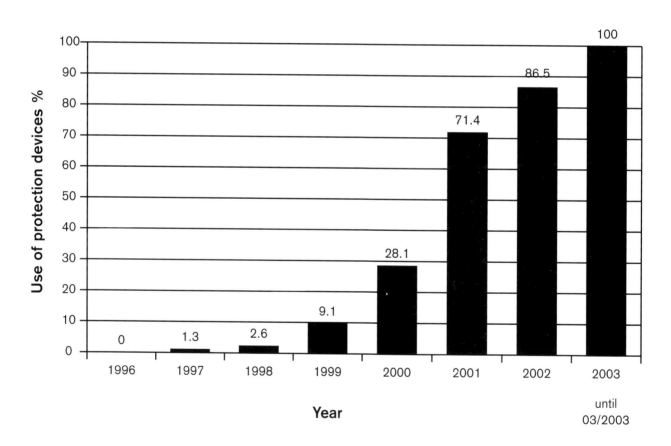

Figure 1. German Cardiology Carotid Stenting Registry (ALKK) [3]: use of protection devices with time. A filter was used in 71% (476/668) and an occlusive system in 27% (181/668).

The filters approved for use within ICSS are given in Table 1.

Name of filter	Manufacturer/distributor
NeuroShield	MedNova/Abbott Vascular
EmboShield	Abbott Vascular
Angioguard	Cordis
Accunet	Guidant
EPI (FilterWire EX)	Boston Scientific
FilterWire EZ	Boston Scientific

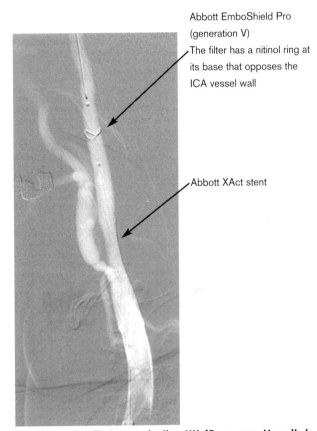

Abbott EmboShield Pro (generation V)
The filter has a nitinol ring at its base that opposes the ICA vessel wall

Abbott XAct stent

Figure 2. The first case in the UK (Freeman Hospital, Newcastle) utilising a generation-V EmboShield Pro cerebral protection filter. Unhindered cerebral perfusion is demonstrated.

The NeuroShield was an earlier iteration of the EmboShield device which is currently enjoying its fifth reincarnation (EmboShield Pro) and the EPI was an earlier version of the FilterWire EZ. Figure 2 demonstrates the first case in the UK (Freeman Hospital, Newcastle) utilising a generation-V EmboShield Pro.

At least three other CE-marked filters are available, to include the Microvena Trap™, which was granted its CE mark in October 2000, the SpideRX™ and the Interceptor™ (Medtronic), which both received their CE marks in July 2004. Although all these devices are readily available to experienced centres, in reality, distributing companies will often mandate that experienced operators support inexperienced centres before unconditional release of equipment is granted. Furthermore, many carotid-stent registries mandate the use of cerebral protection. These are often industry-supported and a number are North American and, therefore, arguably subject to reimbursement and litigation issues that may be less relevant elsewhere. At least one trial comparing CAS and CEA, EVA-3S, dictated that cerebral protection was an absolute requirement for the CAS-limb of the trial [4]. This trial has been suspended. In other trials such as the ICSS, cerebral protection is recommended, but not mandated; this accepted, the highest recruiting centre for the trial, Utrecht, does not routinely employ cerebral protection during CAS.

Evidence

Evidence that filters trap macroemboli

There is substantial circumstantial and level IV and level V evidence (from uncontrolled case-series) that filters are capable of trapping debris when used during CAS. A number of early experiences report pathological analysis of filter findings retrieved *in vivo.* Debris including fibrin, cholesterol clefts, red and white cell aggregates and organised thrombus may be recovered [5]. It is thought that this material is likely to have been liberated by the endovascular manipulation of the carotid bifurcation plaque and subsequently caught in the filter rather than the alternative, i.e. that

Although the threshold of damage to the micro- and macrovasculature of the human brain remains unknown, particles of the type and size that are retrieved from filters will clearly impact on deep perforators and larger debris may easily cause devastating proximal middle cerebral artery occlusion. At the current time, with a number of technical refinements in addition to enhanced filters, to include advances in our understanding of pharmacological support, dedicated carotid stents and low profile rapid-exchange systems, one may encounter larger debris infrequently. Accepting this fact, macroemboli are still encountered in filters during contemporary practice. Figure 3 is a contemporary image elegantly displaying entrapped macroembolus in a SpideRx filter. This debris is of such a size as to pose a considerable threat to the ipsilateral middle cerebral artery (MCA) and may cause devastating stroke if it embolised to the brain.

Impact of filters on procedural microemboli

Preliminary *ex vivo* work on filters indicated that 88% of the total procedural embolic load is trapped. However, the actual *in vivo* percentage is unknown, as particles smaller than the pores may pass through or around the filter. It has been clear for some time that there is a degree of inefficiency when filters are employed, but there is also some more recent data suggesting that filters may be associated with increased numbers of microemboli.

These data focus largely on microemboli measured by surrogate markers such as Transcranial Doppler (TCD) or diffusion-weighted imaging of the brain (DWI).

Prospective cohort analyses comparing unprotected CAS with cases protected by means of distal balloon occlusion demonstrated a significant reduction in microembolic signals (MES) when a distal balloon was used (164 +/-108 MES in the control versus 68 +/-83 in the protected group; p=0.002) [6]. The use of filters, however, has been shown to increase the numbers of distal microemboli. Within a clinical randomised trial, performed at the Sheffield Vascular Institute, there were significantly more MES

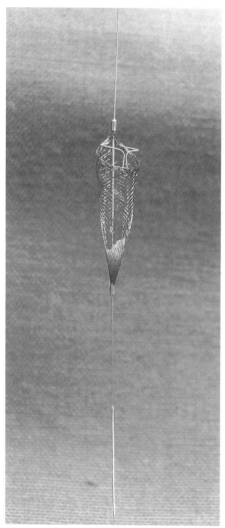

Figure 3. A contemporary image elegantly displaying entrapped macroembolus in a SpideRx filter. This debris is of such a size as to pose a considerable threat to the ipsilateral middle cerebral artery (MCA) and may cause devastating stroke if passing unhindered to the brain.

this material has formed on the filter device *in situ*. The reported mean size of trapped particles ranges from 201-5043 microns and the numbers released range from 26-174. It has to be borne in mind that the pore size of the currently available devices ranges from 80-150 microns and *ex vivo* work suggests that substantial numbers of microemboli, i.e. particles smaller than 60 microns simply pass unhindered to the brain with a filter in place.

Table 2. Comparing new white lesions on diffusion-weighted imaging MRI of the brain for protected and unprotected CAS.

Worker	Incidence of new white lesions (unprotected)	Incidence of new white lesions (protected)
Jaeger et al [9, 10]	29% (20/70)	15% (3/20)
Macdonald et al [7]	18% (4/22)	29% (7/24)

in patients 'protected' by means of a filter-type cerebral protection device (EmboShield™). Furthermore, off-site analysis determined that a substantial proportion of these MES corresponded to particulate matter and could not be simply dismissed as air, due to agitated contrast injection [7].

A Dutch single centre prospective analysis of microembolic signals on procedural TCD for unprotected CAS and filter-protected CAS recently reported [8]. Patients were divided into three groups: 161 patients treated before filters had become available (group 1), 151 patients treated with filters (group 2), and 197 patients treated without filters after these devices had become available (group 3). The authors concluded that carotid angioplasty and stent placement yielded more microemboli in patients treated with filters than in unprotected procedures; however, the infrequent occurrence of cerebral sequelae did not allow comprehensive statistical comparison between groups.

With respect to evidence that these liberated microemboli reach the brain, the literature highlights that there is a 15%-29% incidence of new white lesions detected on diffusion-weighted MRI of brain following protected CAS [7, 9]. Within the randomised trial, there were more new white lesions on TCD in protected cases compared with unprotected cases. This did not reach statistical significance, perhaps because the trial was powered for the TCD findings; however, two prospective cohort analyses from a German institution showed the complete opposite.

The discrepancy between the Sheffield randomised trial and the German prospective cohort analyses must be examined.

A comparison of the randomised trial results (for the procedural time-frame) and the German cohort analyses of unprotected and protected series [9, 10] is given in Table 2.

The use of historical controls has allowed confounding variables to influence outcome. The differences between Jaeger's unprotected and protected populations are of crucial importance. These are a prime consideration when the numbers of cases are relatively small.

Firstly, 25% (18/70) of the unprotected group were asymptomatic and 35% (7/20) of the protected group were asymptomatic. It is known that symptomatic patients have a higher incidence of new white lesions following unprotected carotid stenting than asymptomatic patients (23% versus 12%) [11]. This is borne out by Jaeger's own experience in the unprotected population; 76% (38/70) symptomatic patients had positive DWI scans, whilst only 24% (12/70) asymptomatic patients had positive scans. This would tend to lower the incidence of new white lesions in the protected group.

Secondly, 90% of the unprotected population had atherosclerotic disease with its propensity to embolise, compared with only 70% of the protected group, the remainder comprising post-radiotherapy and restenotic lesions with arguably lower emboligenic potential.

Thirdly, an arch aortogram was performed prior to selective carotid arteriography at the same sitting as unprotected carotid stenting, whereas only selective carotid arteriography was reported as being performed at the same sitting as protected carotid stenting, thus eliminating a potentially emboligenic stage in the protected series.

Fourthly, two different procedural methods are described for the unprotected series: the 'over-the-wire' and the 'long sheath' method, whilst only the 'long sheath' method was utilised in the protected series, adding variability to the outcomes.

Lastly, three types of stent were used in the unprotected group: in 63% of cases, an Easy WallStent™ (Boston Scientific Corporation, Natick MA 01760, USA) was used; in 14%, a Rolling Membrane WallStent was used; and in only 23% of cases, was an over-the-wire (OTW) Carotid WallStent™ (Boston Scientific) used. The Easy WallStent™ is a relatively high-profile (7 French) non-dedicated device, i.e. one that has been adapted from peripheral use, and thus has the potential for greater procedural embolisation. The Rolling Membrane is a precursor to the Easy WallStent. The Carotid WallStent™ is a dedicated carotid stent with a lower crossing profile (5.6 French for the 7mm iteration and 5.9 French for the 9mm iteration). In the protected series, an OTW Carotid WallStent (a dedicated device) was used in 95% of cases.

It is possible that all these differences increased the incidence of new white lesions in the unprotected group and confounding variables of this type are commonplace in non-randomised studies. Clearly, none of these factors are relevant to a randomised trial in which standardised methodology is mandatory.

So, it can be shown that use of a filter-type device can significantly increase MES on TCD of the ipsilateral MCA and may substantially increase new white lesions on diffusion-weighted MRI of the brain, both representing surrogate markers of microembolisation. The reasons for this are not clear and may include fragmentation of larger debris causing showers of smaller material or 'seeding' of formed elements off the exterior filter surface.

Evidence of clinical benefit from the use of cerebral protection

From July 1996 to March 2003, 1483 patients from 26 hospitals were included in the prospective CAS Registry of the ALKK (German cardiology clinic study) group [3]. A protection device was used in 668 of 1483

patients (45%). The use of a protection device grew rapidly from 2000 and reached 100% in 2003. Patients treated with a protection device had prior carotid artery dilatation more often (3.5% versus 1%, p<0.001), a prior myocardial infarction (34% versus 27.4%, p=0.007) and a history of arterial hypertension (89.9% versus 78.6%, p=0.007), compared to patients treated without a protection device. Thrombus was more often visible in patients treated with distal protection (16.5% versus 8%, p<0.001). The use of a protection device led to a 10-minute longer intervention (45 minutes versus 35 minutes, median, p<0.001). Patients treated with a protection device had a lower rate of ipsilateral stroke (1.7% versus 4.1%, p=0.007) and a lower rate of all non-fatal strokes and all deaths (2.1% versus 4.9%, p=0.004) during the hospital stay. This was confirmed by multiple logistic regression analysis (adjusted OR=0.45, 95% CI: 0.23-0.91, p=0.026). A similar reduction could be found for symptomatic as well as asymptomatic carotid artery stenoses.

However, this registry incorporates the shifting technical landscape that was prevalent during the time frame of introduction of protection devices.

A systematic review of studies reporting on the incidence of minor stroke, major stroke or death within 30 days after CAS reported recently [12]. In 2357 patients, 2537 CAS procedures were performed without protection and in 839 patients, 896 CAS procedures were performed with protection, albeit with a mixture of devices. The groups were similar with respect to age, sex distribution, cerebrovascular risk factors and indicators for CAS. However, somewhat disappointingly for a systematic review, randomised trial data were not evaluated, perhaps because there are no such data available. The studies included in the review were often small (some as small as ten cases, raising the question of the operators' learning curves), self-audited and heterogeneous with respect to study design, lesion type, clinical indication, methods and techniques employed. The authors themselves concluded that "increasing expertise within institutions might influence complication rates". If the analysis is limited to those studies reporting after 2002, after which time more homogeneity with respect to technical aspects of the procedure may be expected, the all-stroke/death rate was 2% for the protected series and 3.2% for the unprotected series. This difference is not statistically significant.

In prospective cohort analyses, Cremonesi et al [13] reported a periprocedural embolic rate of 3.2% (4/125) in the unprotected cohort and 0.7% (1/150) in the protected cohort; however, it was recognised that a long learning curve may exist with some of the protection devices. This represents level IV evidence; protected stenting was compared with historical controls of unprotected stenting.

Indeed, a critical evaluation of all these reports will highlight that the protected patients in each of these reviews have been compared with historical controls. The influence of dedicated stents, learning curves, improved pharmacological support and lower profile systems, which were developed in parallel with protection devices, is easily overlooked. Each of these additional technical refinements may be individually shown to have a profound influence on outcome. Stents adapted from peripheral or coronary designs were used in earlier evaluations of unprotected CAS cohorts, as their use predates the availability of protection devices. The use of dedicated carotid stents significantly improves outcomes with respect to all-stroke/death and major disabling stroke/death when compared to adapted stents [14]. The influence of learning curves can readily be appreciated within the randomised trial setting of CAVATAS. With increasing throughput within the trial, both angioplasty (predating the availability of protection devices) and CEA got safer [15]. The influence of contemporary pharmacological support in the form of the dual antiplatelet regime (aspirin plus clopidogrel) significantly improves outcome over the historical standard of care at the time of CAVATAS (aspirin plus heparin infusion). A recent randomised trial was stopped prematurely because of the size of the significant difference in the aspirin/clopidogrel and aspirin/heparin limbs of the trial [16].

The German Pro-CAS registry evaluated patients treated with and without protection devices between 2000 and 2003; filters were used in 76%. Patients treated before 2000, representing essentially dated endovascular technique were analysed separately. There was no difference in combined mortality and permanent neurological deficit between protected and unprotected populations (20/923, 2.2% unprotected, 33/1609, 2.1% protected) [17]. Interestingly, the total rate of transient neurological symptoms was higher in the protected group (4/923, 4.6% unprotected and 122/1609, 7.6% protected). This included prolonged reversible neurological deficit, transient ischaemic attack and transient monocular blindness. It is possible that this finding is consistent with the known increase in microembolic signals to the brain on TCD when a filter is used.

Overall, the literature is hampered by the lack of a randomised trial powered to make the distinction between protected and unprotected CAS on the basis of clinical outcomes. If the all-stroke/death rates in the systematic review for studies reporting after 2002 are revisited, in order to detect non-inferiority of unprotected CAS when the difference between the two groups is 2% and 3.2%, perhaps more than 2000 patients would be required. If one wished to power a trial to demonstrate superiority of protected CAS based on clinical outcomes, it is clear that one would need to be far more ambitious with respect to numbers recruited.

Prediction of emboligenic risk

The literature abounds with conflicting evidence about the imaging characteristics of vulnerable plaque and features such as hypoechogenicity, hyperechogenicity and degree of stenosis (a surrogate marker of embolic load) have all been postulated to correlate with increasing procedural risk. An ultrasonic parameter, the Grey Scale Median (GSM) has been utilised to determine embolic risk [18]. A GSM ≤25 is thought to be associated with increased risk of stroke during CAS, but the evaluation of this parameter requires software modifications of the ultrasound machine and specific sonographer training and may be difficult, therefore, to incorporate seamlessly into clinical practice.

A recent study aimed to identify the clinical factors predictive for the presence or absence of visible debris captured by filters during CAS [19]. Patients undergoing CAS with the use of a distal filter device (n=279) were prospectively entered into an investigational registry. Recorded variables were classified as patient-, lesion-, or procedure-related. The filter was assessed for visible debris in each case. The odds ratio (OR) and 95% confidence interval (CI) were determined for each variable to predict visible debris. The ability of each variable to predict the absence of visible debris was assessed by calculating the individual negative predictive value (NPV). Visible debris was present in 169 filters (60.3%). There was an increased risk of visible debris found with several variables (OR, 95% CI): hypertension (2.9, 1.7 to 5.2), hypercholesterolemia (2.3, 1.4 to 3.9), stent diameter >9 mm (16.6, 9.0 to 30.0), and any neurologic event (4.2, 1.5 to 9.9). The NPV failed to exceed 0.80 (80%) for any variable. The authors concluded that several clinical variables were associated with the presence of visible debris captured by distal filter devices. The study, however, failed to identify any variables capable of consistently predicting the absence of visible debris. The authors suggested that their findings supported the routine rather than the selective use of cerebral protection during CAS.

Future predictions

The current data seem to be an argument for a randomised trial of protected versus unprotected CAS based on clinical outcomes. The argument that randomised clinical trials of new interventions are unethical, because the new treatment is better than the alternative treatment or no treatment, is based on presumption more than fact, and arguments to the contrary are compelling [1]. However, it is perhaps unlikely that anyone or any group of individuals will have the enthusiasm for such a sizeable trial. The threat of litigation must be appreciated and certainly, in the North American healthcare environment, FDA approval for dedicated carotid stents often mandate use of the manufacturers' protection device. Many industry-sponsored published registries that are easily accessible by patients on the internet emphasise that the CAS procedure was protected.

The available filters have limitations which may be addressed by further technical refinements and this may be the future of protected CAS. Alternatively, other mechanical devices such as 'membrane' stents may supersede currently available mechanical protection devices. These are stents covered with a fine porous mesh that allow perfusion via the ECA origin which is routinely covered during CAS but braces back atheromatous plaque. Supporting experimental work is available [20].

Finally, it remains possible that future advances in pharmacological support may render mechanical techniques of 'protection' obsolete.

Summary

◆ Filters are currently the protection device of choice, used in 90% of CAS treatment episodes.

◆ Substantial *in vivo* analyses demonstrate that filters trap macroemboli thought to have been liberated by endovascular manipulation of plaque.

◆ Filters may generate more microemboli than are demonstrated in unprotected CAS, as shown on procedural TCD and diffusion-weighted MRI of the brain; the clinical relevance of these microemboli is unknown.

◆ There is no level I evidence to support the use of filter-type protection devices.

◆ The available literature is hampered by comparisons against historical controls of unprotected CAS, with many confounding variables that may influence outcome.

◆ Vulnerable plaque may not routinely be reliably predicted.

◆ The pragmatic response would be to routinely employ filters, accepting both a certain learning curve for their safe utilisation and the trade-off in the capture of macroemboli in exchange for increased microemboli.

◆ Future developments may include further technical refinements to filters, to other existing philosophies in cerebral protection, alternative novel protective mechanical elements to include 'membrane' stents or further advances in pharmacological support.

References

1. Wilson CB. Adoption of new surgical technology. *Br Med J* 2006; 332: 112-4.

2. Theron J, Payelle GG, Coskun O, *et al*. Carotid artery stenosis: treatment with protected balloon angioplasty and stent placement. *Radiology* 1996; 201: 627-36.

3. Zahn, R, Mark B, Niedermaier N, *et al*. Embolic protection devices for carotid artery stenting: better results than stenting without protection? *Eur Heart J* 2004; 25: 1550-8.

4. Mas JL, Chatellier G, Beyssen B. EVA-3S Investigators. Carotid angioplasty and stenting with and without cerebral protection: clinical alert from the Endarterectomy Versus Angioplasty in Patients With Symptomatic Severe Carotid Stenosis (EVA-3S) trial. *Stroke* 2004; 35: e18-20.

5. Macdonald S, Venables GS, Cleveland TJ, *et al*. Protected carotid stenting: safety and efficacy of the MedNova neuroShield filter. *J Vasc Surg* 2002; 35(5): 966-72.

6. Al-Mubarak N, Roubin GS, Vitek J, Iyer SS, New G, Leon MB. Effect of the distal balloon protection system on microembolization during carotid stenting. *Circulation* 2001; 104: 1999-2002.

7. Macdonald S. Thesis for the Degree of Doctor of Philosophy: Neuroprotection and flow dynamics in carotid stenting, October 2004. University of Sheffield Main Library, Volumes I & II, 2004 [MO115661SH]. Main LibThesis, 12638.

8. Vos JA, van den Berg JC, Ernst SM, *et al*. Carotid angioplasty and stent placement: comparison of transcranial Doppler US data and clinical outcome with and without filtering cerebral protection devices in 509 patients. *Radiology* 2005; 237: 374-5.

9. Jaeger H, Mathias K, Drescher R, *et al*. Clinical results of cerebral protection with a filter device during stent implantation of the carotid artery. *CVIR* 2001; 24: 249-56.

10. Jaeger H, Mathias K, Elke H, *et al*. Cerebral ischaemia detected with diffusion-weighted MR imaging after stent implantation in the carotid artery. *Am J Neuroradiol* 2002; 23: 200-7.

11. van Heesewijk JMP, Vos JA, Louwerse ES, *et al*. New brain lesions at MR imaging after carotid angioplasty and stent placement. *Radiology* 2002; 224: 361-5.

12. Kastrup A, Groschel K, Krapf H, *et al*. Early outcome of carotid angioplasty and stenting with and without cerebral protection devices: a systematic review of the literature. *Stroke* 2003; 34: 813-9.

13. Cremonesi A, Manetti R, Setacci C, *et al.* Protected carotid stenting. Clinical advantages and complications of embolic protection devices in 442 consecutive patients. *Stroke* 2003; 34: 1936-43.

14. McKevitt F, Macdonald S, Venables G, *et al.* Complications following carotid angioplasty and carotid stenting in patients with symptomatic carotid artery disease. *Cerebrovasc Dis* 2004; 17: 28-34.

15. CAVATAS Investigators. Endovascular versus surgical treatment in patients with carotid stenosis in the Carotid and Vertebral Artery Transluminal Angioplasty Study (CAVATAS): a randomised trial. *Lancet* 2001; 357: 1729-37.

16. McKevitt F, Randall MS, Cleveland TJ, *et al.* The benefits of combined anti-platelet treatment in carotid artery stenting. *Eur J Vasc Endovasc Surg* 2005; 29: 522-7.

17. Theiss, W, Hermanek, P, Mathias, K, *et al,* for the German Societies of Angiology and Radiology. Pro-CAS; a prospective registry of carotid angioplasty and stenting. *Stroke* 2004; 35: 2134-9.

18. Biasi, GM, Froio, A, Diethrich, EB, *et al.* Carotid plaque echolucency increases the risk of stroke in carotid stenting. The Imaging in Carotid Angioplasty and Risk of Stroke (ICAROS) Study. *Circulation* 2004; 110: 756-62.

19. Sprouse LR 2nd, Peeters P, Bosiers MJ. The capture of visible debris by distal cerebral protection filters during carotid artery stenting: is it predictable? *J Vasc Surg* 2005; 41: 950-5.

20. Muller-Hulsbeck S, Husler EJ, Schaffner SR, *et al.* An *in vitro* analysis of a carotid artery stent with a protective membrane. *J Vasc Interv Radiol* 2004; 15: 1295-1305.

Chapter 15

Redo carotid intervention: the role of carotid artery stenting

A Ross Naylor MD FRCS, Professor of Vascular Surgery

Siew Chng MD, Clinical Surgical Fellow

Sherif Awad MB MRCS, Senior House Officer in Surgery

Leicester Royal Infirmary, Leicester, UK

Introduction

"Get your facts first, and then you can distort them as much as you please."

Mark Twain

Despite being one of the most scientifically scrutinised procedures in the history of medicine, carotid endarterectomy (CEA) retains a unique ability to court controversy, none more so than the management of recurrent stenosis. This subject continues to polarise opinions around the world, largely because of a complete lack of randomised trial data to guide practice.

For supporters of intervention, the rationale for treatment is very simple. A recurrent stenosis is associated with an increased risk of late ipsilateral stroke and intervention is, thereafter, justified by the findings of the randomised trials of symptomatic and asymptomatic patients and (more recently) the SAPPHIRE trial [1-3]. Thereafter, the only debate is whether treatment should be surgical or endovascular. Opponents of intervention cite the different pathology associated with recurrent stenosis (myointimal hyperplasia versus atherosclerosis), the low risk of stroke associated with asymptomatic restenosis and question whether the asymptomatic trials can, therefore, be used to justify intervention.

In order to try and formulate a rationale for planning management (based on the little available evidence), the problem will be analysed relative to:

- what is the prevalence of restenosis after CEA;
- do all patients with restenosis face the same risk of stroke; and
- what are the results of published series on intervention (CEA and carotid angioplasty/ stenting [CAS]).

What is the prevalence of restenosis?

Several overviews have been published, but most are now too historical, used (predominantly) retrospective data, involved a variety of imaging modalities (Doppler waveform analysis, angiography, duplex, ocular plethysmography) and were taken from an era when the concept of 'best medical therapy' was rudimentary to say the least. Notwithstanding these limitations, however, Frerick's meta-analysis was important because it demonstrated the temporal pattern of restenosis, which was highest (10%) in the first 12 months after surgery, thereafter falling to 3% in the second year and 2% in the third [4]. This suggests that for those units who do wish to intervene in patients with recurrent disease, it is probably neither clinically nor cost-effective to continue surveillance beyond 12 months.

Table 1. Prevalence of restenosis and ipsilateral stroke following carotid endarterectomy (data derived from prospective, randomised trials).

>50% author	Mean FU	Restenosis prevalence	Redo CEA	Restenosis untreated	Ipsilateral CVA +restenosis >50%	Ipsilateral CVA +restenosis <50%
Ranaboldo [14]	12m	24/186 (12.9%)	0	24	1/24 (4.2%) (*)	0/162 (0.0%)
Hansen [15]	12m	16/220 (8.9%)	0	16	1/16 (6.3%)	21/204 (10.3%)
AbuRahma [5]	12m	33/149 (22.1%)	3	30	2/30 (6.7%)	0/116 (0.0%)
CAVATAS [16]	12m	27/174 (15.5%)	n/a	n/a	n/a	n/a
AbuRahma [17]	26m	34/193 (17.6%)	0	34	1/34 (2.9%)	0/159 (0.0%)
Katz [18]	29m	2/100 (2.0%)	2	0	n/a	0/98 (0.0%)
Gonzalez-Fajardo [19]	29m	2/94 (2.1%)	1	1	0/1 (0.0%)	0/92 (0.0%)
Abu Rahma [20]	29m	35/145 (24.1%)	9	26	0/26 (0.0%)	0/110 (0.0%)
Abu Rahma [21]	30m	55/394 (14.0%)	13	42	0/42 (0.0%)	1/339 (0.3%)
Cao [22]	33m	56/1344 (4.2%)	18	38	1/38 (2.6%) (*)	11/1288 (1.0%)
Ballotta [23]	34m	2/332 (0.6%)	1	1	0/1 (0.0%)	1/330 (0.3%)
Naylor [6]	36m	16/272 (5.9%)	1(**)	15	1/16 (6.3%) (*)	6/256 (2.3%)
Grego [24]	48m	11/159 (6.9%)	1	10	0/10 (0.0%)	5/148 (3.4%)
>60%						
ACAS [25]	31m	105/607 (17.3%)	0	105	4/105 (3.8%)	16/502 (3.2%)
O'Hara [26]	34m	8/125 (6.4%)	0	8	0/8 (0.0%)	0/117 (0.0%)
Ballotta [23]	34m	2/3232 (0.6%)	1	1	0/1 (0.0%)	1/322 (0.3%)
Naylor [6]	36m	10/272 (3.7%)	1(**)	9	1/9 (11.1%) (*)	6/262 (2.3%)
>70%						
CAVATAS [16]	12m	9/174 (5.2%)	0	9	0/9 (0.0%)	5/165 (3.0%)
AbuRahma [27]	21m	6/200 (3.0%)	4	2	0/2 (0.0%)	0/194 (0.0%)
AbuRahma [17]	26m	16/193 (8.0%)	0	16	1/16 (6.3%)	0/177 (0.0%)
Cao [22]	33m	29/1344 (2.2%)	18	11	1/11 (9.1%) (*)	11/1315 (0.9%)
Ballotta [23]	34m	1/332 (0.3%)	1	0	n/a	1/330 (0.3%)
Naylor [6]	36m	8/272 (2.9%)	1 (**)	7	1/7 (14%) (*)	6/264 (2.3%)

(*) patient found to have occlusion at time of imaging after stroke had occurred

(**) suffered stroke after angioplasty

In order to evaluate contemporary practice, a new overview (for this chapter) was undertaken that was restricted to prospective, randomised trials involving CEA patients (all published ≥1993), where a decision was made at the outset to undertake serial surveillance in as many patients as possible.

The principal data are summarised in Table 1. The prevalence of restenosis after CEA is presented according to degree of restenosis (>50%, >60%, >70%) and length of follow-up. In the group comprising 'restenosis >50', it is immediately apparent that there is still a wide variation in findings. For example, AbuRahma observed a 22% prevalence of restenosis >50% in 149 patients at 12 months [5], while Naylor reported a 5.9% prevalence in 276 patients at three years [6]. Notwithstanding the potential for varying diagnostic criteria, 'restenosis >50%' on its own is pretty meaningless as few clinicians would advocate secondary intervention unless the degree of stenosis was more severe. Table 1, therefore, presents additional data on the prevalence of restenosis >70% (including occlusion). Six studies (all containing >100 patients and including two international trial databases) observed a restenosis rate >70% of ≤8% (most were <3%). Importantly, four had follow-up >24 months (i.e. well beyond the 'high-risk' period identified by Frerick). This suggests that the overall prevalence of clinically significant restenosis in contemporary CEA practice is relatively low. This should be borne in mind when determining whether a surveillance programme could ever prove cost-effective.

Do all patients have the same stroke risk?

Clearly the answer is no, but there is a tendency to 'lump' all patients together as if they were a homogenous group. First and foremost, the highest risk subgroup comprises patients who present with ipsilateral carotid territory symptoms. Few would dispute that these patients warrant secondary intervention.

Asymptomatic patients, however, continue to pose a management dilemma, although one (often forgotten) subgroup probably should be surveyed and treated. These are patients who underwent CEA under locoregional anaesthesia and who suffered a neurological deficit during test clamping of the internal carotid artery (ICA). Clearly, these patients will not tolerate carotid occlusion during follow-up. In Leicester, where CEA is still performed under general anaesthesia, a similar strategy (surveillance and secondary intervention) would be advocated for the small number of patients who had mean middle cerebral artery velocities ≤10cm/sec during ICA clamping.

Notwithstanding these two subgroups, the majority of restenoses will be asymptomatic. Table 1 details the prevalence of stroke ipsilateral to stenosed and non-stenosed arteries, having excluded patients who underwent a redo CEA or CAS. It is highly likely that all (or most) of these non-operated patients will be asymptomatic.

At first sight, there would appear to be an association between increasing stenosis severity and late ipsilateral stroke. However, the reader should take note of the data highlighted by an asterisk (*) in Table 1. These patients suffered an ipsilateral stroke, but were found to have an occluded ICA when imaged. None had any evidence of restenosis at their preceding surveillance scan. If these (occlusions) are excluded, there is no obvious association between restenosis (whatever the degree) and late stroke risk. This is particularly well demonstrated by the ACAS findings [1]. Here, 607 surgical patients underwent serial surveillance. Although the prevalence of restenosis >60% was 17% at 31 months, the incidence of late ipsilateral stroke was only 3.8% in patients with a restenosis >60%, as compared with 3.2% in patients with no significant restenosis. Unfortunately, it is difficult to evaluate parallel data for patients with ≥70% restenoses (i.e. the most clinically important). This is because the actual numbers of patients at risk were small and they were more likely to be offered redo CEA.

The available data (although not as statistically robust as one would wish) suggest that patients undergoing CEA in the current era of improved statin therapy and better antiplatelet agents face a low risk of stroke in the long term. Accordingly, indiscriminate treatment of asymptomatic restenoses cannot simply be justified on the available evidence.

Table 2. Outcomes for surgical intervention for recurrent stenosis after CEA (ranked by morbidity and mortality).

Study	n=	30d m&m	% asymp	Rec sten/mths FU	CNI
Hill [28]	40	0.0%	50%	-	7.2%
Hobson [29]	16	0.0%	44%	12.5% at 30m (>50%)	6.2%
Dillavou [30]	27	0.0%	48%	21% at 54m (>50%)	0.0%
Harris [31]	24	0.0%	50%	8% at 84m (>50%)	4.2%
Stoner [32]	153	1.9%	64%	9.2% at 52m (>50%)	1.3%
Archie [33]	69	2.9%	52%	13% at 50m (>50%)	4.3%
AbuRahma [34]	41	2.4%	29%	0% at 60m (>50%)	12%
Ballinger [35]	74	2.8%	35%	7.3% at 48m (>50%)	2.7%
Cho [36]	64	3.1%	52%	8% at 27m (>50%)	9.4%
AbuRahma [37]	58	3.4%	21%	0.0% at 42m (>50%)	17.2%
Rockman [38]	82	3.7%	59%	11% at 35m (>50%)	1.2%
Bowser [39]	27	3.7%	37%	25% at 39m (>50%)	3.7%
Coyle [40]	69	4.3%	46%	-	0.0%
O'Hara [41]	206	4.5%	57%	11% at 60m (>80%)	1.0%
Mehta [42]	59	4.5%	69%	4.5% at 48m (>50%)	4.5%
AbuRahma [43]	124	4.3%	22%	9% at 60m (>50%)	17%
Mansour [44]	82	4.8%	34%	8% at 60m (>80%)	7.3%
Maxwell [45]	63	4.8%	30%	-	
Abou-Zamzam [46]	56	5.4%	27%	5.4% at 29m (>80%)	1.8%
Rockman [47]	89	5.6%	56%	6.3% at 35m (>50%)	7.9%
Kresowik [11]	401	5.7%	not available	-	-
Kresowik [10]	380	6.3%	not available	-	-
AbuRahma [48]	46	7.0%	28%	2% at 31m (>80%)	-

30d m+m = 30-day death/stroke risk; Rec sten/mths FU = prevalence of recurrent stenosis at X months follow-up; CNI = cranial nerve injury

Some clinicians will still prefer to justify intervention on the basis of either the ACAS/ACST findings or the conclusions from SAPPHIRE [1-3]. However, clinicians who do advocate this evidence base to justify practice should take note of important data from these trials. Firstly, women did not gain significant benefit from CEA in the asymptomatic trials and, therefore, it would be inappropriate to intervene on every asymptomatic female with a recurrent stenosis. Although the ACST paper in the *Lancet* reported

benefit in asymptomatic females, the data only included successful CEA patients beyond the first 30 days [2]. When the operative risk was included (and the ACAS data combined with ACST), women did not appear to derive benefit from CEA [7, 8]. The exception, however, might be the younger female (perhaps <65 years). This is because emerging evidence [9] suggests that there may be some benefit in the younger female (probably after eight years of follow-up). Finally, ACST showed no benefit for CEA in patients aged >75

Table 3. Outcomes for carotid angioplasty for recurrent stenosis after CEA (ranked by morbidity and mortality).

Study	n=	30d m&m	% asymp	Rec sten/mths FU
Miotto [49]	20	0.0%	-	15% at 37m (>50%)
Alric [50]	17	0.0%	76%	0.0% at 17m (>50%)
Koebbe [51]	23	0.0%	-	4.5% at 36m (>50%)
Hobson [29]	19	0.0%	53%	0.0% at 11m (>50%)
Lanzino [52]	25	0.0%	-	16% at 27m (>50%)
Leger [53]	8	0.0%	75%	75% at 12m (>50%)
McDonnell [54]	30	0.0%	80%	10% at 20m (>90%)
Cohen [55]	10	0.0%	-	-
Hobson [56]	54	1.9%	65%	0.0% (>50%)
New [13]	342	3.7%	61%	6% at 14m (>50%)
Yadav [57]	25	4.0%	23%	0% at 8m (>50%)
Vitek [58]	110	4.0%	40%	no data
AbuRahma [34]	22	4.5%	23%	48% at 60m (>50%)
Bowser [39]	52	5.7%	40%	43% at 26m (>50%)
Rockman [47]	16	6.3%	69%	14% at 14m (>50%)
Bergeron [59]	15	13%	7%	0.0% at 37m (>50%)
AbuRahma [37]	25	16%	28%	56% at 42m (>50%)

30d m+m = 30-day death/stroke risk; Rec sten/mths FU = prevalence of recurrent stenosis at X months follow-up

years. Accordingly, patients of this age group with asymptomatic restenoses should probably be reassured and thereafter treated with best medical therapy.

What are the results of secondary intervention?

If having decided that the patient does require some form of secondary intervention, what evidence is there to guide whether this should be surgical or endovascular? Unfortunately, there are no randomised trials to guide decision-making. Traditionally, redo CEA/bypass has been the gold standard, but CAS has emerged as an important alternative. As noted earlier, older meta-analyses were limited by their historical nature and it would, therefore, be inappropriate to compare these older series with more recent CAS studies. To enable more meaningful interpretation of the data, a second systematic review was undertaken from 36 studies published between 1994-2005 which detailed outcomes following redo CEA (Table 2) and CAS (Table 3).

Surgical results

As with all retrospective data, the reader should not overinterpret the findings. For example, the prevalence of cranial nerve injury will always be under-reported in retrospective studies and outcomes must take into account the cohort of patients under study. For example, the data from Table 2 suggest that the lowest 30-day rates of death/stroke following redo surgery were generally seen in series with the highest proportion of asymptomatic patients.

Not surprisingly, the results in Table 2 are very heterogeneous. Four series (107 patients) encountered no deaths/strokes in the peri-operative period, while eight (444 patients) reported an operative risk <3%. To put this into context, the latter results are superior to the 4.3% death/stroke rate observed in eight studies on primary CEA for asymptomatic, atherosclerotic disease (published between 1990-2000) where assessment was done by a neurologist [7]. Accordingly, exceptional as these results are, they will inevitably be prone to bias (retrospective, indeterminate number of patients lost to follow-up, less likely to publish bad results). The two most important studies in Table 2, however, are the two sequential, multistate audits by Kresowik [10,11]. These involved large reviews of outcome in ten States in North America over a one-year period. The first (published in 2001) included 380 redo CEAs with a 30-day death/stroke rate of 6.3% [10]. Three years later, a second one-year audit of 401 redo CEAs observed a slight fall in risk to 5.7% [11]. Inevitably, these data are more likely to reflect true practice in the 'real world'.

However, if Kresowik's audit data are a truer reflection of the actual risk, what evidence is there that at this level of risk, redo CEA confers clinical benefit? In this respect, simple extrapolation of these data into the ACAS findings (where there was a 2.3% operative risk) means that with a 6% procedural risk, you will only be preventing 22 strokes at five years by treating 1000 patients. This is hardly supportive of re-intervention to 'all comers'. As will be seen, a similar observation will also become apparent for advocates of CAS for restenosis.

Table 2 summarises other important complications of redo CEA. First, a significant proportion will develop a recurrent restenosis during follow-up. It is not possible to evaluate these data statistically as the studies were too heterogeneous in terms of reporting standards. Interestingly, however, the desire to intervene on a recurrent restenosis did not appear to be as great the second time round! Moreover, where these data were documented, few (if any) of the

recurrent restenoses treated conservatively suffered a late stroke. Finally, notwithstanding the likelihood of missing data, Table 2 does suggest that redo CEA is associated with a higher risk of cranial nerve injury than after primary CEA. Although this is often ignored in the discussion of risk, some of these injuries can be as disabling as a stroke.

Endovascular results

Table 3 presents parallel data from 17 studies on the role of CAS for treating restenosis. As with redo CEA, the reader is advised to exercise caution when interpreting the findings. Eight series (152 patients) reported zero strokes/deaths after CAS, while nine (206 patients) documented a 30-day death/stroke rate of <2%. This is considerably less than the 2.95% risk reported in 4581 asymptomatic patients undergoing CAS for primary atherosclerotic disease in the International Stent Registry [12]. The largest study on CAS for restenosis (342 patients) was a multicentre registry of outcomes (30-day death/stroke = 3.7%), where it was noted by the authors that their good results probably reflected the fact that CAS had been performed in tertiary centres of excellence [13]. No national or multistate audits of CAS for recurrent stenoses have been reported.

In summary, the published procedural risks following CAS for restenosis are broadly similar to those following redo CEA (note again that the best results following CAS were generally seen in studies with the highest proportion of asymptomatic patients). Moreover, note the trend for higher rates of secondary restenosis after CAS. No CAS patient has suffered a cranial nerve injury, although many will have suffered groin and other access complications not seen in CEA patients. These were not, however, systematically reported in these 17 CAS series.

Further evidence for justifying the use of CAS in recurrent stenosis might be used (by some) from the recently published SAPPHIRE trial [3]. Here 'non-inferiority to CEA' regarding CAS in 'high-risk' patients was demonstrated. However, readers of the paper will have observed that 78% of the SAPPHIRE patients were asymptomatic in whom restenoses after CEA were a major subgroup. In these asymptomatic patients, both CAS and CEA were associated with an approximate 6% 30-day rate of death/stroke. As was observed in the section on redo CEA, at this level of risk, there is little evidence of clinical benefit long term.

Conclusions

In our opinion, the true role of stenting for the treatment of recurrent carotid stenosis will not be determined unless randomised trials are performed. This is, unfortunately, highly unlikely. The available evidence suggests that the risk of severe restenosis in the current era of 'best medical therapy' is low. Redo intervention is, however, entirely justified in symptomatic patients and those with intolerance of ICA clamping at the time of the original procedure. In

Leicester, we do not currently recommend re-intervention in the remaining patients with asymptomatic, recurrent stenoses. For those of you who feel that the international trials justify a more liberal approach than ours, the available evidence suggests that re-intervention should probably be restricted to asymptomatic male patients <75 years and asymptomatic females <65 years.

The choice of re-intervention (CEA or CAS) is inevitably based on individual clinical/imaging criteria and the experience of each unit. Our current preference is for redo surgery in patients who are highly symptomatic, who are young (<60 years) or who have evidence of intraluminal thrombus. For the remainder (especially those who are asymptomatic or have a contralateral cranial nerve injury or previous neck irradiation), CAS is the preferred option.

Summary

◆ The prevalence of clinically significant restenosis (>70%) after CEA is low.

◆ Restenosis after CEA is rarely symptomatic.

◆ There is no compelling evidence that significant restenosis increases late stroke risk.

◆ Redo CEA/CAS is clearly justified in symptomatic patients.

◆ Surveillance and redo CEA/CAS is appropriate in patients developing a neurological deficit when CEA is performed under locoregional anaesthesia.

◆ Routine redo CEA/CAS cannot be justified in all patients with an asymptomatic recurrent stenosis.

References

1. Executive Committee for the Asymptomatic Carotid Atherosclerosis Study. Endarterectomy for asymptomatic carotid artery stenosis. *JAMA* 1995; 273: 1421-8.

2. Asymptomatic Carotid Surgery Trial Collaborators. The MRC Asymptomatic Carotid Surgery Trial (ACST): carotid endarterectomy prevents disabling and fatal carotid territory strokes. *Lancet* 2006: in press.

3. Yadav JS, Wholey MH, Kuntz RE, *et al.* Protected carotid artery stenting versus endarterectomy in high-risk patients. *New Engl J Med* 2004; 351: 1493-1501.

4. Frerick H, Kievit J, van Baalen JM, van Bockel JH. Carotid recurrent stenosis and risk of ipsilateral stroke: a systematic review of the literature. *Stroke* 1998; 29: 244-50.

5. AbuRahma AF, Robinson PA, Hannay RS, Hudson J, Cutlip L. Prospective controlled study of carotid endarterectomy with Hemashield patch: is it thrombogenic? *Vascular Surgery* 2001; 35: 167-74.

6. Naylor AR, Hayes PD, Payne DA, Allroggen H, Steele S, Thompson MM, London NJM, Bell PRF. A randomised trial of vein versus Dacron patching during carotid endarterectomy: (ii) long-term results. *J Vasc Surg* 2004; 39: 985-93.

7. Rothwell PM, Goldstein LB. Carotid endarterectomy for asymptomatic carotid stenosis: Asymptomatic Carotid Surgery Trial. *Stroke* 2004; 35: 2425-7.

8. Rothwell PM. ACST: which subgroups will benefit most from carotid endarterectomy? *Lancet* 2004; 364: 1122-3.

9. ACST Writing Committee. ACST: which subgroups will benefit most from carotid endarterectomy? *Lancet* 2004; 364: 1125-6.

10. Kresowik TF, Bratzler DW, Karp HR, *et al.* Multistate utilization, processes, and outcomes of carotid endarterectomy. *J Vasc Surg* 2001; 33(2): 227-34; discussion 234-5.

11. Kresowik TF, Bratzler DW, Kresowik RA, *et al.* Multistate improvement in process and outcomes of carotid endarterectomy. *J Vasc Surg* 2004; 39(2): 372-80.

12. Wholey MH, Al-Mubarek N, Wholey MH. Updated review of the global carotid artery stent registry. *Cath Cardiovasc Intervent* 2003; 60: 259-66.

13. New G, Roubin GS, Iyer SS. Safety, efficacy, and durability of carotid artery stenting for restenosis following carotid endarterectomy: a multicenter study. *J Endovasc Ther* 2000; 7(5): 345-52.

14. Ranaboldo CJ, Barros DS'a AAB, Bell PRF, Chant ADB, Perry PM. Randomised controlled trial of patch angioplasty for carotid endarterectomy *Br J Surg* 1993; 80: 1528-30.

15. Hansen F, Lindblad B, Perrson NH, Bergqvist D. Can recurrent stenosis after carotid endarterectomy be prevented by low-dose acetylsalicylic acid: a double-blind randomised and placebo controlled study. *Eur J Vasc Surg* 1993; 7: 380-5.

16. McCabe DJH, Pereira A, Clifton A, *et al.* Restenosis after carotid angioplasty, stenting or endarterectomy in the Carotid and Vertebral Artery Transluminal Angioplasty Study (CAVATAS). *Stroke* 2005; 36: 281-6.

17. AbuRahma AF, Hopkins ES, Robinson PA, Deel JT, Agarwal S. Prosepctive randomised trial of carotid endarterectomy with PTFE versus collagen impregnated Dacron (Hemashield) patching: late follow-up. *Ann Surg* 2002: 237: 885-93.

18. Katz D, Snyder SO, Gandhi RH. Long-term follow-up for recurrent stenosis: a prospective randomised study of expanded PTFE patch angioplasty versus primary closure after carotid endarterectomy. *J Vasc Surg* 1994; 19: 198-205.

19. Gonzalez-Fajardo JA, Perez JL, Mateo AM. Saphenous vein patch versus PTFE patch after carotid endarterectomy. *J Cardiovasc Surg* 1994; 35: 523-8.

20. AbuRahma AF, Robinson PA, Saiedy S, Richmond BK, Khan J. Prospective randomised trial of bilateral carotid endarterectomies: primary closure versus patching. *Stroke* 1999; 30: 1185-9.

21. AbuRahma AF, Robinson PA, Saiedy S, Khan J, Boland JP. Prospective randomised trial of carotid endarterectomy with primary closure and patch angioplasty with saphenous vein, jugular vein and PTFE: long-term follow-up. *J Vasc Surg* 1998; 27: 222-34.

22. Cao P, Giordano G, DeRango P, *et al.* Eversion versus conventional carotid endarterectomy: late results of a prospective multicentre randomised trial. *J Vasc Surg* 2000; 31: 19-30.

23. Ballotta E, DaGiau G, Saladini M, *et al.* Carotid endarterectomy with patch closure versus carotid eversion endarterectomy and reimplantation: a prospective randomized study. *Surgery* 1999; 125(3): 271-9.

24. Grego F, Antonello M, Lepidi S, Bonvini S, Deriu GP. Prospective randomised study of external jugular vein patch versus PTFE during carotid endarterectomy: peri-operative and long-term results. *J Vasc Surg* 2003; 38: 1232-40.

25. Moore WS, Kempezinski RF, Nelson JJ, Toole JF. Recurrent carotid stenosis: results of the Asymptomatic Carotid Atherosclerosis Study. *Stroke* 1998; 29: 2018-25.

26. O'Hara PJ, Hertzer NR, Masch EJ, *et al.* A prospective randomised study of saphenous vein patching versus synthetic patching during carotid endarterectomy. *J Vasc Surg* 2002; 35: 324-32.

27. AbuRahma AF, Stone PA, Welch CA, *et al.* Prospective study of carotid endarterectomy with modified polytetrafluoroethylene (ACUSEAL) patching: early and late results. *J Vasc Surg* 2005; 41(5): 789-93.

28. Hill BB, Olcott C, Dalman RL, Harris EJ, Zarins CK. Reoperation for carotid stenosis is as safe as primary carotid endarterectomy. *J Vasc Surg* 1999; 30(1): 26-35.

29. Hobson RW, Goldstein JE, Jamil Z, *et al.* Carotid restenosis: operative and endovascular management. *J Vasc Surg* 1999; 29(2): 228-35.

30. Dillavou ED, Kahn MB, Carabasi RA, Smullens SN, DiMuzio PJ. Long-term follow-up of reoperative carotid surgery. *Am J Surg* 1999; 178(3): 197-200.

31. Harris RA, Stow N, Fisher CM, Neale ML, Appleberg M. Carotid redo surgery: both safe and durable. *ANZ J Surg* 2003; 73(12): 1000-3.

32. Stoner MC, Cambria RP, Brewster DC, *et al.* Safety and efficacy of reoperative carotid endarterectomy: a 14-year experience. *J Vasc Surg* 2005; 41(6): 942-9.

33. Archie JP. Restenosis after carotid endarterectomy in patients with paired vein and Dacron patch reconstruction. *Vasc Surg* 2001; 35(6): 419-27.

34. AbuRahma AF, Bates MC, Wulu JT, Stone PA. Early postsurgical carotid restenosis: redo surgery versus angioplasty/stenting. *J Endovasc Ther* 2002; 9(5): 566-72.

35. Ballinger BA, Money SR, Chatman DM, Bowen JK, Ochsner JL. Sites of recurrence and long-term results of redo surgery. *Ann Surg* 1997; 225(5): 512-5.

36. Cho JS, Pandurangi K, Conrad MF, Shepard AS, Carr JA, Nypaver TJ, Reddy DJ. Safety and durability of redo carotid operation: an 11-year experience. *J Vasc Surg* 2004: 39: 155-61.

37. AbuRahma AF, Bates MC, Stone PA, Wulu JT. Comparative study of operative treatment and percutaneous transluminal angioplasty/stenting for recurrent carotid disease. *J Vasc Surg* 2001; 34(5): 831-8.

38. Rockman CB, Riles TS, Landis D. Redo carotid surgery: an analysis of materials and configurations used in carotid reoperations and their influence on perioperative stroke and subsequent recurrent stenosis. *J Vasc Surg* 1999; 29(1): 72-80.

39. Bowser AN., Bandyk DF, Evans A. Outcome of carotid stent-assised angioplasty versus open surgical repair of recurrent carotid stenosis. *J Vasc Surg* 2003; 38(3): 432-8.

40. Coyle KA, Smith RB, Gray BG, *et al.* Treatment of recurrent cerebrovascular disease. Review of a 10-year experience. *Ann Surg* 1995; 221(5): 517-21.

41. O'Hara PJ, Hertzer NR, Karafa MT, *et al.* Reoperation for recurrent carotid stenosis: early results and late outcome in 199 patients. *J Vasc Surg* 2001; 34(1): 5-12.

42. Mehta M, Roddy SP, Darling RC, *et al.* Safety and efficacy of eversion carotid endarterectomy for the treatment of recurrent stenosis: 20-year experience. *Ann Vasc Surg* 2005; 19(4): 492-8.

43. AbuRahma AF, Jennings TG, Wulu JT, Tarakji L, Robinson PA. Redo carotid endarterectomy versus primary carotid endarterectomy. *Stroke* 2001; 32: 2787-92.

44. Mansour MA, Kang SS, Baker WH. Carotid endarterectomy for recurrent stenosis. *J Vasc Surg* 1997; 25(5): 877-83.

45. Maxwell JG, Maxwell BG, Brinker CC, Covington DL, Weatherford D. Carotid endarterectomy reoperations in a regional medical center. *Am Surg* 2000; 66(8): 773-80.

46. Abou-Zamzam AM, Moneta GL, Landry GJ. Carotid surgery following previous carotid endarterectomy is safe and effective. *Vasc Endovasc Surg* 2002; 36(4): 263-70.

47. Rockman CB, Bajakian D, Jacobowitz GR, *et al.* Impact of carotid artery angioplasty and stenting on management of recurrent carotid artery stenosis. *Ann Vasc Surg* 2004; 18(2): 151-7.

48. AbuRahma AF, Snodgrass KR, Robinson PA. Safety and durability of redo carotid endarterectomy for recurrent carotid artery stenosis. *Am J Surg* 1994: 168(2): 175-8.

49. Miotto D, Picchi G, Rettore C. Endovascular treatment for recurrent carotid stenosis. *Radiol Med* 2001; 101(5): 355-9.

50. Alric P, Branchereau P, Berthet JP, Mary H, Marty-Ane C. Carotid artery stenting for stenosis following revascularization or cervical irradiation. *J Endovasc Ther* 2002; 9(1): 14-9.

51. Koebbe CJ, Liebman K, Veznedaroglu E, Rosenwasser R. The role of carotid angioplasty and stenting in carotid revascularization. *Neurol Res* 2005; 27 Suppl 1: S53-8.

52. Lanzino G, Mericle RA, Lopes DK. Percutaneous transluminal angioplasty and stent placement for recurrent carotid artery stenosis. *J Neurosurg* 1999; 90(4): 688-94.

53. Leger AR, Neale M, Harris JP. Poor durability of carotid angioplasty and stenting for treatment of recurrent artery stenosis after carotid endarterectomy: an institutional experience. *J Vasc Surg* 2001; 33(5): 1008-14.

54. McDonnell CO, Legge D, Twomey E, *et al.* Carotid artery angioplasty for restenosis following endarterectomy. *Eur J Vasc Endovasc Surg* 2004; 27(2): 163-6.

55. Cohen JE, Gomori JM, Ratz G, Ben Hur T, Umansky F. Protected stent-assisted carotid angioplasty in the management of late post-endarterectomy restenosis. *Neurol Res* 2005; 27 Suppl 1: S64-8.

56. Hobson RW, Lal BK, Chakhtoura EY, *et al.* Carotid artery closure for endarterectomy does not influence results of angioplasty-stenting for restenosis. *J Vasc Surg* 2002; 35(3): 435-8.

57. Yadav JS, Roubin GS, King P, Iyer S, Vitek J. Angioplasty and stenting for restenosis after carotid endarterectomy. Initial experience. *Stroke* 1996; 27(11): 2075-9.

58. Vitek JJ, Roubin GS, New G, Al-Mubarek N, Iyer SS. Carotid angioplasty with stenting in post-carotid endarterectomy restenosis. *J Invasive Cardiol* 2001; 13(2): 123-5.

59. Bergeron P, Chambran P, Benichou H, Alessandri C. Recurrent carotid disease: will stents be an alternative to surgery? *J Endovasc Surg* 1996; 3(1): 76-9.

Chapter 16

Asymptomatic carotid stenoses: evidence for treatment and recommendations

Peter Gaines FRCP FRCR, Consultant Vascular Radiologist

Sheffield Vascular Institute, The Northern General Hospital, Sheffield, UK

Introduction

Arterial disease is the most common chronic disease affecting the developed world [1, 2], resulting in carotid atherosclerosis being present in 0.5% of the population in their 50s increasing to 10% in the over 80s [3]. Although carotid disease is responsible for 20-30% of the patients suffering from a stroke [4, 5], unfortunately only approximately 17% of patients have any symptoms prior to the first cerebral catastrophe [6]. The outcome for stroke is not only poor for the patient, but also for society as a whole; it is the second leading cause of death worldwide and survivors carry a high residual deficit with half being left dependant upon others for everyday activities [1, 7].

In summary, carotid atherosclerosis is a common but insidious manifestation of a systemic disorder with potentially disastrous outcome for the patient and society. It would seem reasonable that any patient with known asymptomatic carotid disease should have good primary prevention. For any intervention over and above best medical therapy to be justified, the risk of that intervention needs to be balanced against the expected outcome for a patient with an asymptomatic carotid stenosis.

Natural history

It is not the intention or remit to detail best medical therapy for aymptomatic carotid disease. The estimated risk of stroke in the presence of an asymptomatic carotid stenosis is approximately 2-3% per year [3, 8, 9]. This, however, needs some qualification. These data are in patients not taking the current standard of best medical therapy (BMT). Indeed, the current data available from the UK would strongly indicate that at a community level, BMT is having a major effect on the incidence of stroke. Rather than the expected rise the incidence of stroke as a function of obesity, diabetes etc, Rothwell and colleagues have demonstrated that there has been a 40% fall in the age-specific incidence of stroke over the last 40 years [10].

Carotid endarterectomy (CEA)

There have now been four randomised trials of carotid endarterectomy for patients with asymptomatic carotid disease of which two are recent and sizeable.

The Asymptomatic Carotid Atherosclerosis Study (ACAS) [8] randomised 1662 patients with an asymptomatic angiographic 60% carotid stenosis to carotid endarterectomy or best medical therapy. The study was stopped prematurely because it showed a projected significant benefit at five years in favour of CEA. The combined risk of ipsilateral stroke and perioperative stroke and death was reduced from 11.0% to 5.1% at five years, a relative risk reduction of 53%, and absolute reduction of 5.9%. It did not show reduction in major stroke or any benefit for women.

The MRC Asymptomatic Carotid Surgery Trial (ACST) [11] randomised 3120 patients with ultrasound-confirmed 60% asymptomatic stenosis and demonstrated remarkably similar results. On this occasion there was a significant reduction in any stroke and peri-operative death at five years from 11.8% to 6.4% (RRR 46%, ARR 5.4%). There was a demonstrable reduction in fatal or disabling stroke but once again the benefit occurred in men rather than women.

What are the problems with these data?

- Best medical therapy was not identified and defined at the start of the trials and was not as we know it today. Not only may the risk of stroke be reduced by contemporary BMT, but it should be noted that the risk of death after CEA is more likely by a factor of ten to be non-stroke related. The majority of these are other cardiovascular deaths and are highly likely to be reduced by statins, ACE inhibitors etc.
- The absolute risk reduction is small: 50 patients needed to be operated upon to prevent one stroke at three years [12, 13]. That is to say that 49 patients will undergo non-beneficial surgery with all its attendant risk to benefit that one patient by three years. If all asymptomatic stenoses >60% in a community were to be treated by CEA this would result in only a 4% reduction in the expected number of initial strokes [3].
- There appears to be no definite benefit for women [14].
- Benefit is dependent upon a risk of peri-operative stroke and death being less than 3%. Even in the major trials this was not always possible [15] and within the community, away from major high volume centres, these figures are unlikely to be achieved [16-18].

- It has been argued that benefit would be most apparent for those patients with an 80% stenosis because they are at higher risk [19-21]. That risk is difficult to quantify and be certain about. At least one study demonstrated that with high-grade disease (>80%), any increase in stroke was on the contralateral side [22], and another demonstrated that half the events in patients with 60-99% disease are not due to the carotid disease itself but are either cardiogenic or lacunar [23]. Any therapy directed at the carotid disease will therefore have no effect on 50% of the ipsilateral disease and no effect on the contralateral strokes. ACAS and ACST did not stratify their outcomes by the degree of stenosis and indeed, contrary to the symptomatic surgical trials, failed to show any incremental benefit according to the degree of stenosis. In addition, it is likely that those patients with a high-grade stenosis will be older with an increased burden of atherosclerosis. Such features will increase the risk of CEA and the likely benefit is not guaranteed.

Carotid stenting

There are ample data to indicate that carotid artery stenting (CAS) is an effective alternative to CEA for the management of symptomatic disease, and indeed, national stroke guidelines recognise CAS as a suitable form of therapy for high-grade carotid disease [24]. The majority of stenting, however, is performed for asymptomatic disease. In the global carotid registry [25] asymptomatic patients accounted for 47% of those reported, but a simple review of the published literature indicates that in some centres patients with asymptomatic carotid disease accounted for 74% of treatments. Similarly in the SAPPHIRE Trial [26], 70.1% of patients in the randomised group were asymptomatic. What then is the quality of the data to support this treatment?

There is only one randomised trial of CAS versus CEA for asymptomatic carotid disease [27]. This was published on-line, contained only 85 patients and concluded that stenting was equally as efficacious as endarterectomy. The only other trial has been

SAPPHIRE [26] that randomised 334 surgically high-risk patients (70.1% of patients were asymptomatic) between CEA and CAS. Of the asymptomatic patients, 5.4% who received a stent suffered post-procedural death, stroke or MI. This is nearly twice the recommended maximum major adverse event rate recommended by the AHA [6]. In those published articles where asymptomatic patients have been reported separately from symptomatic patients the serious adverse event rate lies anywhere between 0-11.1% [28-51]. Long-term outcomes are sparse. The one-year follow-up data reported in SAPPHIRE [27] showed a 9.9% rate of adverse event at one year following CAS in asymptomatic patients compared to 21.5% following CEA. This high surgical event rate is to be expected since patients were only included in the study if they were at high surgical risk. Initial inspection of the one-year stent outcomes would suggest that they are 2-3 times worse than the expected event rate if nothing had been done to the asymptomatic stenosis. Some latitude should be given since it is possible that the outcomes for this surgically high-risk subgroup of patients is worse than the general outcomes detailed in natural history studies. Away from SAPPHIRE, there are no long-term outcomes published, and because these data are largely from single institutional observational studies it is impossible to know if CAS is better than doing nothing more than offering BMT.

The way forward

Clinicians are dearly in need of good data to indicate whether, in patients with asymptomatic carotid disease, it is reasonable to offer CEA in the face of modern BMT, and whether to offer CAS at all. There are now two randomised trials on the verge of recruitment that will go a long way towards answering these doubts.

The Asymptomatic Carotid Surgical and Stenting Trial (ACST-II) will compare the outcomes in patients who are randomised between CEA and CAS. There is no medical arm.

TACIT (the Trans-Atlantic Carotid Intervention Trial) is a European/North American collaboration which will randomise 2400 patients between BMT and intervention. Intervention will be randomised between CEA and CAS. Best medical therapy will be prescribed for all patients and sub-studies aim to investigate the role of plaque characterisation, change in cognitive function, etc.

Even should the major trials indicate CEA or CAS confers benefit to patients over and above best medical therapy, the number needed to treat (NNT) will remain high. It is, therefore, of major importance that research identifies sub-groups of patients who are at high risk of stroke from a carotid lesion that previously was asymptomatic.

Summary

♦ Asymptomatic carotid atherosclerosis is a common and potentially devastating disease.

♦ Carotid endarterectomy is an effective treatment when offered to males with a relatively good life expectancy by technically good surgeons with a surgical complication rate of less than 3%, but remains a labour intensive and costly form of treatment.

♦ Little good evidence supports the use of stents to manage asymptomatic carotid disease in most patients.

♦ Neither endarterectomy nor stents have been tested against current concepts of best medical therapy.

♦ Research is required to identify sub-groups of patients most likely to gain major benefit from either CEA or CAS.

♦ Clinicians are encouraged to enrol patients in the proposed trials.

References

1. Murray CJL, Lopez AD. Mortality by cause for eight regions of the world: global burden of disease study. *Lancet* 1997; 349: 1269-76.

2. Fuster V. Epidemic of cardiovascular disease and stroke: the three main challenges. *Circulation* 1999; 99: 1132-37.

3. Warlow C. Endarterectomy for asymptomatic carotid stenosis? *Lancet* 1995; 345: 1254-5.

4. Zhu CZ, Norris JW. Role of carotid stenosis in ischemic stroke. *Stroke* 1990; 21: 1131-4.

5. Timsit S, Sacco R, Mohr J, et al. Early clinical differentiation of cerebral infarction from severe atherosclerotic stenosis and cardioembolism. *Stroke* 1992; 23: 486-91.

6. Moore W, Barnett H, Beebe H, Bernstein E, Brener B, Brott T, et al. Guidelines for carotid endarterectomy. A multidisciplinary consensus statement from the ad hoc Committee, American Heart Association. *Stroke* 1995; 26: 188-201.

7. Wolfe CDA. The impact of stroke. *Br Med Bull* 2000; 56: 275-86.

8. Executive Committee for the Asymptomatic Carotid Atherosclerosis Study. Endarterectomy for Asymptomatic Carotid Artery Stenosis. *JAMA* 1995; 273(18): 1421-8.

9. Toole JF, Chambless LE, Heiss G, et al. Prevalence of stroke and transient ischemic attacks in the Atherosclerosis Risk in Communities (ARIC) study. *Ann Epidemiol* 1993; 3: 500-3.

10. Rothwell PM, Coull AJ, Giles MF, Howard SC, Silver LE, Bull LM, et al. Change in stroke incidence, mortality, case-fatality, severity, and risk factors in Oxfordshire, UK from 1981 to 2004 (Oxford Vascular Study). *Lancet* 2004; 363: 1925-33.

11. Halliday A, Mansfield A, Marro J, Peto C, Peto R, Potter J, et al. Prevention of disabling and fatal strokes by successful carotid endarterectomy in patients without recent neurological symptoms: randomised controlled trial. *Lancet* 2004; 363(9420): 1491-502.

12. Warlow C. Carotid endarterectomy for asymptomatic carotid stenosis. *Br Med J* 1998; 317: 1468.

13. Benavente O, Moher D, Pham B. Carotid endarterectomy for asymptomatic carotid stenosis: a meta-analysis. *Br Med J* 1998; 317: 1477-80.

14. Rothwell PM. ACST: which subgroups will benefit most from carotid endarterectomy? *Lancet* 2004; 364: 1122-3.

15. Hobson RIW, DG, Fields WS, Goldstone J, Moore WS, Towne JB, Wright CB and the Veterans Affairs Cooperative Study Group. Efficacy of carotid endarterectomy for asymptomatic carotid stenosis. *N Engl J Med* 1993; 328: 221-7.

16. Stukenborg GJ. Comparison of carotid endarterectomy outcomes from randomized controlled trials and Medicare administrative databases. *Arch Neurol* 1997; 54: 826-32.

17. Wong JF, JM, Suarez-Almazor ME. Regional performance of carotid endarterectomy. *Stroke* 1997; 28: 891-8.

18. Hsai DC, Moscoe LM, Krushat WM. Epidemiology of carotid endarterectomy among Medicare beneficiaries: 1985-1996 update. *Stroke* 1998; 29(2): 346-50.

19. Roederer GO, Langlois YE, Jager KA, Primozich JF, Beach KW, Phillips DJ, et al. The natural history of carotid arterial disease in asymptomatic patients with cervical bruits. *Stroke* 1984; 15(4): 605-13.

20. Chambers BR, Norris JW. Outcome in patients with asymptomatic neck bruits. *N Engl J Med* 1986; 315: 860-5.

21. Norris JW, Zhu CZ. Stroke risk and critical carotid stenosis. *J Neurol Neurosurg Psychiatry* 1990; 53: 235-7.

22. BockRG-W, AC, Mock PA, Robinson DA, irwig L, Lusby RJ. The natural history of asymptomatic carotid artery disease. *J Vasc Surg* 1993; 17(1): 160-71.

23. Inzitari D, Eliasziw M, Gates P, Sharpe BL, Chan RKY, Meldrum HE, et al. The causes of stroke in patients with asymptomatic internal carotid artery stenosis. *N Engl J Med* 2000; 342(23): 1693-700.

24. Intercollegiate Stroke Working Party. National Clinical Guidelines for Stroke. 2nd edition. 2004: 43.

25. Wholey MH, Al-Mubarak N. Update review of the global carotid stent registry. *Catheterization and Cardiovascular Interventions* 2003; 60: 259-66.

26. Yadav JS, Wholey MH, Kuntz RE, Fayad P, Katzen BT, Mishkel GJ, et al. Protected carotid-artery stenting versus endarterectomy in high-risk patients. *N Engl J Med* 2004; 351(15): 1493-501.

27. Brooks W, McClure R, Jones M, Coleman T, Breathitt L. Carotid angioplasty and stenting versus carotid endarterectomy for treatment of asymptomatic carotid stenosis: a randomized trial in a community hospital. *Neurosurgery Online* 2004; 54(2): 318-25.

28. Yadav JS, Roubin GS, Iyer S, Vitek J, King P, Jordan WD, et al. Elective stenting of the extracranial carotid arteries. *Circulation* 1997; 95(2): 376-81.

29. Waigand J, Gross CM, Uhlich F, Kramer J, Tamaschke C, Vogel P, et al. Elective stenting of carotid artery stenosis in patients with severe coronary artery disease. *Eur Heart J* 1998; 19(9): 1365-70.

30. Lanzino GM, RA, Lopes DK, Wahkloo AK, Guterman LR, Hopkins LN. Percutaneous transluminal angioplasty and stent placement for recurrent carotid artery stenosis. *J Neurosurg* 1999; 90: 688-94.

31. Mericle RK, SH, Lanzino G, Lopes DK, Wakhloo AK, Guterman LR, Hopkins LN. Carotid artery angioplasty and use of stents in high-risk patients with contralateral occlusions. *J Neurosurg* 1999; 90: 1031-6.

32. Henry M, Amor M, Klonaris C, Henry I, Masson I, Chati Z, et al. Angioplasty and stenting of the extracranial carotid arteries. *Texas Heart Institute Journal* 2000; 27(2): 150-8.

33. Ahmadi R, Willfort A, Lang W, Schillinger M, Alt E, Gschwandtner M, et al. Carotid artery stenting: effect of learning curve and intermediate-term morphological outcome. *J Endovasc Ther* 2001; 8: 539-46.

34. Kirsch EC, Khangure MS, van Schie GP, Lawrence-Brown MM, Stewart-Wynne EG, McAuliffe W. Carotid arterial stent placement: results and follow-up in 53 patients. *Radiology* 2001; 220(3): 737-44.

35. Roubin GS, New G, Iyer SS, Vitek JJ, Al-Mubarak N, Liu M, et al. Immediate and late clinical outcomes of carotid artery stenting in patients with symptomatic and asymptomatic carotid artery stenosis. A 5-year provective analysis. *Circulation* 2001; 103: 532-7.

36. Dietz A, Berkefeld J, Theron JG, Schmitz-Rixen T, Zanella FE, Turowski B, et al. Endovascular treatment of symptomatic carotid stenosis using stent placement: long-term follow-up of patients with a balanced surgical risk/benefit ratio. *Stroke* 2001; 32(8): 1855-9.

37. Jaeger H, Mathias K, Drescher R, Hauth E, Bockisch G, Demirel E, et al. Clinical results of cerebral protection with a filter device during stent implantation of the carotid artery. *Cardiovasc Intervent Radiol* 2001; 24(4): 249-56.

38. Criado FJ, Lingelbach JM, Ledesma DF, Lucas PR. Carotid artery stenting in a vascular surgery practice. *J Vasc Surg* 2002; 35(3): 430-4.

39. Kao HL, Lin LY, Lu CJ, Jeng JS, Yip PK, Lee YT. Long-term results of elective stenting for severe carotid artery stenosis in Taiwan. *Cardiology* 2002; 97(2): 89-93.

40. Madyoon H, Braunstein E, Callcott F, Oshtory M, Gurnsey L, Croushore L, et al. Unprotected carotid artery stenting compared to carotid endarterectomy in a community setting. *J Endovasc Ther* 2002; 9(6): 803-9.

41. Adami CA, Scuro A, Spinamano L, Galvagni E, Antoniucci D, Farello GA, et al. Use of the Parodi anti-embolism system in carotid stenting: Italian trial results. *J Endovasc Ther* 2002; 9(2): 147-54.

42. Whitlow PLM. Carotid artery stenting protected with an emboli containment system. *Stroke* 2002; 33(5): 1308-14.

43. Cremonesi A, Manetti R, Setacci F, Setacci C, Castriota F. Protected carotid stenting: clinical advantages and complications of embolic protection devices in 442 consecutive patients. *Stroke* 2003; 34(8): 1936-41.

44. Bush RL, Lin PH, Bianco CC, Lawhorn TI, Hurt JE, Lumsden AB. Carotid artery stenting in a community setting: experience outside of a clinical trial. *Ann Vasc Surg* 2003; 17(6): 629-34.

45. Kastrup A, Groschel K, Krapf H, Brehm BR, Dichgans J, Schulz JB. Early outcome of carotid angioplasty and stenting with and without cerebral protection devices. A systematic review of the literature. *Stroke* 2003; 34: 813-9.

46. Maleux G, Bernaerts P, Thijs V, Vaninbroukx J, Daenens K, Fourneau I, et al. Extracranial carotid artery stenting in surgically high-risk patients using the carotid wallstent endoprosthesis: midterm clinical and ultrasound follow-up results. *Cardiovasc Intervent Radiol* 2003; 26(4): 340-6.

47. Terada T, Tsuura M, Matsumoto H, Masuo O, Yamaga H, Tsumoto T, et al. Results of endovascular treatment of internal carotid artery stenoses with a newly developed balloon protection catheter. *Neurosurgery* 2003; 53(3): 617-23.

48. Eskandari MK, Longo GM, Vijungco JD, Morasch MD, Pearce WH. Does carotid stenting measure up to endarterectomy? A vascular surgeon's experience. *Arch Surg* 2004; 139(7): 734-8.

49. Debette S, Henon H, Gauvrit JY, Haulon S, Mackowiak-Cordoliani MA, Gautier C, et al. Angioplasty and stenting for high-grade internal carotid artery stenosis: safety study in 39 selected patients. *Cerebrovasc Dis* 2004; 17(2-3): 160-5.

50. Theiss W, Hermanek P, Mathias K, Ahmadi R, Heuser L, Hoffmann FJ, et al. Pro-CAS: a prospective registry of carotid angioplasty and stenting. *Stroke* 2004; 35(9): 2134-9.

51. Yen MH, Lee DS, Kapadia S, Sachar R, Bhatt DL, Bajzer CT, et al. Symptomatic patients have similar outcomes compared with asymptomatic patients after carotid artery stenting with emboli protection. *Am J Cardiol* 2005; 95(2): 297-300.

Chapter 17

Carotid plaque morphology: can endovascular success be predicted?

Colin Bicknell MD MRCS, Specialist Registrar, North West Thames

Nick Cheshire MD FRCS, Professor of Vascular Surgery

St. Mary's Hospital, London, UK

Introduction

Carotid endoluminal intervention has developed quickly over the last few years, but is regarded with scepticism by many, due to the potential for embolisation during the procedure. It seems logical to assume that the morphology of the carotid plaque can be used specifically to determine the risk during endovascular intervention, with soft friable plaques being more liable to embolise. The evidence for this can be indirectly studied by examining morphological aspects of the plaque and the relationship with spontaneous embolisation and symptoms. More directly, evidence for this can be obtained by assessing the risk of neurological events during procedures for different morphological subtypes and the potential for embolisation of different carotid plaques.

Stratification of the risks of carotid stenting and the potential for embolisation will help the clinician calculate the risk/benefit ratio for the individual patient and allow the patient to make an informed decision. In addition, the technique and stent used can be modified to suit each particular plaque, such as the use of closed cell configuration stents for plaques likely to embolise.

Morphological aspects

Mature atheromatous plaques are a heterogeneous group of lesions. Typically, the atherosclerotic lesion consists of a well-defined, raised plaque with a lipid and necrotic-filled central core with an overlying fibrous cap. These characteristics are often shared, but plaques may develop in many different ways. The differing morphology of atherosclerotic plaques may explain the reason for the varying behaviour of carotid lesions during endovascular treatment.

The American Heart Association[1] considers lesions advanced by histological criteria when accumulations of lipid, cells and matrix components that make up the plaque are associated with intimal thickening and deformity of the arterial wall. These advanced lesions are defined as Type IV-VI. Type IV lesions are characterised by the presence of a pool of extracellular lipid, occupying a significant proportion of the atheromatous plaque. Type V lesions are characterised by the formation of prominent fibrous tissue within the plaque. Type VI lesions are often referred to as complicated lesions. They are Type IV or Type V lesions that have developed plaque surface disruptions in the form of ulcerations or fissuring (Type VIa), contain haematoma or haemorrhage (Type VIb) or lesions on which thrombotic deposits have formed

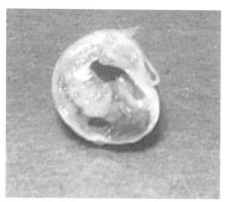

Figure 1. A transverse section through a carotid plaque demonstrating the soft lipid core and ulceration, which may be liable to freely embolise during endoluminal intervention.

(Type VIc). Once a lesion exhibits one or more of these features, its potential for spontaneous embolisation and causing symptomatic disease in the carotid and coronary circulation increases.

It is reasonable to suggest that plaques with significant, soft lipid cores (Type IV) and thin-walled or ulcerated lesions (Type VIa) may be more liable to fragment and embolise during endovascular treatment. In the same way, it may be hypothesised that plaques with thrombotic deposits (Type VIc) on their surface may also break up and more commonly give rise to thrombo-emboli. There is a relationship between these factors, which may compound the problem. The atheromatous core is the most thrombogenic substrate within the plaque, as demonstrated by *ex vivo* studies of different coronary plaque components exposed to flowing blood [2]. Consequently, there is a strong association between plaque ulceration and thrombosis of the carotid plaque [3]. Figure 1 shows a carotid plaque in transverse section. The plaque contains a soft necrotic core and is ulcerated, which may make this lesion liable to break up and embolise during endoluminal intervention. By studying plaque morphological features, we can speculate whether these lesions actually pose more of a risk during carotid endoluminal intervention; nevertheless, this relationship needs further exploration.

Spontaneous embolisation

The morphology of the carotid plaque is a major factor in spontaneous embolisation. Histological examination of carotid endarterectomy specimens demonstrates a relationship between symptomatic plaques and morphological features such as plaque surface fissuring or ulceration [3-6], fibrous cap thinning [4], luminal thrombus [3], haemorrhage within the plaque [7-9], and an increased volume of the lipid core [10]. It is, therefore, likely that these features are all associated with an increase in spontaneous embolisation and that this is the cause of transient ischaemic attack (TIA) and stroke in these patients. Pre-operatively, spontaneous emboli can be more commonly demonstrated in the ipsilateral middle cerebral artery from plaques that are later shown to demonstrate similar characteristics [3].

Histological analysis following endarterectomy is an efficient method of determining plaque morphology and its relationship to symptomatic disease, but the relationship can also be demonstrated *in vivo* using various imaging modalities. Duplex has shown that echolucent plaques, which are predominantly soft with a rich lipid component often containing haemorrhage [11, 12], are significantly more common in symptomatic patients [13-18]. Echolucent plaques are also associated with increased numbers of infarcts shown on computed tomographic (CT) imaging [19, 20] and increased numbers of emboli detected during transcranial Doppler (TCD) [21]. Some have attempted to study the relationship between ulceration and symptomatic disease using computer-assisted duplex plaque analysis and magnetic resonance imaging (MRI). Plaque surface disruption is significantly associated with symptomatic disease [22, 23].

There is, therefore, convincing evidence that the morphology of individual plaques is related to spontaneous embolisation and symptoms, but whether these data can be used to stratify the risks during endoluminal intervention is debatable.

Neurological events during carotid endoluminal intervention

Angiography is considered as one of the most accurate methods of determining the anatomy and pathological changes at the level of the carotid bifurcation. Retrospective studies of case series have shown that long and multiple stenoses are significantly associated with neurological events during and after carotid artery stenting (CAS) [24, 25]. There was no increase in events around the time of endoluminal intervention in either of these studies in patients with ulcerated, irregular or tightly narrowed plaques. Those with plaques that extended into the common carotid bifurcation were also not shown to be more at risk.

Study of the morphology of the carotid bifurcation, in relation to symptoms after CAS, relies on the accuracy of *in vivo* imaging of the plaque. Irregularity of the luminal border of the stenosis suggests ulceration or superimposed thrombosis. However, whilst some cases are clearly ulcerated on angiography (Figure 2), others are difficult to judge and reports have demonstrated that the sensitivity and specificity of angiography to determine ulceration and thrombosis is relatively poor. Irregularity on angiographic images has a sensitivity of 45.9% and a specificity of 74.1% for the detection of ulcerated atherosclerotic plaques identified at surgery [26]. In addition to these shortcomings, angiography can show only an outline of the plaque and gives no account of internal plaque morphology. Examination of retrospective series that examine the effect of morphology as a predictor of outcome during CAS must take these findings into consideration.

Duplex examination of plaques is widely used to show, not only the degree of stenosis, but also gives an idea of the histological subtype of the plaque (Figure 3). The ICAROS Registry (Imaging in Carotid Angioplasties and Risk Of Stroke) is one of the only prospective studies of carotid plaque morphology and its relationship to periprocedural neurological events during CAS. It was designed to study the role of duplex imaging and determine which patients can safely undergo carotid endoluminal intervention [27]. Four hundred and eighteen CAS procedures were registered. The overall cerebral complication rate was 3.6%. Analysis of duplex information showed that 155

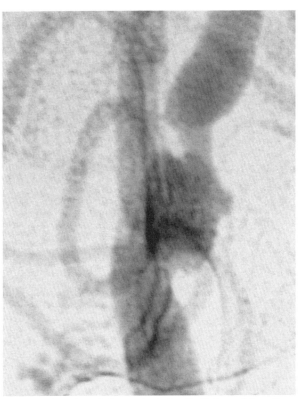

Figure 2. An intra-arterial digital subtraction angiogram of the carotid bifurcation, demonstrating an ulcerated carotid plaque.

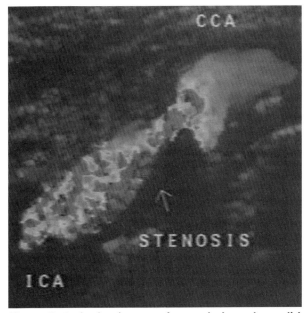

Figure 3. A duplex image of an echolucent carotid plaque, indicating a soft core. These have been shown to be more likely to produce neurological events during carotid endoluminal intervention.

of the patients had plaques with a calculated gray scale median (GSM) of less than 25 (indicating soft plaques with a large lipid core containing haemorrhage). Eleven of these plaques (7.1%) gave rise to cerebral complications compared to four strokes in 263 procedures (1.5%) involving plaques with a GSM of over 25. This finding suggests that duplex plaque characterisation may have a strong role in predicting those at high risk of complications during carotid stenting and that those patients with soft plaques may be more at risk.

It must be remembered, however, that these are registry data and not a consecutive trial, which may lead to under-reporting of events. In addition, the patients in this study were a mixed group, and 54.3% of plaques were restenoses after carotid surgery, which may be echogenic and give rise to less emboli.

Embolisation during carotid endoluminal intervention

Embolisation is the major cause of temporary and permanent neurological defects seen both during and following intervention. Embolic particles are produced in all procedures and at all stages during CAS, and can be demonstrated using transcranial Doppler insonation of the distal vessels. This occurs even with the use of distal protection devices [28, 29]. Embolisation originating from the carotid plaque in the external carotid territory can also be seen directly in the retinal vessels of patients following CAS [30]. The embolic potential of carotid plaques is most probably the most important factor in determining the risk of stroke.

There are no direct comparisons between embolisation or events during CAS and histology, as the plaque is left in situ in this procedure. Emboli from the plaque may, however, be captured and studied. During CAS, the use of distal protection devices and collection of emboli can be employed. Samples obtained after stent deployment in the pooled blood below an inflated protection balloon show large numbers of lipid particles [31-33], whilst examination of distal protection device filters has shown predominantly cholesterol masses, as well as thrombotic material and foam cells [34]. Intervention in the coronary circulation and collection of emboli

reveals similar material collected in distal filters [35]. Since emboli are composed mainly of thrombotic, lipid and necrotic material, it may be that the plaques with the greatest potential for embolisation, and hence stroke, are those with large volume lipid cores, overlying thrombus or those which are unstable with a thin or ulcerated fibrous cap. If this is true, then the results of CAS may be predicted by examining the morphology of the individual plaque.

Models of the CAS procedure are able to directly study the relationship between morphology and the number and size of emboli. These studies use carotid plaques obtained from human carotid endarterectomy procedures and collect emboli following endoluminal intervention using an ex vivo model. One of the first studies of this type involved only five plaques [36]. This showed that emboli were produced at all stages of the angioplasty procedure. Two of these plaques had an irregular, ulcerated surface on pre-operative angiography, which produced a greater number of emboli of a larger size. In a further study, Ohki performed carotid artery stenting in an ex vivo model using 24 circumferentially intact plaques. The study examined embolisation during the procedure and its relationship to morphology. Morphological features associated with higher numbers of emboli were high-grade stenoses and echolucent plaques [37].

At St. Mary's Hospital, we have also studied embolisation and its relationship to the morphological features of the plaque in an ex vivo model. A pulsatile ex vivo carotid angioplasty model was developed in which flow, pressure, velocity, temperature and viscosity were similar to in vivo parameters. Circumferentially intact carotid endarterectomy specimens underwent a standardised angioplasty procedure and emboli were collected in distal filters. These emboli were counted and sized, using microscopy and related to morphological features of the plaque. Thirty-eight specimens were successfully angioplastied in our model. Emboli were produced during the procedure in all cases, with a wide variation in number and size. The median number of emboli was 104 (IQR 33.75-242.5, min 13, max 1090). The greatest numbers of emboli were found during the balloon stage of the procedure. Thirty-five of 38 plaques produced emboli greater than 200 microns in size, and eight of 38 plaques produced emboli greater than 1mm in length. Carotid endarterectomy specimens within this model, therefore, produce a variable number of emboli of different sizes, suggesting the embolic potential of different plaques is varied.

Using duplex, plaque morphological features were examined. Highly stenosed plaques (greater than 90%) generated significantly larger maximum sizes of emboli, 1500 microns (IQR 1150-1850, range 400-2200) versus 500 microns (IQR 200-1250, range 75-2800) for plaques with a stenosis of less than 90%. In addition, there were significantly greater numbers of emboli produced by plaques graded as echolucent (median 182, IQR 93.5-421, range 32-1090) when compared to echogenic plaques (median 29, IQR 27-39, range 18-97) [38].

One other study of embolisation during CAS has used human carotid arteries *in situ* within cadavers [39]. Nineteen arteries from ten cadavers were angioplastied, emboli collected distally and the post-angioplasty plaques examined histologically. The presence of intraplaque haemorrhage was associated with increased numbers of emboli collected during the procedure. Interestingly, there was no association between plaque stenosis or echolucency on pre-procedure duplex examination and embolisation as has been shown in previous studies. This may be due to the low number of high-grade, echolucent plaques. The diameter of stenoses ranged from 32-85%, and there were only four echolucent plaques.

Embolisation within other vascular territories

Within the coronary circulation, the morphology of the atherosclerotic plaque is also important in the development of disease. A thin fibrous cap overlying a large, lipid-rich core is associated with plaque rupture, thrombosis and myocardial infarction [40]. During interventional procedures, plaque features can be directly visualised using coronary angioscopy. Plaque disruption, yellow colour and thrombus overlying the lesion are associated with early complications after coronary angioplasty [41].

Distal embolisation is known to be an important complication of intervention in saphenous vein bypass grafts that have stenosed. Multiple emboli are collected during angioplasty of these grafts using a distal protection device [35]. Rises in creatinine kinase (CK) and troponin-I levels following angioplasty, with no obvious major vessel occlusion, may be suggestive of distal embolisation. Using angiographic data, features noted to be associated with distal embolisation (measured by a rise in CK levels) include diffusely diseased vein grafts, ulcerated lesions, overlying thrombus, a large plaque volume and marked eccentricity of the plaque [42]. Again this suggests a role for the morphology of the plaque in determining the potential for embolisation.

Morphological features of the plaque in the native and grafted coronary circulation are, therefore, associated with outcome after angioplasty. Whether data from these studies can be extrapolated to treatment of carotid disease remains to be seen.

Conclusions

The morphology of carotid plaques is varied. Whilst some contain high amounts of fibrous material and are relatively stable, others contain large lipid-filled atheromatous cores, may be ulcerated with thrombosis overlying the fibrous cap defect and are unstable. It is clear that these plaques give rise to spontaneous emboli and symptoms more commonly than stable lesions. These unstable plaques may be liable to increased embolisation during endovascular intervention. The evidence to date suggests that some morphological features, such as high-grade stenosis, long or multiple lesions and echolucent plaques, are more liable to embolise and cause symptoms. However, the embolic potential of the carotid plaque during endoluminal intervention may be determined by many factors such as technique, operator experience and arterial anatomy, as well as plaque morphology, which may confuse the picture. Despite this, there does seem to be a role for morphology in determining the risk of embolisation and stroke during the procedure. This may be useful in stratifying risk for individual patients.

Summary

◆ Carotid lesions are varied in their morphological substance, with some lesions exhibiting features that lead to instability.

◆ Spontaneous embolisation and symptoms from plaques are closely related to plaque morphology. Ulceration, a thin fibrous cap, thrombosis, intraplaque haemorrhage and a large volume lipid core make up lesions most at risk.

◆ *In vivo* studies have shown that neurological events during carotid artery stenting occur more commonly in long, multiple, echolucent lesions.

◆ Embolisation seems to occur more commonly during endovascular procedures from lesions that are tightly stenosed and are echolucent in character.

◆ There may be a role for stratification of the risk of carotid endoluminal intervention using plaque morphology, but other factors such as technique, operator experience and arterial anatomy must be taken into account.

References

1. Stary HC, Chandler AB, Dinsmore RE, *et al*. A definition of advanced types of atherosclerotic lesions and a histological classification of atherosclerosis. A report from the Committee on Vascular Lesions of the Council on Arteriosclerosis, American Heart Association. *Arterioscler Thromb Vasc Biol* 1995; 15(9): 1512-31.

2. Fernandez-Ortiz A, Badimon JJ, Falk E, *et al*. Characterization of the relative thrombogenicity of atherosclerotic plaque components: implications for consequences of plaque rupture. *J Am Coll Cardiol* 1994; 23(7): 1562-9.

3. Sitzer M, Muller W, Siebler M, *et al*. Plaque ulceration and lumen thrombus are the main sources of cerebral microemboli in high-grade internal carotid artery stenosis. *Stroke* 1995; 26(7): 1231-3.

4. Carr S, Farb A, Pearce WH, *et al*. Atherosclerotic plaque rupture in symptomatic carotid artery stenosis. *J Vasc Surg* 1996; 23(5): 755-65; discussion 765-6.

5. Park AE, McCarthy WJ, Pearce WH, *et al*. Carotid plaque morphology correlates with presenting symptomatology. *J Vasc Surg* 1998; 27(5): 872-8; discussion 878-9.

6. Ballotta E, Da Giau G, Renon L. Carotid plaque gross morphology and clinical presentation: a prospective study of 457 carotid artery specimens. *J Surg Res* 2000; 89(1): 78-84.

7. Lusby RJ, Ferrell LD, Ehrenfeld WK, *et al*. Carotid plaque hemorrhage. Its role in production of cerebral ischemia. *Arch Surg* 1982; 117(11): 1479-88.

8. Imparato AM, Riles TS, Mintzer R, *et al*. The importance of hemorrhage in the relationship between gross morphologic characteristics and cerebral symptoms in 376 carotid artery plaques. *Ann Surg* 1983; 197(2): 195-203.

9. Persson AV, Robichaux WT, Silverman M. The natural history of carotid plaque development. *Arch Surg* 1983; 118(9): 1048-52.

10. Feeley TM, Leen EJ, Colgan MP, *et al*. Histologic characteristics of carotid artery plaque. *J Vasc Surg* 1991; 13(5): 719-24.

11. Gronholdt ML. Ultrasound and lipoproteins as predictors of lipid-rich, rupture-prone plaques in the carotid artery. *Arterioscler Thromb Vasc Biol* 1999; 19(1): 2-13.

12. Schulte-Altedorneburg G, Droste DW, Haas N, *et al*. Preoperative B-mode ultrasound plaque appearance compared with carotid endarterectomy specimen histology. *Acta Neurol Scand* 2000; 101(3): 188-94.

13. Langsfeld M, Gray-Weale A, Lusby R, *et al*. The role of plaque morphology and diameter reduction in the development of new symptoms in asymptomatic carotid arteries. *J Vasc Surg* 1989; 9(4): 548-57.

14. Geroulakos G, Ramaswami G, Nicolaides A, *et al*. Characterization of symptomatic and asymptomatic carotid plaques using high-resolution real-time ultrasonography. *Br J Surg* 1993; 80(10): 1274-7.

15. El-Barghouty N, Geroulakos G, Nicolaides A, *et al*. Computer-assisted carotid plaque characterisation. *Eur J Vasc Endovasc Surg* 1995; 9(4): 389-93.

16. Elatrozy T, Nicolaides A, Tegos T, *et al*. The objective characterisation of ultrasonic carotid plaque features. *Eur J Vasc Endovasc Surg* 1998; 16(3): 223-30.

17. Sabetai MM, Tegos TJ, Nicolaides AN, *et al*. Hemispheric symptoms and carotid plaque echomorphology. *J Vasc Surg* 2000; 31(1 Pt 1): 39-49.

18. Mathiesen EB, Bonaa KH, Joakimsen O. Echolucent plaques are associated with high risk of ischemic cerebrovascular events in carotid stenosis: the tromso study. *Circulation* 2001; 103(17): 2171-5.

19. Geroulakos G, Domjan J, Nicolaides A, *et al*. Ultrasonic carotid artery plaque structure and the risk of cerebral infarction on computed tomography. *J Vasc Surg* 1994; 20(2): 263-6.

20. Tegos TJ, Sabetai MM, Nicolaides AN, *et al*. Patterns of brain computed tomography infarction and carotid plaque echogenicity. *J Vasc Surg* 2001; 33(2): 334-9.

21. Tegos TJ, Sabetai MM, Nicolaides AN, *et al*. Correlates of embolic events detected by means of transcranial Doppler in patients with carotid atheroma. *J Vasc Surg* 2001; 33(1): 131-8.

22. Pedro LM, Pedro MM, Goncalves I, *et al*. Computer-assisted carotid plaque analysis: characteristics of plaques associated with cerebrovascular symptoms and cerebral infarction. *Eur J Vasc Endovasc Surg* 2000; 19(2): 118-23.

23. Troyer A, Saloner D, Pan XM, *et al*. Major carotid plaque surface irregularities correlate with neurologic symptoms. *J Vasc Surg* 2002; 35(4): 741-7.

24. Mathur A, Roubin GS, Lyer SS, *et al*. Predictors of stroke complicating carotid artery stenting. *Circulation* 1998; 97(13): 1239-45.

25. Qureshi AI, Luft AR, Janardhan V, *et al*. Identification of patients at risk for periprocedural neurological deficits associated with carotid angioplasty and stenting. *Stroke* 2000; 31(2): 376-82.

26. Streifler JY, Eliasziw M, Fox AJ, *et al*. Angiographic detection of carotid plaque ulceration. Comparison with surgical observations in a multicenter study. North American Symptomatic Carotid Endarterectomy Trial. *Stroke* 1994; 25(6): 1130-2.

27. Biasi G, Froio A, Diethrich EB, *et al*. Carotid plaque echolucency increases the risk of stroke in carotid stenting: the Imaging in Carotid Angioplasty and Risk of Stroke (ICAROS) study. *Circulation* 2004; 110(6): 756-62.

28. Markus HS, Clifton A, Buckenham T, *et al*. Carotid angioplasty. Detection of embolic signals during and after the procedure. *Stroke* 1994; 25(12): 2403-6.

29. Orlandi G, Fanucchi S, Fioretti C, *et al*. Characteristics of cerebral microembolism during carotid stenting and angioplasty alone. *Arch Neurol* 2001; 58(9): 1410-3.

30. Wilentz JR, Chati Z, Krafft V, *et al*. Retinal embolization during carotid angioplasty and stenting: mechanisms and role of cerebral protection systems. *Catheter Cardiovasc Interv* 2002; 56(3): 320-7.

31. Martin J-B, Pache J-C, Treggiari-Venzi M, *et al*. Role of the distal balloon protection technique in the prevention of cerebral embolic events during carotid stent placement. *Stroke* 2001; 32(2): 479-84.

32. Reimers B, Corvaja N, Moshiri S, *et al*. Cerebral protection with filter devices during carotid artery stenting. *Circulation* 2001; 104(1): 12-5.

33. Whitlow PL, Lylyk P, Londero H, *et al*. Carotid artery stenting protected with an emboli containment system. *Stroke* 2002; 33(5): 1308-14.

34. Angelini A, Reimers B, Barbera MD, *et al*. Cerebral protection during carotid artery stenting: collection and histopathologic analysis of embolized debris. *Stroke* 2002; 33(2): 456-61.

35. Webb JG, Carere RG, Virmani R, *et al*. Retrieval and analysis of particulate debris after saphenous vein graft intervention. *J Am Coll Cardiol* 1999; 34(2): 468-75.

36. Coggia M, Goeau-Brissonniere O, Duval J-L, *et al*. Embolic risk of the different stages of carotid bifurcation balloon angioplasty: an experimental study. *J Vasc Surg* 2000; 31(3): 550-7.

37. Ohki T, Marin M, Lyon R, *et al*. *Ex vivo* human carotid artery bifurcation stenting: correlation of lesion characteristics with embolic potential. *J Vasc Surg* 1998; 27(3): 463-71.

38. Bicknell CD, Cowling MG, Clark MW, *et al*. Carotid angioplasty in a pulsatile flow model: factors affecting embolic potential. *Eur J Vasc Endovasc Surg* 2003; 26: 22-31.

39. Manninen HI, Rasanen HT, Vanninen RL, *et al*. Stent placement versus percutaneous transluminal angioplasty of human carotid arteries in cadavers *in situ*: distal embolization and findings at intravascular US, MR Imaging, and histopathologic analysis. *Radiology* 1999; 212(2): 483-92.

40. Falk E, Shah PK, Fuster V. Coronary plaque disruption. *Circulation* 1995; 92(3): 657-71.

41. Waxman S, Sassower MA, Mittleman MA, *et al*. Angioscopic predictors of early adverse outcome after coronary angioplasty in patients with unstable angina and non-Q-wave myocardial infarction. *Circulation* 1996; 93(12): 2106-13.

42. Liu MW, Douglas JS, Jr., Lembo NJ, *et al*. Angiographic predictors of a rise in serum creatine kinase (distal embolization) after balloon angioplasty of saphenous vein coronary artery bypass grafts. *Am J Cardiol* 1993; 72(7): 514-7.

Chapter 18

Evidence for the use of stents in the superficial femoral artery

Nick Chalmers FRCR, Consultant Vascular Radiologist

David Thompson FRCR, Specialist Registrar in Radiology

Manchester Royal Infirmary, Manchester, UK

Introduction

The superficial femoral artery (SFA) is a common site for the development of peripheral vascular disease. Disease localised to this segment frequently presents with intermittent claudication. When SFA disease is found in tandem with either proximal or distal disease, critical ischaemia with rest pain, ulceration or gangrene may occur. Balloon angioplasty has been a standard treatment for stenoses and short occlusions of the SFA for 30 years. It is the commonest endovascular procedure in the repertoire, constituting nearly 50% of the total UK interventional radiology workload [1]. Despite this, the randomised controlled trial data supporting its use is minimal. A Cochrane Collaboration review of the randomised trial evidence for angioplasty for intermittent claudication highlights the paucity of data, but concludes that there is no worthwhile benefit of balloon angioplasty compared with conservative treatment [2]. Early failure due to flow-limiting dissection and elastic recoil occur in 10%. Long-term patency rates are disappointing because of restenosis and reocclusion.

A number of explanations have been proposed to account for the poorer success rates in the SFA compared with other vessels (iliac, renal and carotid for example). The SFA is a long vessel which often carries a large bulk of disease. Stenotic disease is rarely confined to a single short stenosis. Occlusions are frequently associated with further stenotic disease proximally and distally. Other factors which are known to contribute to poor outcomes of SFA angioplasty are poor calf run-off, diabetes, occlusion versus stenosis and critical ischaemia versus claudication [3]. The SFA is subject to considerable mechanical stress and strain, including axial stretching and shortening, torsion and extrinsic compression. In young and healthy arteries, flexion of the knee produces corresponding smooth flexion of the popliteal artery, several centimetres proximal to the level of the knee joint. Angiograms performed in flexion in older subjects with less elastic arteries show that flexion of the knee produces marked zig-zag angulation in the distal SFA as well as the popliteal. These factors are bound to have an impact on the performance of stents in this region.

Early experience of stenting in the SFA

Arterial stents were initially developed in the late 1980s and, although there have been numerous technical advances in materials, design and delivery systems, there is still limited evidence to show any benefit of stent placement over angioplasty alone.

Part IV Lower Limb Disease

Stent fractures were observed during both the SIROCCO I and II trials. In the former, up to three stents were permitted, whereas in the latter there was a maximum of two. Stent fractures were more frequent when three stents were used. The causes and significance of stent fractures are the subject of much current debate. Some fractures, usually those associated with complete disruption of a stent, are associated with restenosis. On the other hand isolated stent wire fractures may occur without adverse consequences. It is not known whether stent fractures are progressive. Late follow-up of the SIROCCO cohort will provide useful information in this respect.

The FESTO study sought to assess the significance of stent fractures through a systematic prospective radiographic follow-up of SFA stent patients [11]. Radiographic follow-up at a mean of 10.7 months post-stent implantation was performed in 121 limbs, with a mean of 1.9 stents per limb, and a mean stented length of 160mm. Stent fractures were noted in 37.2% of limbs. Fractures were more common in the longer stented lengths. Fractures were associated with stenosis in 33% and occlusion in 34%. There was a highly significant difference in patency between those limbs that had stent fracture and those that did not. There was also a difference between the various designs of stent in the frequency of fracture: the Cordis SMART stent was associated with fewest fractures and the Bard Luminexx stent (Bard Ltd, Crawley, West Sussex, UK) with most.

The best quality evidence to date in favour of stent placement in the SFA comes from the prolific Viennese group [12]. The ABSOLUTE trial is the first randomised trial to show evidence of any benefit of stents compared with balloon angioplasty in the SFA. One hundred and four patients were randomised to either stent placement, using the Guidant Absolute nitinol stent (Guidant, Diegem, Belgium), or balloon angioplasty (with optional stent placement in case of suboptimal angioplasty). Primary endpoint was >50% restenosis at six months. Stents were used in 32% of the angioplasty group. Restenosis was seen in 12/51 of the stent group (23.5%) compared with 23/53 (43.4%) of the angioplasty group (p=0.032). Patients in the stent group also had a greater maximum treadmill walking distance.

A similar study, the FAST trial, comparing the Bard Luminexx stent with balloon angioplasty in 244 patients, has failed to duplicate these results. Restenosis (on duplex ultrasound) was less common in the stent group (25.5%) than in the angioplasty group (38.3%), but not significantly so [13].

A number of other randomised controlled trials of stenting versus angioplasty in the SFA are ongoing. The SUPER trial is a UK-based multicentre trial comparing the Cordis SMART stent with balloon angioplasty in SFA occlusions. Quality of life and health economic analysis will be included. SUPER-SL is a head-to-head comparison of the SMART stent with the Bard Luminexx stent. This will contribute valuable information about the clinical impact of subtle differences in nitinol stent design.

The RESILIENT study is a comparison of the Edwards Lifesciences (Saint-Prex, Switzerland) LifeStent NT with angioplasty in SFA disease. Phase I, a non-randomised feasibility study, has shown 100% clinical success at six months. Phase II, a multicentre randomised trial, is underway.

Additional measures to reduce restenosis

Drug-eluting stents

The SIROCCO trials had the effect of stimulating interest in bare-metal nitinol stents and at the same time damping enthusiasm for drug-eluting stents in the SFA. It seems likely that the effect of the drug on the neointima is relatively small. It is, therefore, unlikely to be useful in a large vessel such as the SFA, but may be worthwhile in the calf vessels, where even a small reduction in the thickness of the neointimal layer may have a significant impact on patency. This issue is the subject of the ongoing BELOW trial being conducted in Tübingen.

Covered stents and stent grafts

Early attempts to overcome in-stent neointimal hyperplasia, using various designs of stent graft, did not proceed beyond initial feasibility studies. The Gore Hemobahn (WL Gore, Livingston, Scotland), recently renamed Viabahn, is the first commercially produced device to show significant promise in the SFA. It consists of a self-expanding nitinol stent interwoven

The TransAtlantic Intersociety Consensus (TASC) document on the management of peripheral vascular disease was published in 2001 [6]. The literature on femoropopliteal intervention was reviewed and a number of recommendations and observations were made (TASC). In summary, of the papers reviewed, stents were placed in 600 limbs (585 patients, 80% claudicants) with a technical success rate of 98% and one and three-year primary patency rates of 67% and 58%, respectively. Comparative data for 1469 limbs (1241 patients, 72% claudicants) treated with angioplasty alone were a technical success rate of 90% and one and three-year primary patency rates of 61% and 51%. Recommendation 35 stated: "Endovascular procedure is the treatment of choice for type A lesions (single stenosis <3cm), and surgery is the procedure of choice for type D lesions (complete segmental occlusion)". Critical Issue 14 stated: "More evidence is needed to make firm recommendations about the best treatment for type B and C lesions (all the others)". Recommendation 36 stated: "Femoropopliteal stenting as a primary approach to the treatment of intermittent claudication or CLI is not indicated. However, stents may have a limited role in salvage of acute PTA failures or complications". It was also stated that the use of self-expanding stents in this area seemed advisable due to potential compressive forces in the adductor canal. In addition, it was also stated that covered stents may have a future role in reducing restenosis rates.

In 2001, Muradin et al published a meta-analysis of long-term results of balloon dilatation and stent implantation for the treatment of femoropopliteal arterial disease [7]. English-language literature was searched between 1993 and 2000. Nineteen of 118 studies met the inclusion criteria, representing 923 balloon dilatations and 473 stent implantations. Combined three-year patency rates after PTA were 61% for stenosis and claudication, 48% for occlusion and claudication, 43% for stenosis and critical ischaemia and 30% for occlusion and critical ischaemia. The three-year patency rates after stent implantation were 63-66% and were independent of clinical indication and lesion type. They concluded that there was little benefit for stent implantation in claudicants, although for more severe disease, stent implantation seemed more favourable. The effect of publication bias could not be ruled out however.

In 2002, Bachoo and Thorpe published a Cochrane Review entitled "Endovascular stents for intermittent claudication" [8]. Of 42 publications reviewed, only two studies satisfied their inclusion criteria. There were a combined total of 104 patients with claudication only, and angioplasty and stenting with the Palmaz stent was compared with PTA alone. When combined, there was no difference in patency rates or secondary outcomes. They concluded that the small number of relevant trials, small sample sizes and methodological weaknesses, limited the review and that there was an urgent need for high quality randomised multicentre trials.

Although excluded from the Cochrane Review, the study by Cejna et al published in 2001 was one of the largest trials in which 154 limbs (141 patients, 77% claudicants) were randomised to either PTA alone or PTA and primary implantation of a Palmaz stent [9]. Stenting had a significantly higher primary success rate than PTA alone (99% against 84%), although cumulative one and two-year angiographic primary patency rates were equivalent (64% and 53% respectively for PTA alone and 63% and 58% for PTA and stenting) and similarly there was no difference in haemodynamic or clinical success.

Recent stent data

Some recent trial data have shown results which are in contrast with the previously reported unimpressive data concerning SFA stents. These recent data give rise to renewed optimism that modern stent designs may improve patency rates in SFA disease. The evidence of clear clinical benefit of drug-eluting stents in the coronary arteries provided the impetus for research into the effect of drug-eluting stents in the femoropopliteal segment [10]. The SIROCCO studies compared the performance of the self-expanding nitinol SMART stent (Cordis Endovascular, South Ascot, Berks, UK) with and without a coating of the cytostatic drug, sirolimus. These prospective randomised studies failed to demonstrate any worthwhile difference in patency rates between the two. The striking finding, however, was the high patency rates in both treatment groups. A total of 57 patients were randomised in the SIROCCO II study. Restenosis of more than 50% was seen in only two cases at six months giving a primary patency of 96%. Some late restenosis has been observed; however, the 18-month patency rates remain impressive at just over 80%.

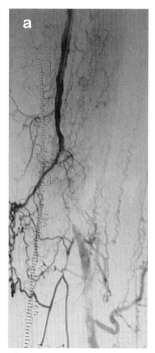
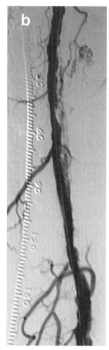
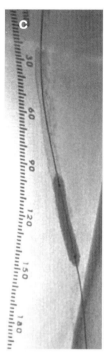
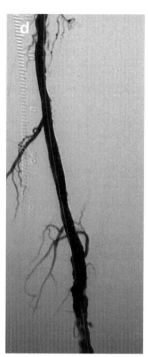

Figure 1. Stent placement following sub-optimal balloon angioplasty in a calcified SFA occlusion. a) Initial angiogram shows a 5cm occlusion of distal SFA. b) Following angioplasty using a 5mm balloon, there is residual stenosis associated with initmal dissection. c) A 7mm-diameter SMART stent has been deployed and post-dilated using a 6mm balloon. d) Final image shows improved appearances.

Stents work initially by preventing elastic recoil and holding back dissection flaps caused by balloon dilatation (Figure 1). Later they may prevent constrictive remodelling. Ideally the stent would be incorporated in the vessel wall and then be covered by endothelium. Unfortunately, this process is usually incomplete which leads to the problems of immediate thrombosis and later restenosis due to neointimal hyperplasia, which occurs either within or immediately adjacent to the stented segment. It is in understanding the processes that lead to failure in which research and development is now being focused.

The ideal stent should be biocompatible, radio-opaque, and flexible with sufficient stiffness to resist compressive forces and a shape-memory so that it recovers its predetermined shape after deforming [4, 5]. Balloon-mounted stents were the first to become commercially available, with most being manufactured from stainless steel. These stents have the advantages of accurate deployment and high radial stiffness, but suffer the disadvantage of being less compliant and may collapse or buckle if undue stress is placed on them, for example in the adductor canal. Self-expanding stents are a newer development and may offer some advantages in the SFA. These stents are manufactured from nitinol or a cobalt alloy. On deployment, they self-expand to their preset diameter. Self-expanding stents have less inherent radial stiffness, but are highly compliant and conformable and are able to recover from buckling or crushing forces.

Although many researchers have addressed the issue of stents in femoropopliteal disease, there are few randomised controlled trials comparing the use of simple balloon angioplasty against primary stenting. There is variation in the reporting of demographic details, clinical and radiological indications and the outcomes. Many of the larger studies involved the use of the Palmaz stent (Cordis Endovascular, South Ascot, Berks, UK), Strecker stent and Wallstent (both Boston Scientific, St. Albans, Herts, UK), and it is not clear if the conclusions can be applied to the newer nitinol stent. In addition, there has been a change in adjunctive medical therapy, particularly with reference to newer antiplatelet therapy.

with a PTFE coating. An international series, that included 80 cases in which the Hemobahn was deployed in the femoral arteries, achieved 79% one-year patency at this site [14]. Jahnke and colleagues undertook a prospective trial of Hemobahn in patients with a minimum lesion length of 3cm (mean lesion length 8.5cm, total occlusion in 82.7%). One and two-year primary patency rates were 78.4% and 74.1% respectively [15].

A multicentre randomised trial of Hemobahn versus balloon angioplasty was performed in the USA. It appears that this study was never published in full. However, the results of a single centre were published. This showed superior primary patency of the PTFE stent graft group compared with the balloon angioplasty group at six months (93% versus 42%) and at two years (87% versus 25%) [16]. The failure to publish the results of the trial as a whole means this finding must be interpreted with caution. The VIBRANT study is comparing the Viabahn PTFE-covered stent graft with bare nitinol stents. This is a multicentre randomised trial which will include 150 patients who will be followed-up for three years.

Pharmacological therapies

Adjunctive measures to reduce thrombosis and restenosis are under investigation. Antiplatelet drugs are generally prescribed during and after stent placement. Many centres advocate the use of dual antiplatelet therapy following stent placement in the SFA, with a four-week course of clopidigrel 75mg daily in addition to lifelong aspirin therapy. However, this practice is based on consensus rather than evidence. A comparative study using historical controls showed no convincing evidence of benefit of clopidogrel [17]. The BLASTER trial was a double blind randomised trial of abciximab (Reopro) versus placebo in femoral artery stenting. It demonstrated no improvement in patency in the active treatment group [18].

Brachytherapy

Brachytherapy offers the potential to reduce restenosis by reducing smooth muscle cell proliferation. All the brachytherapy techniques to date have involved substantial logistical issues which increase the complexity of a simple procedure considerably. Where brachytherapy has been compared with drug-eluting stents, the latter appear to offer greater potential [19]. Outside of the coronary system, high quality evidence to support its use is lacking. The phenomenon of late acute thrombotic occlusion, specifically associated with brachytherapy, has been identified following its use in the coronary arteries. A recent randomised trial of brachytherapy versus placebo to prevent restenosis in femoropopliteal stenting has failed to demonstrate any benefit, mainly due to the high rate of both early and late rethrombosis in the treated group [20].

Biodegradable stents

Biodegradable stents are an attractive concept. The theory is that, once the artery has repaired itself following angioplasty and stent placement, the stent itself is redundant. If the stent were to dissolve, a satisfactory patent lumen would remain. Issues such as stent strut fracture would not arise. The current problem is to identify a suitable material with adequate mechanical properties in the short term, and yet which will slowly dissolve over a period of weeks without toxicity. At least two materials are under current investigation: a magnesium alloy and a poly-lactic acid polymer. Human implantations have been reported in only small numbers to date [21].

Conclusions

Rapid developments are taking place in the field of SFA stenting. Nitinol self-expanding stents appear to offer considerable potential, especially in the patterns of SFA disease that are known to be associated with poor longer-term results from balloon angioplasty. The non-randomised data are encouraging. The randomised data are limited, but supportive. The results of ongoing randomised trials are awaited with interest. Further understanding of the causes and consequences of stent strut fracture will influence the design of the next generation of stents specifically designed for this application. No additional measures have yet been shown to further improve patency rates over those which can be achieved with bare nitinol stents alone.

Summary

◆ Early stent designs were not significantly superior to balloon angioplasty alone in the treatment of SFA disease.

◆ Newer nitinol stents appear to give better results. Limited controlled trial data are available and further trials are in progress.

◆ Stent fractures have been observed. In some cases these are associated with restenosis and occlusion.

◆ There are a small amount of data to support the use of covered stents in the SFA. Further trials are ongoing.

◆ Other adjunctive measures to improve long-term patency have not been shown to be of benefit.

References

1. Interventional Vascular Radiology Report 2000. National Confidential Enquiry into Patient Outcomes and Death (NCEPOD). Accessed at www.ncepod.org.uk/pdf/2000/ir/RadioVasc.pdf on 28th January 2006.

2. Fowkes FGR, Gillespie IN. Angioplasty (versus non-surgical management) for intermittent claudication. *The Cochrane Database of Systematic Reviews* 1998; Issue 2: CD000017.

3. Johnson KW. Femoral and popliteal arteries: reanalysis of results of balloon angioplasty. *Radiology* 1992; 183: 767-71.

4. Jackson RW. The evolution of peripheral arterial stents: are we winning? In: *Endovascular Intervention: Current Controversies*. Wyatt MG, Watkinson AF, Eds. Shrewsbury, UK: tfm publishing Ltd, 2004.

5. Stoeckel D, Bonsignore C, Duda S. A survey of stent designs. *Min Invas Ther & Allied Technol* 2002: 11: 137-47.

6. Dormandy JA, Rutherford RB. Management of peripheral arterial disease (PAD). TASC working group. TransAtlantic Inter-Society Consensus (TASC). *J Vasc Surg* 2000; 31: S1-S296.

7. Muradin GSR, Bosch JL, Stijnen T, Hunink MGM. Balloon dilation and stent implantation for treatment of femoropopliteal arterial disease: meta-analysis. *Radiology* 2001; 221: 137-45.

8. Bachoo P, Thorpe P. Endovascular stents for intermittent claudication. *The Cochrane Database of Systematic Reviews* 2002; Issue 4: CD003228.

9. Cejna M, Thurnher S, Illiasch H, *et al.* PTA versus Palmaz stent placement in femoropopliteal artery obstructions: a multicenter prospective randomized study. *J Vasc Interv Radiol* 2001; 12: 23-31.

10. Duda SH, Bosiers M, Lammer J, *et al.* Sirolimus-eluting versus bare nitinol stent for obstructive superficial femoral artery disease: the SIROCCO II trial. *J Vasc Interv Radiol* 2005; 16: 331-8.

11. Scheinert D, Scheinert S, Sax J, *et al.* Prevalence and clinical impact of stent fractures after femoropopliteal stenting. *J Am Coll Cardiol* 2005; 45: 312-5.

12. Schillinger M, Sabeti S, Loewe C, *et al.* Percutaneous transluminal angioplasty versus stenting in the superficial femoral artery. CIRSE, Nice, September 2005.

13. Krankenberg H. FAST (Femoral Artery Stenting Trial): acute results and 6-month outcomes. Presented at TCT, Washington DC, 2004.

14. Lammer J, Dake MD, Bleyn J, *et al.* Peripheral arterial obstruction: prospective study of treatment with a transluminally placed self-expanding stent-graft. *Radiology* 2000; 217: 95-104.

15. Jahnke T, Andresen R, Müller-Hülsbeck S, *et al.* Hemobahn stent-grafts for treatment of femoropopliteal arterial obstructions: midterm results of a prospective trial. *J Vasc Interv Radiol* 2003; 14: 41-51.

16. Saxon RR, Coffman JM, Gooding JM, *et al.* Long-term results of ePTFE stent-graft versus angioplasty in the femoropopliteal artery: single center experience from a prospective, randomised trial. *J Vasc Interv Radiol* 2003; 14: 303-11.

17. Strecker EPK, Boos IBL, Göttman D, *et al.* Clopidogrel plus long-term aspirin after femoro-popliteal stenting. The CLAFS project: 1- and 2-year results. *Eur Radiol* 2004; 14: 302-8.

18. Ansel GM. Bilateral lower arterial stenting employing Reopro (BLASTER trial). Presented at TCT, Washington DC, 2004.

19. Iofina E, Radke PW, Skurzewski P, *et al.* Superiority of sirolimus eluting stent compared with intracoronary beta radiation for treatment of in-stent restenosis: a matched comparison. *Heart* 2005; 91: 1584-9.

20. Wolfram RM, Budinsky AC, Pokrajac B, *et al.* Vascular brachytherapy with 192Ir after femoropopliteal stent implantation in high-risk patients: twelve-month follow-up results from the Vienna-5 trial. *Radiology* 2005; 236: 343-51.

21. Di Marco C, Griffiths H, Goktekin O, *et al.* Drug-eluting bioabsorbable magnesium stent. *J Interv Cardiol* 2004; 17: 291-5.

Chapter 19

Bypass versus angioplasty in severe ischaemia of the leg (BASIL) trial: how might the results change practice?

Andrew W Bradbury BSc MD MBA FRCS (Ed), Professor of Vascular Surgery

Birmingham University Department of Vascular Surgery

Heart of England NHS Foundation Trust, Birmingham, UK

Introduction

In most developed countries the incidence of severe limb ischaemia (SLI), defined by the presence of rest/night pain and tissue loss (ulceration, gangrene), is estimated at 50-100/100,000 per year and leads to significant morbidity and mortality and the consumption of considerable health and social care resources [1]. The ageing population, increasing prevalence of diabetes [2], and continuing high levels of tobacco consumption mean that, despite advances in medical therapies [3], the numbers of patients requiring lower limb revascularisation for SLI in developed, and increasingly in developing, countries is likely to increase in the foreseeable future.

Numerous previous studies have attempted to compare the clinical and cost-effectiveness of the two currently available treatments; namely, bypass surgery (BSX) and balloon angioplasty (BAP). However, all have had one or more major methodological problems including: a lack of controls; small patient numbers; poorly defined patients and interventions; the inclusion, comparison and combined analysis of patients with intermittent claudication and SLI as well as with aorto-iliac and infra-inguinal disease; retrospective analysis; and short and/or incomplete follow-up [4-32]. The resulting absence of level I evidence meant continuing uncertainty as to whether BSX or BAP is associated

with a better clinical outcome, and a more effective use of healthcare resources, in patients whose leg is threatened by SLI and who are potentially suitable for both treatments [33-39].

The Bypass versus Angioplasty in Severe Ischaemia of the Leg (BASIL) trial compared for the first time within a multi-centre RCT the outcome of a 'BSX first' with a 'BAP first' strategy in terms of amputation-free survival, all-cause mortality, health-related quality of life (HRQL), post-procedure morbidity and mortality, re-interventions and use of hospital resources.

Methods

The detailed methods of the BASIL trial have been published elsewhere [40-42] (Figure 1). Briefly, between August 1999 and June 2004, 452 patients were randomised at one of 27 UK hospitals. Between October 2001 and April 2002 data were also gathered prospectively on all consecutive patients who presented with SLI, and who subsequently underwent diagnostic imaging with a view to revascularisation, at the six top-recruiting trial centres. Centres participating in the BASIL trial were asked to randomise all those patients presenting with SLI due to infra-inguinal atherosclerosis who, in the opinion of

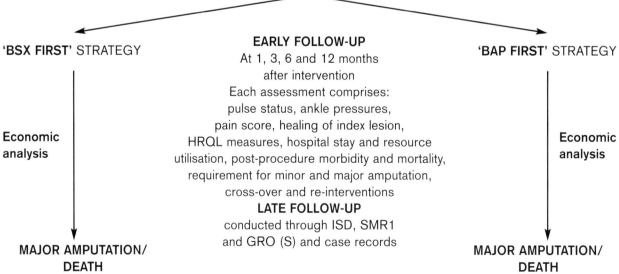

Patient presents with **SEVERE LIMB ISCHAEMIA**
Rest pain and/or tissue loss of presumed arterial aetiology for more than 2 weeks
Supra-inguinal 'inflow' considered capable of supporting infra-inguinal BSX or BAP

Research Nurse discusses trial with patient and distributes
PATIENT INFORMATION SHEET

Research Nurse completes **BASELINE ASSESSMENT FORM**
Patient completes **HRQL FORMS**

Consultant surgeon and radiologist obtain informed consent
PATIENT CONSENT FORM is completed

DIAGNOSTIC IMAGING

CONSULTANT RADIOLOGIST willing to perform infra-inguinal BAP
and **CONSULTANT SURGEON** willing to perform infra-inguinal BSX

RANDOMISATION
Stratified by centre and by clinical presentation into 4 groups

Clinical presentation	Ankle pressure ≥50mmHg	Ankle pressure <50mmHg
Rest/night pain only	A	B
Tissue loss ± rest/night pain	C	D

'BSX FIRST' STRATEGY

Economic analysis

MAJOR AMPUTATION/ DEATH

EARLY FOLLOW-UP
At 1, 3, 6 and 12 months
after intervention
Each assessment comprises:
pulse status, ankle pressures,
pain score, healing of index lesion,
HRQL measures, hospital stay and resource
utilisation, post-procedure morbidity and mortality,
requirement for minor and major amputation,
cross-over and re-interventions
LATE FOLLOW-UP
conducted through ISD, SMR1
and GRO (S) and case records

'BAP FIRST' STRATEGY

Economic analysis

MAJOR AMPUTATION/ DEATH

Figure 1. Flow diagram of BASIL trial methods. *Reproduced with permission from Elsevier* [40].

19 Bypass versus angioplasty in severe ischaemia of the leg (BASIL) trial: how might the results change practice?

155

the responsible consultant vascular surgeon and interventional radiologist, required revascularisation and were suitable for both BSX and BAP. Randomisation to either a 'BSX first' or a 'BAP first' strategy (one-to-one ratio) was stratified by centre, and then by clinical presentation and ankle pressure into four groups (Figure 1). Responsible consultants were encouraged to use their normal preferred techniques and equipment.

The primary endpoint was amputation-free survival (of the trial leg) (AFS) and secondary endpoints were all-cause mortality (ACM), post-procedure morbidity and mortality, re-interventions, health-related quality of life (HRQL), and the use of hospital resources. Self-reported HRQL was measured using the EuroQoL 5-D (EQ5D) and the Short Form 36 (SF-36) at baseline and at three, six and 12 months after randomisation [43-47]. Patient-specific hospital use was measured using the duration of hospital stay as an aggregate unit of services provided in the in-patient hospital setting. Costs were estimated as follows: £421 per vascular ward day, £591 per high dependency unit (HDU) day, £1526 per intensive therapy unit (ITU) days, BSX (£3104) and BAP (£1159) (both average procedure costs) [48-49].

BASIL trial and survey results

In the survey, 456 (272 men and 184 women of median [range] age 75 [33-99] years) consecutive patients presented with SLI due to infra-inguinal disease to the top six recruiting centres (who between them recruited 61% of the trial patients) and underwent diagnostic imaging, usually angiography, with a view to revascularisation either by means of BSX or BAP. Of the 236 (52%) patients who underwent revascularisation, 70 (29%) were considered suitable for randomisation; and of these, 22 refused trial entry and 48 (69%) were randomised.

In the trial, 195/228 (86%) patients randomised to BSX and 216/224 (96%) randomised to BAP underwent an attempt at their allocated treatment at a median (inter-quartile range) of six (3-16) and six (2-20) days (not significant, NS). Patient baseline characteristics are shown in Table 1. By the close of follow-up on 28th February 2005, 99% of patients had been followed-up for one year, 74% for two years, 48% for three years, 22% for four years and

8% for five years. At that point, 248 (55%) patients were alive with their trial leg intact, 38 (8%) were alive with their trial leg amputated, 36 (8%) had died subsequent to having their trial leg amputated and 130 (29%) had died with their trial leg intact.

The 30-day mortality after BSX was 5%, and after BAP was 3%, whether analysed by intention to treat or by first treatment received. A total of 110/195 (57%) BSX patients and 89/216 (41%) BAP patients had one or more complications within 30 days of their intervention. Of the 228 patients randomised to BSX, 195 underwent attempted BSX (Figure 2). The immediate failure rate was 5/195 (2.6%); two bypasses were abandoned and in a further three cases the graft was not running at the end of the procedure. Two patients had successful endarterectomy rather than bypass (Table 2). Four patients who had been randomised to BAP underwent successful BSX as their first intervention. By 12 months, 85/195 attempted BSX had resulted in clinical failure defined by death (n=29), major amputation (n=20) or a return or persistence of symptoms (rest pain, tissue loss) in the trial (operated) leg or the finding of a technical problem with the graft on surveillance (n=36). Of the latter group, 33 went on to have a second intervention, which in most cases was BAP. Further interventions, amputations and deaths over the first 12 months are shown in Figure 2.

Of the 224 patients randomised to BAP, 216 underwent attempted BAP (Figure 3). In the opinion of the vascular interventional radiologist undertaking the procedure, 43 (20%) of these were immediate technical failures. The anatomic extent and type of BAP performed in the 203 patients in whom a guidewire was passed across at least part of the disease to be treated, are shown in Table 3. In addition, 21 patients allocated to BSX crossed over and underwent attempted BAP as their first intervention; of these, five were immediate failures.

By 12 months, 109/216 attempted BAP had resulted in clinical failure as defined by death (n=21), amputation (n=16) or a return or persistence of symptoms (rest pain, tissue loss) (n=72) in the trial leg. Of these, 59 went on to have a second intervention, which in most cases was BSX. Further interventions, amputations and deaths within 12 months of randomisation are shown in Figure 3. Following randomisation to, and attempted BSX,

Table 1. Baseline characteristics of patients randomised in the BASIL trial. *Reproduced with permission from Elsevier* [40].

Allocated strategy		BAP first	BSX first
Characteristic		n=224	n=228
Male		57%	62%
Age	under 70 years	30%	35%
	70-79 years	46%	39%
	80 years or more	24%	26%
Trial leg = right		46%	43%
Smoking status	Never smoked	21%	18%
	Current smoker	32%	40%
	Ex-smoker (not smoked for >1 yr)	46%	42%
Diabetes	Not known to be diabetic	58%	58%
	Insulin-dependent	17%	17%
	Non-insulin-dependent	25%	25%
Angina		19%	18%
Previous myocardial infarction		20%	15%
Previous stroke/transient ischaemic attack		18%	25%
Previous intervention in trial leg		18%	12%
Previous intervention in other leg		16%	21%
Symptomatic arterial disease in other leg?	No	67%	64%
	Yes - intermittent claudication*	9%	11%
	Yes - severe limb ischaemia	23%	26%
Rest/night pain only in trial leg		92%	90%
Tissue loss (ulcer and/or gangrene) in trial leg		75%	73%
Randomisation stratification group			
A: rest/night pain only; ankle pressure ≥50mmHg		20%	21%
B: rest/night pain only; ankle pressure <50mmHg		4%	6%
C: tissue loss ± rest/night pain; ankle pressure ≥50mmHg		48%	50%
D: tissue loss ± rest/night pain; ankle pressure <50mmHg		27%	23%
On a statin**		34%	33%
On drug treatment for hypertension		63%	59%
On antiplatelet agent***		54%	62%
Mean creatinine (standard deviation) (μmol/l)		113 (62)	116 (95)

* Intermittent claudication refers to pain in leg on walking but not at rest or at night, no tissue loss;

** for hypercholesterolaemia;

*** in most cases aspirin 75mg daily

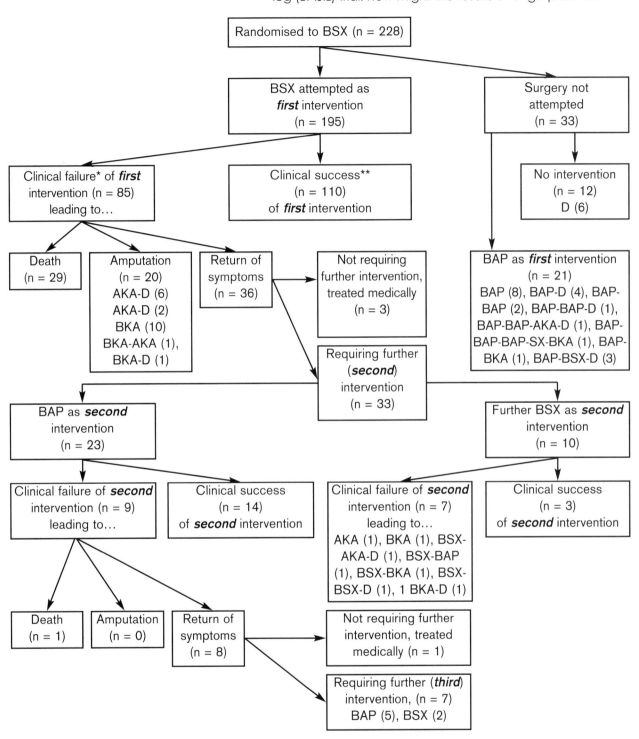

*Clinical failure of an intervention is defined as death, amputation of trial leg, return or persistence of symptoms (rest pain/tissue loss), whether or not further intervention is required, by 12 months from randomisation

**Clinical success of an intervention is defined as patient alive with trial leg intact without further intervention at 12 months

Figures in italics describe all patient events (BSX, bypass surgery; BAP, balloon angioplasty; BKA, below knee amputation; AKA, above knee amputation; D, death; NI, no intervention) during the first 12 months from randomisation. A dash is used to separate the stages, so for example, in the bottom box of Figure 3 entitled "Requiring further (third) intervention, (n = 9)", the term "2 BSX-BSX-BKA" means that of those who require a third intervention two had further surgery (3rd intervention), then more surgery (4th intervention), then a BKA (5th intervention). Then, because there is no "-D" at the end, these 2 patients were alive at 12 months after randomisation.

Figure 2. Trial profile of patients randomised to BSX: early (12-month) follow-up. *Reproduced with permission from Elsevier* [40].

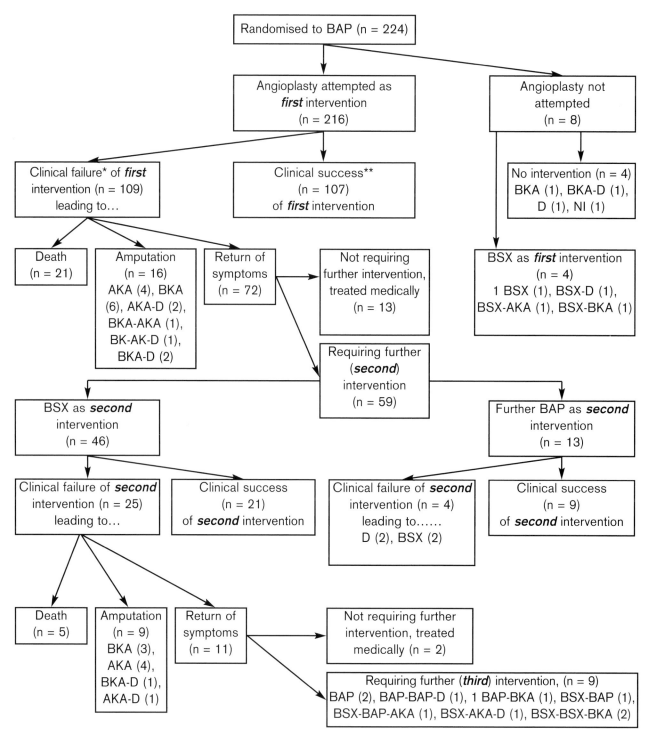

Figure 3. Trial profile of patients randomised to BAP: early (12-month) follow-up. *Reproduced with permission from Elsevier* [40].

*Clinical failure of an intervention is defined as death, amputation of trial leg, return or persistence of symptoms (rest pain/tissue loss), whether or not further intervention is required, by 12 months from randomisation

**Clinical success of an intervention is defined as patient alive with trial leg intact without further intervention at 12 months

Figures in italics describe all patient events (BSX, bypass surgery; BAP, balloon angioplasty; BKA, below knee amputation; AKA, above knee amputation; D, death; NI, no intervention) during the first 12 months from randomisation. A dash is used to separate the stages, so for example, in the bottom box of Figure 3 entitled "Requiring further (third) intervention, (n = 9)", the term "2 BSX-BSX-BKA" means that of those who require a third intervention two had further surgery (3rd intervention), then more surgery (4th intervention), then a BKA (5th intervention). Then, because there is no "-D" at the end, these 2 patients were alive at 12 months after randomisation.

Table 2. Anatomic extent and type of BSX. *Reproduced with permission from Elsevier* [40].

	Prosthetic (ePTFE or Dacron) bypass	Ipsilateral GSV non-reversed vein bypass	Ipsilateral GSV reverse vein bypass	Non-ipsilateral GSV vein bypass	Composite (prosthetic and vein) bypass	Total
Femoral-AK-PA	23	5	30	0	4	62
Femoral-BK-PA	11	17	33	1	2	64
Femoral-CA	1	22	20	3	5	51
PA-CA	0	1	6	2	0	9
AK-to-BK-PA	0	0	1	0	0	1
IA-AKP	1	0	0	0	0	1
	36	45	90	6	11	188

GSV = great saphenous vein; ePTFE = Expanded PolyTetraFluoroEthylene; AK = above knee; BK = below knee; PA = popliteal artery; IA = iliac artery

Four patients randomised to angioplasty crossed over to surgery: Fem-BKPA PTFE bypass graft; Fem-BKPA *in situ* vein graft; CIA-BKPA Dacron bypass graft; Fem-AKPA reverse vein graft

Table 3. Anatomic extent and type of BAP. *Reproduced with permission from Elsevier* [40].

Vessel(s) treated	Transluminal	Sub-intimal	Combined	Total
SFA only	22	31	4	57
PA only	8	9	2	19
CA only	2	2	0	4
SFA + PA	22	44	6	72
SFA + PA + CA	8	9	10	27
SFA + CA	3	1	3	7
PA + CA	8	5	3	16
PFA	1	0	0	1
	74	101	28	203

SFA = superficial femoral artery; PA = popliteal artery; CA = crural artery (posterior tibial and/or anterior tibial and/or peroneal arteries); PFA = profunda femoris artery (deep femoral artery)

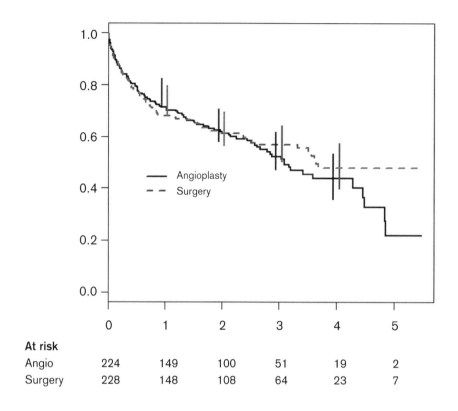

Figure 4. Amputation-free survival following BSX and BAP by intention to treat. *Reproduced with permission from Elsevier* [40].

109/195 (56%) patients were alive with the trial leg intact at 12 months without further intervention. This compares with 107/216 (50%) patients following randomisation to, and attempted BAP. Looking at the follow-up as a whole by intention to treat, BSX was associated with a lower re-intervention rate (41/224, 18.3%) than BAP (59/228, 25.9%); a difference of 7.6% (95% CI 0.04%, 15.12%). When analysed by the first intervention received, the difference between re-intervention following BSX (33/199, 16.6%) and BAP is greater (67/237, 28.3%); a difference of 11.7% (95% CI 3.9%, 19.2%).

Figures 4 and 5 show Kaplan-Meier survival curves to the primary endpoint (AFS) and the secondary endpoint of ACM. Up to six months, there was a trend towards an increased hazard with BSX relative to BAP in terms of ACM, whereas after six months there was a trend towards a reduced hazard with BSX in terms of AFS and ACM (Table 4). In the period beyond two years from randomisation, there was a

significantly reduced hazard in terms of AFS (adjusted HR 0.37 [95% CI 0.17, 0.77], p=0.008) and ACM (adjusted HR 0.34 [95% CI, 0.17, 0.71], p=0.004) for BSX relative to BAP.

Patients in both treatment groups reported improved EQ5D and SF36 physical component summary scores by three months [8]. Although this was largely sustained during follow-up, little further improvement was observed beyond three months. There were no significant differences in HRQL when the two treatment groups are compared. This finding is consistent across the three HRQL scores. In terms of hospital resources used during the first 12 months, although there was no difference in the number of hospital admissions, patients randomised to BSX spent significantly longer in hospital and required significantly more HDU and ITU care than those randomised to BAP. Thus, 23% of patients randomised to BSX required HDU and 4% required ITU care during the first 12 months of follow-up

19 Bypass versus angioplasty in severe ischaemia of the
leg (BASIL) trial: how might the results change practice?

161

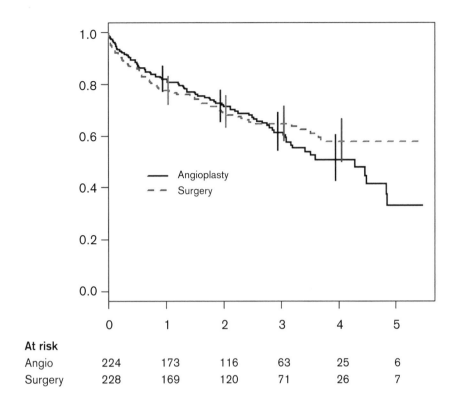

Figure 5. All-cause mortality following BSX and BAP by intention to treat. *Reproduced with permission from Elsevier* [40].

At risk

Angio	224	173	116	63	25	6
Surgery	228	169	120	71	26	7

Table 4. Comparison of hazard of AFS and ACM. *Reproduced with permission from Elsevier* [40].

	Number of events		Hazard ratio from Cox regression model (95% CI)	
	BAP	BSX	surgery relative to angioplasty	
Amputation-free survival (primary endpoint)				
Period	n=224	n=228	Unadjusted	Adjusted*
Whole follow-up period	106	98	0.89 (0.68, 1.17)	0.88 (0.66, 1.16)
Up to 6 months	46	50	1.07 (0.72, 1.6)	1.04 (0.69, 1.56)
After 6 months	60	48	0.75 (0.51, 1.1)	0.73 (0.49, 1.07)
After 2 years**	28	16	0.44 (0.22, 0.88)	0.37 (0.17, 0.77)
All-cause mortality (secondary endpoint)				
Period	n=224	n=228	Unadjusted	Adjusted*
Whole follow-up period	87	79	0.90 (0.66, 1.22)	0.95 (0.69, 1.29)
Up to 6 months	26	31	1.20 (0.71, 2.02)	1.27 (0.75, 2.15)
After 6 months	61	48	0.78 (0.53, 1.13)	0.81 (0.55, 1.19)
After 2 years**	27	11	0.38 (0.19, 0.77)	0.34 (0.17, 0.71)

* adjusted for age, sex, stratification group, BMI, current or ex-smoker, creatinine, diabetes, statin use at baseline

** *post hoc* analysis conducted after examination of the survival curves

compared with 0.5% and 7% of patients randomised to BAP. The mean cost of in-patient hospital treatment during the first 12 months of follow-up in patients randomised to a BSX first strategy has been estimated as £23,322 (£20,096 hospital stay and £3,225 procedure costs), which is approximately a third higher than the £17,419 (£15,381 hospital stay and £2,039 procedure costs) for patients randomised to a BAP first strategy.

How should these new data affect practice?

The principal finding of the BASIL trial is that, up to two years, BSX and BAP first strategies appear to be associated with broadly similar outcomes in terms of AFS, ACM and HRQL. However, this equivalence does not necessarily mean that the two strategies are equal, or equally appropriate for every patient. In the short term, a BSX first strategy is associated with significantly increased morbidity and length of stay in hospital, resulting in higher hospital costs in the first 12 months. However, the 30-day mortality was low and not significantly higher than that observed following BAP. The 30-day technical failure rate was also very low. Furthermore, after two years, BSX appeared to be associated with a significantly reduced risk of future amputation and/or death. This suggests that, despite the increased short-term morbidity, patients may enjoy a more durable benefit from a BSX than a BAP first strategy. In addition, although surgery may be more expensive in the short term, if BSX is associated with fewer re-interventions and amputations, then it may well represent the cheaper option in the long term. By contrast, a BAP first strategy was associated with a much higher immediate failure (c.20%) and re-intervention rate than BSX. Overall, approximately a half of the attempted BAP failed within the first 12 months and over half of these patients went on to have BSX as a second procedure. As such, the intention to treat nature of the primary analyses may make the short-term results of a BAP first strategy appear at first sight considerably better than they really are. Thus, it would appear that a significant number of patients treated primarily with BAP, had to cross over to surgery shortly afterwards in order to keep their limb.

Although not primarily the subject of the trial, it is worth noting how few patients were on antiplatelet

agents and statin therapy, and how many patients were still smoking, upon entry to the trial. This is an observation that has been made and commented upon in other recent studies looking at similar groups of patients [51]. There is clear evidence that so-called best medical therapy (BMT) comprising antiplatelet agents, smoking cessation and lipid lowering therapy can halt, even reverse, the development and progression of lower limb arterial disease and is associated with a significant reduction in future cardiovascular events, including the need for limb-salvage intervention (BSX and BAP) and amputation [3]. One can only speculate as to how many of the BASIL trial patients, had they been receiving BMT, would have avoided developing SLI and its consequences. It is also probable that more aggressive BMT would have improved the results of the trial interventions. Improving the medical management of patients with, and at risk of developing, SLI would seem to be an urgent priority in primary and secondary care.

In summary, the short to medium-term results of the BASIL trial indicate that patients presenting with SLI due to infra-inguinal atherosclerosis, and who appear technically suitable for both BSX and BAP, can reasonably be treated with either modality in the first instance, depending on individual patient characteristics and local expertise. However, notwithstanding the high failure and re-intervention rate associated with BAP, one could argue that patients who are expected to live for only one to two years, have no vein, but do have significant comorbidity, should be offered BAP first. If the procedure fails (a one in five risk), the patient may not be disadvantaged and can go on to have BSX if it is considered appropriate. It also appears to be a less expensive option in this patient group, at least in the short term. By contrast, in patients expected to live more than one to two years, and who are considered fit for surgery, and who have a useable vein, the low mortality, low technical failure rate, superior durability, and reduced re-intervention rate associated with BSX probably outweighs short-term considerations of increased morbidity and cost. Indeed, BSX may turn out to be the cheaper option in the longer term. It is intended to follow-up this unique cohort of patients for another 30 months (August 2007) so that these provisional conclusions can be refined and made with greater certainty or, alternatively, refuted.

19 Bypass versus angioplasty in severe ischaemia of the leg (BASIL) trial: how might the results change practice?

163

The BASIL trial also clearly indicates that, almost regardless of what treatment is received, many patients with SLI have an extremely poor prognosis in terms of major limb amputation, death and HRQL. Furthermore, the BASIL survey suggests that almost a half of all patients presenting with SLI due to infra-inguinal disease to major UK vascular units, and who undergo angiography with a view to revascularisation, are considered unsuitable and/or unfit for either BSX or BAP. Thus for many patients, SLI is essentially an untreatable condition with a prognosis similar to that of metastatic carcinoma. As in oncology, it seems clear that the only way of improving the overall burden of SLI is to diagnose and treat, largely medically, lower limb ischaemia at a much earlier stage.

Summary

◆ The numbers of patients presenting with severe limb ischaemia and requiring revascularisation is likely to grow substantially worldwide in the future.

◆ The BASIL trial is the first randomised controlled trial to compare a surgery first with an angioplasty first strategy for severe limb ischaemia.

◆ The BASIL trial has shown that angioplasty is associated with less morbidity and cost in the short term, but a significantly higher immediate and short-term failure rate than surgery.

◆ By contrast, surgery is associated with a lower technical failure rate and better durability, but is associated with a greater use of hospital resources over the first 12 months.

◆ In patients with limited life expectancy and significant comorbidity, angioplasty is probably the first treatment of choice.

◆ However, in patients expected to live more that two years and who have useable vein for a bypass, surgery is associated with a better medium to long-term outcome in terms of all-cause mortality and amputation-free survival.

◆ The medical management of patients with severe limb ischaemia is often inadequate in both primary and secondary care.

References

1. TASC. Management of peripheral arterial disease (PAD). TransAtlantic Inter-Society Consensus (TASC). Section D: chronic critical limb ischaemia. *Eur J Vasc Endovasc Surg* 2000; 19: Suppl A: S144-243.

2. Cavanagh PR, Lipsky BA, Bradbury AW, Botek G. Treatment for diabetic foot ulcers. *Lancet* 2005: 366(9498):1725-35.

3. Burns P, Gough S, Bradbury AW. Management of peripheral arterial disease in primary care. *Br Med J* 2003; 326: 584-8.

4. Alber M, Romiti M, Brochado-Neto FC, Pereira CAB. Meta-analysis of alternate autogenous vein bypass grafts to infrapopliteal arteries. *J Vasc Surg* 2005; 42: 449-55.

5. Wolfle KD, Bruijnen H, Loeprecht H, Rumenapf G, Schweiger H, Grabitz K, Sandmann W, Lauterjung L, Largiader J, Erasmi H, Kasprzak PM, Raithel D, Allenberg JR, Lauber A, Berlakovich GM, Kretschmer G, Hepp W, Becker HM, Schulz A. Graft patency and clinical outcome of femorodistal arterial reconstruction in diabetic and non-diabetic patients: results of a multi-centre comparative analysis. *Eur J Vasc Endovasc Surg* 2003; 25: 229-34.

6.   van der Zaag ES, Legemate DA, Prins MH, Reekers JA, Jacobs MJ. Angioplasty or bypass for superficial femoral artery disease? A randomised controlled trial. *Eur J Vasc Endovasc Surg* 2004; 28: 132-7.

7.   Hobbs SD, Yapanis M, Burns PJ, Wilmink AB, Bradbury AW, Adam DJ. Peri-operative myocardial injury in patients undergoing surgery for critical limb ischaemia. *Eur J Vasc Endovasc Surg* 2005; 29: 301-4.

8.   Giswold ME, Landry GJ, Sexton GJ, Yeager RA, Edwards JM, Taylor LM Jr, Moneta GL. Modifiable patient factors are associated with reverse vein graft occlusion in the era of duplex scan surveillance. *J Vasc Surg* 2003; 37: 47-53.

9.   Nguyen LL, Conte MS, Menard MT, Gravereaux EC, Chew DK, Donaldson MC, Whittemore AD, Belkin M. Infrainguinal vein bypass graft revision: factors affecting long-term outcome. *J Vasc Surg* 2004; 40: 916-23.

10. Ishii Y, Gossage JA, Dourado R, Sabharwal T, Burnand KG. Minimum internal diameter of the greater saphenous vein is an important determinant of successful femorodistal bypass grafting that is independent of the quality of the runoff. *Vascular* 2004; 12: 225-32.

11. Papavassiliou VG, Walker SR, Bolia A, Fishwick G, London N. Techniques for the endovascular management of complications following lower limb percutaneous transluminal angioplasty. *Eur J Vasc Endovasc Surg* 2003; 25: 125-30.

12. Lipsitz EC, Ohki T, Veith FJ, Rhee SJ, Kurvers H, Timaran C, Gargiulo NJ, Suggs WD, Wain RA. Fate of collateral vessels following subintimal angioplasty. *J Endovasc Therapy* 2004; 11: 269-73.

13. Lipsitz EC, Veith FJ, Ohki T. The value of subintimal angioplasty in the management of critical lower extremity ischemia: failure is not always associated with a rethreatened limb. *J Cardiovasc Surg* 2004; 45: 231-7.

14. Bates MC, Aburahma AF. An update on endovascular therapy of the lower extremities. *J Endovasc Therapy* 2004; 11 Suppl 2: 107-27.

15. Baird RN, Bradley MD, Murphy KP. Tibioperoneal angioplasty and bypass. *Acta Chirurg Belgica* 2003; 103: 383-7.

16. Bradbury AW. Angioplasty is the first-line treatment for critical limb ischaemia: the case against. In: *Vascular and Endovascular Controversies*. Greenhalgh RM, Ed. WB Saunders, 2003: 295-307 (25th Charing Cross International Symposium 2003).

17. Loftus IM, Hayes PD, Bell PR. Subintimal angioplasty in lower limb ischaemia. *J Cardiovasc Surg* 2004; 45: 217-29.

18. Salas CA, Adam DJ, Papavassiliou VG, London NJ. Percutaneous transluminal angioplasty for critical limb ischaemia in octogenarians and nonagenarians. *Eur J Vasc Endovasc Surg* 2004; 28: 142-5.

19. Treiman GS. Subintimal angioplasty for infrainguinal occlusive disease. *Surg Clin N Am* 2004; 84: 1365-80.

20. Wolf GL, Wilson SE, Cross AP. Percutaneous transluminal angioplasty versus operation for peripheral arteriosclerosis. *J Vasc Surg* 1989; 9: 1-9.

21. Holm J, Arfridsson B. Chronic lower limb ischaemia. A prospective randomised controlled trial comparing the 1-year results of vascular surgery and percutaneous transluminal angioplasty (PTA). *Eur J Vasc Surg* 1991; 5: 517-22.

22. Nasr MK, McCarthy RJ, Hardman J, Chalmers A, Horrocks M. The increasing role of percutaneous transluminal angioplasty in the primary management of critical limb ischaemia. *Eur J Vasc Endovasc Surg* 2002; 23: 398-403.

23. Roddy SP, Darling RC 3rd, Maharaj D, Chang BB, Paty PS, Kreienberg PB, Lloyd WE, Ozsvath K, Shah DM. Gender-related differences in outcome: an analysis of 5880 infrainguinal arterial reconstructions. *J Vasc Surg* 2003; 37: 399-402.

24. Al-Omran M, Tu JV, Johnston KW, Mamdani MM, Kucey DS. Outcome of revascularization procedures for peripheral arterial occlusive disease in Ontario between 1991 and 1998: a population-based study. *J Vasc Surg* 2003; 38: 279-88.

25. Saketkhoo RR, Razavi MK, Padidar A, Kee ST, Sze DY, Dake MD. Percutaneous bypass: subintimal recanalization of peripheral occlusive disease with IVUS guided luminal re-entry. *Tech Vasc Intervent Radiol* 2004; 7: 23-7.

26. Desgranges P, Boufi M, Lapeyre M, Tarquini G, van Laere O, Losy F, Melliere D, Becquemin JP, Kobeiter H. Subintimal angioplasty: feasible and durable. *Eur J Vasc Endovasc Surg* 2004; 28: 138-41.

27. Clair DG, Dayal R, Faries PL, Bernheim J, Nowygrod R, Lantis JC 2nd, Beavers FP, Kent KC. Tibial angioplasty as an alternative strategy in patients with limb-threatening ischemia. *Ann Vasc Surg* 2005; 19: 63-8.

28. Atar E, Siegel Y, Avrahami R, Bartal G, Bachar GN, Belenky A. Balloon angioplasty of popliteal and crural arteries in elderly with critical chronic limb ischemia. *Eur J Radiol* 2005; 53: 287-92.

29. Surowiec SM, Davies MG, Eberly SW, Rhodes JM, Illig KA, Shortell CK, Lee DE. Waldman DL, Green RM. Percutaneous angioplasty and stenting of the superficial femoral artery. *J Vasc Surg* 41: 269-78.

30. Trocciola SM, Chaer R, Dayal R, Lin SC, Kumar N, Rhee J, Pierce M, Ryer EJ, McKinsey J, Morrissey NJ, Bush HL, Kent KC, Faries PL. Comparison of results in endovascular interventions for infrainguinal lesions: claudication versus critical limb ischemia. *American Surgeon* 2005; 71: 474-80.

31. Tefera G, Hoch J. Turnipseed WD. Limb-salvage angioplasty in vascular surgery practice. *J Vasc Surg* 2005; 41: 988-93.

32. Tartari S, Zattoni L, Rolma G, Sacco A. Subintimal angioplasty of infrapopliteal artery occlusions in the treatment of critical limb ischaemia. Short-term results. *Radiologia Medica* 2004; 108: 265-74.

33. Leng GC, Davis M, Baker D. Bypass surgery for chronic lower limb ischaemia. *Cochrane Database of Systematic Reviews* 2000; (3): CD002000.

34. Jackson MJ, Wolfe JH. Are infra-inguinal angioplasty and surgery comparable? *Acta Chirurgica Belgica* 2001; 101: 6-10.

35. Bradbury AW, Ruckley CV. Angioplasty for lower limb ischaemia: time for randomised controlled trials. *Lancet* 1996; 347: 277-8.

36. Bradbury AW, Bell J, Lee AJ, Prescott RJ, Gillespie I, Stansby G, Fowkes FG. Bypass or angioplasty for severe limb ischaemia? A Delphi Consensus Study. *Eur J Vasc Endovasc Surg* 2002; 24: 411-6.

19 Bypass versus angioplasty in severe ischaemia of the leg (BASIL) trial: how might the results change practice?

165

37. Schermerhorn ML, Cronenwett JL, Baldwin JC. Open surgical repair versus endovascular therapy for chronic lower-extremity occlusive disease. *Ann Rev Med* 2003; 54: 269-83.

38. Bradbury A, Wilmink T, Lee AJ, Bell J, Prescott R, Gillespie I, Stansby G, Fowkes FG. Bypass versus angioplasty to treat severe limb ischemia: factors that affect treatment preferences of UK surgeons and interventional radiologists. *J Vasc Surg* 2004; 39: 1026-32.

39. Tsetis D, Belli AM. The role of infrapopliteal angioplasty. *Br J Radiol* 2004; 77:1007-15.

40. The BASIL Trial Participants. Bypass versus angioplasty in severe ischaemia of the leg (BASIL): multi-centre, randomised controlled trial. *Lancet* 2005; 366: 1925-34.

41. Wolfe JHN, Wyatt MG. Critical and sub-critical limb ischaemia. *Eur J Vasc Endovasc Surg* 1997; 13: 578-82.

42. Caruana MF. Bradbury AW. Adam DJ. The validity, reliability, reproducibility and extended utility of ankle to brachial pressure index in current vascular surgical practice. *Eur J Vasc Endovasc Surg* 2005; 29: 443-51.

43. EuroQol Group. EuroQol: a new facility for the measurement of health-related quality of life. *Health Policy* 1990; 16: 199-208.

44. Ware JE, Sherbourne CD. The MOS 36-item short-form health survey (SF-36): conceptual framework and item selection. *Med Care* 1992; 30: 473-83.

45. Dolan P. Modeling valuations for EuroQol health states. *Med Care* 1997; 35: 1095-108.

46. Ware JE, Kosinski M, Dewey JE. *How to score version two of the SF-36® health survey*. Lincoln, RI: Quality Metric, 2000.

47. Abadie A, Drukker D, Herr JL, Imbens GW. Implementing matching estimators for average treatment effects in Stata. *The Stata Journal* 2004; 4: 290-311.

48. NHS National Services Scotland. Scottish Health Service Costs, Year Ended 31st March, 2004. Edinburgh: Information Services Division, NHS National Services Scotland, 2004.

49. Michaels J, Brazier J, Palfreyman S, Shackley P, Slack R. Cost and outcome implications of the organisation of vascular services. *Health Technology Assessment* 2000; 4: 11.

50. Hernandez-Osma E, Cairols MA, Marti X, Barjau E, Riera S. Impact of treatment on the quality of life in patients with critical limb ischaemia. *Eur J Vasc Endovasc Surg* 2002; 23: 491-4.

51. Conte MS, Bandyk DF, Clowes AW, Moneta GL, Namini H, Seely L. Risk factors, medical therapies and peri-operative events in limb salvage surgery: observations from the PREVENT III multicentre trial. *J Vasc Surg* 2005; 42: 456-65.

Chapter 20

CryoPlasty and pharmacomanipulation: current evidence and future developments

Ralph W Jackson MB BS MRCP FRCR, Consultant Vascular and Interventional Radiologist
Northern Vascular Centre, Freeman Hospital, Newcastle-upon-Tyne, UK
James E McCaslin MB BS MRCS (Eng), Vascular Research Fellow
Queen Elizabeth Hospital, Gateshead, UK

Introduction

This chapter will discuss two very different approaches to the continuing problem of restenosis following femoropopliteal angioplasty and stenting. The ultimate aim is to stop vascular smooth muscle cell (VSMC) proliferation to prevent neointimal hyperplasia (NIH). CryoPlasty is the application of cold thermal energy to the vessel wall during conventional angioplasty. The evidence for its use, possible mechanisms of action and applications will be described. For the purposes of this chapter, pharmacomanipulation will include the evidence for local and systemic delivery of drugs with particular reference to drug-eluting stents (DES).

CryoPlasty

Equipment and technique

There is currently only one commercially available system for CryoPlasty. The PolarCath™ was developed by Cryovascular Systems Inc. (Los Gatos, Ca, USA), which has recently been acquired by Boston Scientific. The system consists of a balloon catheter, nitrous oxide cylinder and an inflation unit (Figure 1). The balloon catheter has a coaxial shaft with two concentric, non-compliant balloons, 'balloon within a balloon design'. A vacuum is applied between the two layers. Nitrous oxide is used to inflate the balloon which has radio-opaque markings to aid balloon placement and help visualise proper

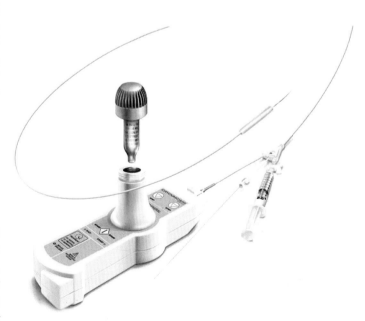

Figure 1. PolarCath™ peripheral dilatation system.
Courtesy of Boston Scientific.

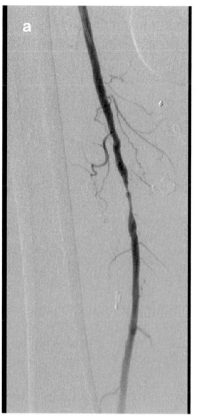 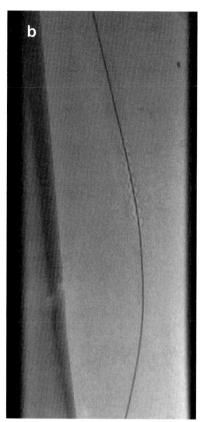 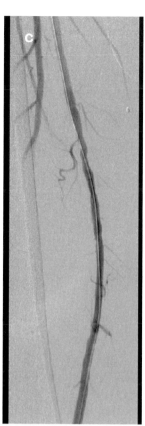

Figure 2. a) Straightforward recurrent mid-SFA stenosis. b) The markers on the balloon make it visible during inflation with nitrous oxide. c) Following CryoPlasty there is an excellent result.

expansion of the inflated balloon. This is because the nitrous oxide is a negative contrast agent (Figure 2). The microprocessor controlled inflation unit regulates inflation pressure which is stepped up to 8 atmospheres. The nitrous oxide enters the balloon as a liquid and then changes to a gas causing an endothermic reaction resulting in a balloon surface temperature of minus 10°C. The dilating and cooling phase lasts 20 seconds. There is then a passive warming phase after which the balloon is manually deflated and removed. Each inflation of the balloon requires a new nitrous oxide cylinder.

The PolarCath™ is indicated to treat iliac, femoral, popliteal, infrapopliteal, renal and subclavian arteries. It is also indicated for the treatment of polytetrafluoroethylene (PTFE) access grafts and native arteriovenous dialysis fistulae. The catheters for femoropopliteal applications use a standard 0.035" wire and come in 4-8mm diameters. Sheath requirements are between 5 and 8 French and

balloon lengths are 2, 4 and 6cm on 80 or 120cm shafts. The tibial balloons use an 0.014" wire, have diameters of 2.5 to 4mm and are 135cm long.

Proposed mechanisms of action for CryoPlasty

It has been proposed by the manufacturers that CryoPlasty may have a beneficial effect when compared with conventional angioplasty by being a more benign way of dilating vessels. The three main mechanisms are:

- altered plaque response due to ice formation weakening the plaque, allowing a more uniform vessel dilatation and less medial injury;
- reduced elastic recoil and significant dissection because of temporary vessel 'solidification', reducing elasticity and therefore a lower need for stenting;

♦ induction of apoptosis in VSMCs, leading to reduced NIH and negative remodelling.

What evidence is there for these claims and why may apoptosis be important?

Effect of freezing injury on arteries

The practice of freezing tissues to very low temperatures either for preservation (e.g. sperm donation) or ablation (e.g. liver metastases) is well established. Many factors determine the tissue response to freezing, including the rate of freezing and thawing, final temperature and duration, presence of cryoprotectants and the specific properties of the tissue. There is less knowledge about the effect on the arteries and much of it comes from animal or *in vitro* experiments. Initial cryotherapy studies *in vivo* by Gage *et al* showed the response to arterial freezing in dogs to be benign and largely devoid of neointimal proliferation [1]. Cheema *et al* studied rabbit iliac arteries treated with CryoPlasty at minus 26°C compared to standard angioplasty [2]. There was early arterial wall cell loss, but late intimal hyperplasia and vascular fibrosis, with no late beneficial effects on lumen area compared to balloon angioplasty alone. Grassl and Bischof examined the response to CryoPlasty between human, pig and rat VSMCs, either in suspension or a tissue-equivalent model [3]. They found that pig and human cells responded similarly and that cells in the tissue-equivalent model were more sensitive than in suspension after treatment at minus 11°C (30% vs. 70% viability). Tatsutani *et al* evaluated *in vitro* human coronary endothelial cell and SMC survival and apoptosis rates in response to hypothermia and freezing [4]. Below 20°C most cells were killed. Cell proliferation was largely unaffected by temperatures ranging from zero to minus 10°C and between minus 15 and minus 20°C, proliferation was reduced. Apoptosis rates of 20-40% were seen at minus 10°C.

Apoptosis

Apoptosis, or programmed cell death, describes the ordered process of dismantling and phagocytosis of cell structures, based on morphological events that distinguish it from necrosis. There is overlap between the two processes, but due to minimal disruption of cell membranes or release of lysosomal enzymes during apoptosis, there is little inflammation. Necrosis may, however, follow on if there is a failure to clear the apoptotic bodies. Normal human vessels show very low rates of VSMC apoptosis and proliferation. In atherosclerotic arteries, however, the presence of inflammatory cells and cytokines and changes in blood flow alter the balance and apoptosis may become predominant. VSMC apoptosis has, therefore, been implicated in plaque rupture, due to thinning of the cap, and aneurysm formation. Apoptosis, however, can be localised within the vessel wall due to heterogeneous sensitivity of the VSMCs [5, 6].

Acute vascular injury causes apoptosis and this is not unique to CryoPlasty. In humans, where there has been restenosis after conventional angioplasty, both increased and decreased rates of apoptosis have been found. Statins are also able to induce apoptosis [7]. There is some evidence that neointimal cells are more susceptible than media VSMCs to apoptosis and that statins preferentially induce apoptosis in neointimal VSMCs. A peak of VSMC apoptosis in animal models is seen within hours of angioplasty with a second peak days to weeks later. Using an atherosclerotic rabbit model, however, Durand found the peak of neointimal and medial apoptosis at seven days preceded by cell proliferation [8]. The presence of apoptosis was inversely related to restenosis due to positive remodeling, possibly because of reduced collagen synthesis.

Clinical use in humans

There are two fully published human studies of CryoPlasty in the femoropopliteal segment [9, 10]. Table 1 shows a summary of the findings of the two trials. The initial report consisted of 15 patients treated with an early model of the CryoPlasty system [9]. A lower inflation pressure of six atmospheres was used. The majority of patients were claudicants (13/15) with predominantly stenoses (10/15). The proportion of diabetics was high at 60%. Fourteen of the 15 lesions (93%) were successfully treated with CryoPlasty alone. One patient was left with a 50% residual stenosis and significant dissection. Two patients were

Table 1. Summary of human trials of CryoPlasty.

	M Fava JVIR 2004 [9]	J Laird JVIR 2005 [10]
Number of patients	15	102
Claudicants	87%	100%
Diabetics	60%	31%
Occlusions	33%	15%
CryoPlasty alone success	93%	85%
Primary patency		
6 month Angio n=14	100%	
9 month Doppler n=90		70%
14 month Angio n=9	83%	

excluded from follow-up, due to other procedural complications. Twelve patients, therefore, had six-month angiography revealing no 'binary restenosis', meaning less than 50%. The actual degree of stenosis was 21% compared to the immediate residual stenosis of 16%. Nine patients had further follow-up angiography at nine to 24 months (mean 14 months). In these nine patients, there was a primary patency rate of 83.3% (8/9).

The second paper reports on a prospective multicentre registry of 102 claudicants treated with the current version of the CryoPlasty system which inflates to eight rather than six atmospheres [10]. Patients were pre-treated with both aspirin and clopidogrel. A smaller proportion, 31%, had diabetes. A range of lesions (40% TASC C [11]) were treated, including 15 occlusions. 84.3% of the lesions were in the superficial femoral artery. CryoPlasty alone was successful in 85%. There was a 6.9% rate of significant dissection and an 8.8% bailout stent rate. Ninety patients were followed to nine months. Two

had died due to unrelated causes but the fate of the other ten is unknown. Clinical patency, as defined by no need for revascularisation of the index lesion, was 82.2%. The primary patency of the treated segment was assessed with duplex ultrasound. Restenosis was defined as a peak systolic velocity ratio of greater than two with respect to the proximal normal segment. The primary patency rate was 70.1%. Interestingly, all of the nine stented segments remained clinically patent and, of the 15 occlusions, five of which were stented, the clinical patency rate was 92.3%.

Two further CryoPlasty studies have only been published in abstract form [12, 13]. Twenty patients, 17 of whom had diabetes, underwent tibial vessel CryoPlasty for critical ischaemia with a 95% rate of limb salvage and freedom from major amputation [12]. Six patients, however, had adjunctive atherectomy as part of their primary treatment. A trial of below-the-knee CryoPlasty ('BTK CHILL') is currently recruiting. In the other study, 18 patients with in-stent restenosis or occlusion (n=6) were treated with a procedural success rate of 94% [13]. Atherectomy was used for the patients with occluded stents. Clinical patency at ten months was 78%, based on target lesion revascularisation and duplex ultrasound.

Discussion

The evidence so far indicates that CryoPlasty is a safe and practicable option for many femoropopliteal lesions including in-stent restenosis. No procedure-specific complications have been reported. Whilst the preliminary data are encouraging, are they better than reported results for conventional angioplasty and if they are, why?

Comparison with previous studies is difficult, as no two studies are the same in terms of case mix, revascularisation technique and lesion characteristics. Follow-up is not standardised. Multiple endpoints are used including clinical assessment, ABPI, duplex ultrasound and angiography. Even angiographic results can be expressed in different ways e.g. 'binary' restenosis rather than the actual luminal diameter change. The patients in the multicentre registry were treated with both aspirin and clopidogrel which is not standard therapy and may be an important factor in its own right.

Outcomes in claudicants are better than in those with critical ischaemia, as the disease is usually more limited. The TASC document in 2000 summarised the studies available and derived a one-year primary patency rate of 61% for femoropopliteal angioplasty (1241 patients, 72% claudicants) [11]. In 2001, a meta-analysis of 12 studies published between 1994 and 2000 estimated one-year primary patency rates of 77% and 65% for stenoses and occlusions respectively [14]. Whilst the CryoPlasty primary patency results from the multicentre registry are similar to these (71% at nine months), only 77 of the patients had adequate duplex follow-up. The threshold peak systolic velocity ratio of 2.0 to indicate significant restenosis may be too sensitive and reduce the primary patency rate unreasonably. Clearly, however, it is the clinical outcome that counts. The clinical patency rate (82%) was based on the lack of need for revascularisation. What is not known is how many of the patients had recurrent symptoms, but declined further intervention or the fate of the ten patients lost to follow-up.

Because there is no standardised technique for angioplasty, could the computer-controlled balloon inflation be important? The overall inflation/deflation cycle lasts between 40 and 60 seconds. It is, therefore, a reasonably prolonged inflation at a standard pressure. This in itself may be an independent factor and may be partly responsible for the relatively low dissection rate reported. The bailout stent rate was 8.8%, or nine patients, five of whom had had occlusions. Whilst this is stated to be a low stenting rate, this may not be the case in the UK. It is interesting to note that none of these nine patients required revascularisation during the trial. One could surmise that CryoPlasty may provide a favourable environment for stenting, but based on the numbers treated so far, this would be speculation.

Freezing the artery during angioplasty is peculiar to CryoPlasty. Immediate changes to the vessel wall during treatment and longer-term inhibition of smooth muscle hyperplasia via stimulation of apoptosis are hoped to result in improved clinical outcomes. Currently, the human data are lacking and only longer-term follow-up and randomised trials will define the importance of CryoPlasty.

Pharmacomanipulation

As stated in the introduction, this section will focus on drugs used to reduce NIH following angioplasty.

Evidence from the cardiology literature

The evidence so far has almost entirely come from the coronary literature. Although many different drugs have and are being trialled, the commonest drugs used in the coronary circulation are sirolimus (Rapamycin) and paclitaxel. Sirolimus is a macrolide antibiotic which inhibits the cell cycle at the transition from G0 to G1, thus preventing cell division. It also has potent anti-inflammatory effects. Paclitaxel promotes the stabilisation of microtubules and alters their function. It inhibits proliferation and migration of vascular VSMCs by its cytotoxic and antineoplastic effects. DES using these agents in trials in the coronary circulation have reduced target-lesion revascularisation (TLR) rates to single figures (4-6%) [15]. Studies comparing the two stent systems have come out marginally in favour of the sirolimus-eluting stent, in terms of less late lumen loss rather than clinical outcomes. Patients at higher risk for restenosis (e.g. diabetics) had a lower TLR rate which was not seen in a population at generally low risk. There may of course be differences in the stents or polymers, which carry the drugs, in addition to the drugs themselves, which could have separate effects. Because DES are expensive, there have been trials of oral sirolimus given around the time of the intervention [16, 17]. A variety of peri-procedural drug regimens have been tried resulting in lower restenosis rates when compared with bare metal stents. This approach is clearly attractive, not least in economic terms, but has not been shown to be superior to DES. Whichever drug is given, however, there is a concern about delayed endothelialisation due to the non-specific effect of the drug and possible late stent thrombosis.

Drug-eluting stents in the legs

The evidence for DES in the femoropopliteal segment in humans is largely limited to the SIROCCO trials [18, 19]. The six-month data from the extension trial (SIROCCO II) trial are fully published and the 18-month findings are available in abstract form only. The trial randomised 57 patients with claudication or critical limb ischaemia and stenoses or occlusions (67%) to the SMART (Cordis) bare or slow-eluting sirolimus stents. A maximum of two stents were allowed to treat lesions averaging 8cm in length. At six and 18 months, there were no significant differences in clinical outcomes. At six months, the angiographic mean luminal diameters were 4.94 mm +/- 0.69 versus 4.76 mm +/- 0.54, the binary restenosis rates were zero versus 7.7%, and the late loss values were 0.038mm +/-0.64 versus 0.68mm +/- 0.97 in the sirolimus and bare stent groups, respectively. At 18 months, duplex ultrasound revealed a 20.7% binary restenosis rate in the sirolimus group (six stenoses and no occlusions in 29 patients), versus 17.9% in the bare stent group (four stenoses and one occlusion in 28 patients). As with the SIROCCO I trial, the bare metal stents performed better than expected when compared with older generation stents. To the best of the authors' knowledge there is only one other ongoing trial of DES in the femoropopliteal segment.

The Zilver PTX trial, sponsored by Cook, aims to recruit 480 patients with femoropopliteal lesions less than 7cm (phase 1) or up to 14cm (phase 2). Patients will be randomised either to angioplasty or the paclitaxel-eluting Zilver stent. The primary endpoint will be primary patency at 12 months [20].

There is one study of bailout drug-eluting versus bare metal stents during infrapopliteal angioplasty for critical limb ischaemia [21]. Fifty-eight patients, 75% diabetic, were non-randomly given either a sirolimus-eluting coronary stent (Cypher, Cordis) or one of four bare metal stents. The tibial vessel lesions were generally short, 1-2cm, and around three quarters of patients had inflow femoropopliteal lesions treated at the same time. At six months the primary patency rate for the lesions treated with DES was significantly higher and the TLR correspondingly lower, but the limb salvage was 100% in both groups. DES may, therefore, have a role to play in tibial angioplasty and certainly this would make sense as the vessel sizes treated are similar to the coronary arteries.

Discussion

Whilst DES have become established in coronary artery interventions, there has been little progress in their use in peripheral arteries. Perhaps this is not surprising. Bare stents have been shown to be more effective than angioplasty alone in the coronary arteries and, therefore, DES are a logical next step. Primary stenting, however, has not yet been shown to be effective in the femoropopliteal segment. The reason for this may be due to the different biomechanical characteristics of this area compared to the coronaries. We know that stents improve initial angiographic appearances by limiting elastic recoil and dissection. However, the femoropopliteal segment is subject to many forces such as compression within the adductor canal, torsion and longitudinal flexion and extension. There is also a larger plaque burden and whilst coronary restenosis tends to plateau by 12 months, it is more progressive in the leg. Additionally, stent fractures occur in the longer term and appear to be associated with restenosis [22]. Stent design will have to evolve to combat these factors before DES have a chance to be effective. One way is to make the stent temporary. Biodegradable and absorbable stents are already being studied and therefore could act as a platform for drug elution. Using pig iliac arteries, a dexamethasone-eluting polylactic acid stent was found to cause less neointimal hyperplasia than a Wallstent (Boston Scientific) [23].

Conclusions

It is clear that results from femoropopliteal angioplasty need improving upon. CryoPlasty and drug therapy to prevent neointimal hyperplasia are both promising ways to achieve this. However, due to the complexity of the diseased femoropopliteal segment, neither has yet proven itself to be superior to angioplasty and bailout stenting where needed.

Summary

◆ Cryoplasty freezes the artery to minus 10°C during dilatation, resulting in reduced rates of dissection and stimulating smooth muscle cell apoptosis.

◆ Apoptosis of the smooth muscle cells may reduce neointimal hyperplasia and negative remodelling.

◆ Cryoplasty is safe, but has not yet been shown to be superior to angioplasty alone.

◆ Drug-eluting stents are effective in reducing neointimal hyperplasia in the coronary arteries. However, the sirolimus-eluting SMART stent is no more effective than the bare stent in the femoropopliteal segment.

◆ Stent design for femoropopliteal interventions will need to improve before drug elution has a chance to work.

References

1. Gage A, Fazekas G, Riley E. Freezing injury to large blood vessels in dogs. *Surgery* 1967; 61: 748-54.
2. Cheema AN, Nili N, Li CW, *et al*. Effects of intravascular cryotherapy on vessel wall repair in a balloon-injured rabbit iliac artery model. *Cardiovascular Res* 2003; 59(1): 222-33.
3. Grassl ED, Bischof JC. *In vitro* model systems for evaluation of smooth muscle cell response to cryoplasty. *Cryobiology* 2005; 50: 162-73.
4. Tatsutani KN, Joye JD, Virmani R, *et al*. *In vitro* evaluation of vascular endothelial and smooth muscle cell survival and apoptosis in response to hypothermia and freezing. *Cryo Letters* 2005; 26(1): 55-64.
5. Bennett MR. Apoptosis in the cardiovascular system. *Heart* 2002; 87: 480-7.
6. Walsh K, Smith RC, Kim H-S. Vascular cell apoptosis in remodeling, restenosis, and plaque rupture. *Circ Res* 2000; 87: 184-8.
7. Wolfgang E. Statin-induced vascular smooth muscle cell apoptosis: a possible role in the prevention of restenosis? *Current Drug Targets - Cardiovascular & Hematological Disorders* 2004; 5(2): 135-44.
8. Durand E, Mallat Z, Addad F, *et al*. Time courses of apoptosis and cell proliferation and their relationship to arterial remodelling and restenosis after angioplasty in an atherosclerotic rabbit model. *J Am Coll Cardiol* 2002; 39: 1680-5.
9. Fava M, Loyola S, Polydorou A, *et al*. Cryoplasty for femoropopliteal arterial disease: late angiographic results of initial human experience. *J Vasc Interv Radiol* 2004; 15: 1239-43.
10. Laird J, Michael RJ, Biamino G, *et al*. Cryoplasty for the treatment of femoropopliteal arterial disease: results of a prospective, multicenter registry. *J Vasc Interv Radiol* 2005; 16: 1067-73.
11. Dormandy JA, Rutherford RB. Management of peripheral arterial disease (PAD). TASC Working Group. Trans-Atlantic

Inter-Society Consensus (TASC). *J Vasc Surg* 2000; 31(suppl): S1-S296.

12. Moran M, Joye J, St Goar F. Cryoplasty for critical limb ischaemia: initial below-the-knee results. *Am J Cardiol* 2004; 94 (suppl 6A): 7E.

13. Joye J. Initial results using CryoPlasty to treat lower extremity in-stent restenosis. Abs 71. Presented at the Society of Interventional Radiologists annual meeting, 2004.

14. Muradin GS, Bosch JL, Stijnen T, *et al.* Balloon dilation and stent implantation for treatment of femoropopliteal arterial disease: meta-analysis. *Radiology* 2001; 221: 137-45.

15. Moliterno DJ. Healing Achilles - Sirolimus versus Paclitaxel. *N Engl J Med* 2005; 353: 724-7.

16. Rodriguez AE, Alemparte MR, Vigo CF, *et al.* Pilot study of oral rapamycin to prevent restenosis in patients undergoing coronary stent therapy: Argentina Single-Center Study (ORAR Trial). *J Invasive Cardiol* 2003; 15: 581-4.

17. Hausleiter J, Kastrati A, Mehilli J, *et al.* Randomized, double-blind, placebo-controlled trial of oral sirolimus for restenosis prevention in patients with in-stent restenosis. *Circulation* 2004; 110: 790-5.

18. Duda SH, Pusich B, Richter G, *et al.* Sirolimus eluting stents for the treatment of obstructive superficial femoral artery disease: 6-months results. *Circulation* 2002; 106: 1505-9.

19. Duda SH, Bosiers M, Lammer J, *et al.* Sirolimus-eluting versus bare nitinol stent for obstructive superficial femoral artery disease: the Sirocco II trial. *J Vasc Interv Radiol* 2005; 16: 331-8.

20. Zilver PTX trial at: http://clinicaltrials.gov/ct/show/NCT00 120406?order=6.

21. Siablis D, Kraniotis P, Karnabatidis D, *et al.* Sirolimus-eluting versus bare stents for bailout after suboptimal infrapopliteal angioplasty for critical limb ischemia: 6-month angiographic results from a nonrandomized prospective single-center study. *J Endovasc Ther* 2005; 12: 685-95.

22. Allie DE, Hebert CJ, Walker CM. Nitinol stent fractures in the SFA. Endovascular Today, July/August 2004. Available at: http://www.evtoday.com/PDFarticles/0704/et0704_vu_allie. pdf.

23. Uurto I, Mikkonen J, Parkkinen J, *et al.* Drug-eluting biodegradable poly-D/L-lactic acid vascular stents: an experimental pilot study. *J Endovasc Ther* 2005; 12: 371-9.

Chapter 21

Cutting balloon angioplasty in the lower limb: current evidence and recommendations

Ian Gillespie MB ChB DMRD FRCSE FRCR, Consultant Vascular Radiologist
Edinburgh Royal Infirmary, Edinburgh, Scotland

Introduction

Conventional percutaneous balloon angioplasty (PTA) has been found to be effective in treating focal lower limb arterial stenoses and occlusions. However, some lesions are resistant to conventional balloon angioplasty due to their complex morphology or the presence of calcification, and this may result in primary technical failure or subsequent restenosis. Similarly, recurrent disease, in-stent restenosis, and stenoses at vascular bypass graft anastomoses may not respond well to treatment with standard or even high-pressure balloons.

The use of cutting balloons to treat recurrent disease or in-stent restenosis in the coronary circulation has been well described and it has been suggested that this could be extrapolated into use in the peripheral circulation. Indeed, cutting balloon angioplasty (CBA) has now been reported in the following anatomical sites and clinical situations:

- coronary ostial and non-ostial disease;
- coronary in-stent restenosis;
- renal in-stent restenosis;
- peripheral in-stent restenosis;
- vascular graft anastomotic restenosis;
- haemodialysis fistula-related stenosis;
- resistant paediatric renal artery stenosis (FMD, neurofibromatosis, vasculitis);
- endourology (pyelotomy, ureterotomy);
- biliary strictures;
- oesophageal strictures;
- arterial stenoses in Takayasu's arteritis;
- fenestration of endografts.

Conventional balloon angioplasty

The primary technical success and long-term patency after conventional angioplasty varies according to anatomical level and disease morphology. The TASC document describes meta-analysis of results as follows [1].

- Weighted average primary technical success:
  - iliac stenosis   95%
  - iliac occlusion   82%
  - femoropopliteal stenosis   90%
  - femoropopliteal occlusion   80-85%
- Weighted average five-year patency (ABPI-based):
  - iliac   61%
  - femoropopliteal   48%

Rutherford and Durham produced composite patency curves for iliac and femoropopliteal PTA of 70% and 52% respectively [2]. It is clear that results of balloon angioplasty are better in the iliac segment than in the femoropopliteal segment.

Selective stenting may improve both primary success and long-term patency in iliac disease, but is still the subject of investigation in the femoropopliteal segment, where long-term results have been much less impressive. Some authors have achieved excellent results using subintimal angioplasty in long segment disease, especially in the infrainguinal circulation [3].

Other factors which have been shown to affect outcome include:

- length of disease segment;
- presence of diabetes;
- quality of run-off;
- clinical indication (claudication vs limb salvage);
- residual stenosis post-PTA.

It is against this complex clinical background that cutting balloons must demonstrate improvement in primary technical success and ultimately, in improved patency, in order to justify a place on the shelf in departments of interventional radiology. In addition, they must be compared with the results of other recently available techniques which are also currently under investigation. These include atherectomy, drug-eluting stents, cryotherapy, brachytherapy, stem cell therapy etc.

Percutaneous transluminal angioplasty

Conventional balloon angioplasty causes uncontrolled cracks and fissures in the intima and media with stretching and expansion of the arterial wall, sometimes associated with dissection. Barotrauma is caused as the pressure required to expand the vessel is applied to the whole surface area and length of the artery in contact with the inflated balloon. The natural response to this vessel wall trauma leads to a proliferative process, resulting in neointimal hyperplasia which is proportional to the severity of injury and results in late restenosis. Schillinger et al has attempted to quantify acute vascular inflammation by serial measurement of acute phase reactants (C-reactive protein, fibrinogen, serum amyloid A) after PTA and has related this to the subsequent development of restenosis [4].

Cutting balloon design and mechanism of action

The cutting balloon is a non-compliant balloon which has 3-4 blades or atherotomes mounted on its surface. The exposed height of each atherotome is 0.127mm and is designed to incise the surface endothelium and thus to disrupt the elastic and fibrotic continuity of the vessel wall and fibrous plaque. The microtomes are covered by sleeves or folds within the balloon profile prior to inflation and again on deflation which protects the vessel wall during insertion and removal.

Cutting balloons (Boston Scientific; Figures 1-3) are now available in diameters ranging from 2-8mm, although sizes above 4mm in diameter have only been available relatively recently. Small balloon sizes (2-4mm) are 1.5mm in length, available on a monorail system and utilise an 0.014" guidewire. The 5-8mm sizes are available in 1cm or 2cm lengths, on an over the wire system and utilise an 0.018" guidewire. The rated burst pressure for all cutting balloons is 10ATM. Low balloon pressures in the 4-8ATM range are recommended for inflation. The larger balloon sizes require a 7 French sheath and are mounted on a 4.2 French catheter shaft.

When a cutting balloon is inflated, the major forces are only applied to the arterial wall at the site of the blades and this atherotomy makes small controlled microincisions in the intima and plaque. Subsequent gentle dilatation of these microincisions by the non-compliant balloon produces controlled longitudinal fracture lines at lower balloon pressures than are used with conventional angioplasty and so reduces hoop stress.

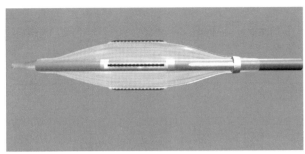

Figure 1. Atherotomes exposed when balloon inflated. *Courtesy of Boston Scientific.*

known to initiate the proliferative process of neointimal hyperplasia which compromises the outcome of both angioplasty and vascular surgical grafting [6].

This has been further supported by Inoue who measured significantly reduced inflammatory markers after CBA, in patients randomised to either coronary CBA or PTA [7].

Historically, the availability of only 2-4mm diameter cutting balloons restricted their use in the legs to

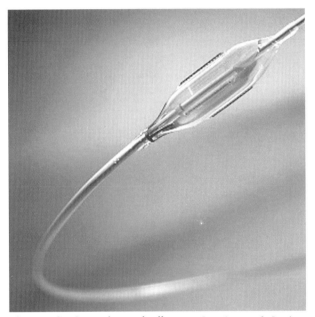

Figure 2. 1cm long balloon. *Courtesy of Boston Scientific.*

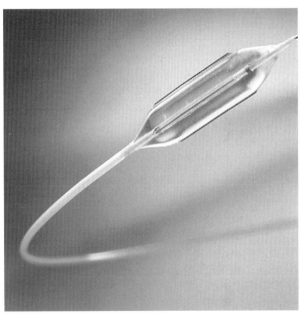

Figure 3. 2cm long balloons now available. *Courtesy of Boston Scientific.*

There is, therefore, minimal stretching and expansion of the vessel wall and less barotrauma. Less elastic recoil occurs and there is less perivascular injury.

Several studies utilising intravascular ultrasound in the coronary circulation have demonstrated that cutting balloons achieve similar luminal dimensions, but with greater plaque reduction and less vessel expansion than with conventional angioplasty [5]. Animal experiments suggest that this reduction in vessel wall trauma will reduce the release of factors

infrainguinal disease, but the more recent introduction of larger diameters enables their application also in suprainguinal vessels. The short length of the atherotomes (max. 2cm) is a major factor limiting the use of CBA in long segment disease, as is often found when treating patients with lower limb ischaemia.

There are few reports of significant complications relating to cutting balloons. These include vessel rupture, coronary stent damage due to blade dislodgement, and coronary aneurysm formation. No complications have so far been reported with

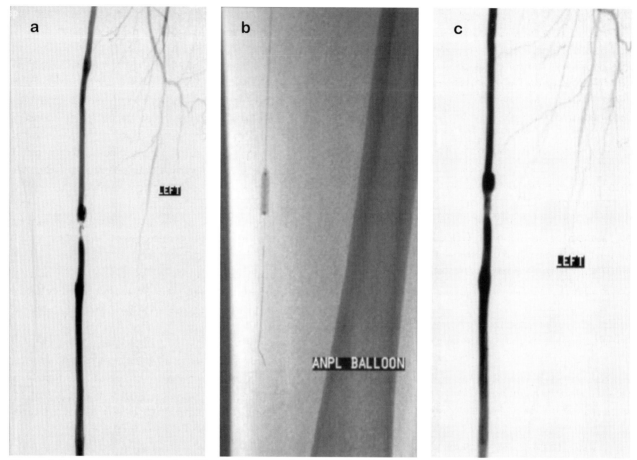

Figure 4. Images pre and post-cutting balloon angioplasty of an *in situ* vein graft stenosis. a) Digital subtraction angiography of an infrainguinal *in situ* vein femoropopliteal bypass graft, demonstrating a 90% mid-graft stenosis. This was picked up during graft surveillance and was causing significant turbulence, despite the patient being asymptomatic. b) Via a 6 French sheath in the left groin, using an antegrade approach, the lesion was traversed using an 0.018" guidewire. After 5000 iu heparin intra-arterially, 5mm cutting balloon angioplasty was performed (Boston Scientific, St. Albans, Hertfordshire, UK) with slow inflation of the balloon to 4 atmospheres. c) Digital subtraction angiography post-dilatation demonstrates a good radiological result with rapid flow, smooth contour of the dilated arterial walls and preservation of run-off. The graft remains patent with no recurrence of stenosis 2½ years later with no further intervention. *Courtesy of Professor Tony Watkinson and Mr Andrew Cowan from the Royal Devon and Exeter Hospital, Exeter, UK.*

reference to use in lower limb arteries. Figure 4 illustrates a case of pre- and post-cutting balloon angioplasty of an *in situ* vein graft stenosis.

Evidence

Coronary circulation

CBA was initially developed by Barath for use in the coronary circulation in 1991 [8]. It has since been utilised in both ostial and non-ostial coronary disease, small vessel disease, calcified coronary stenoses, and in-stent coronary stenosis and most of the available literature relates to coronary applications [9]. Some of this evidence derived from coronary use will be presented, as it forms the only largescale data on which the use of CBA depends.

Ergene *et al* reported a randomised trial of CBA vs PTA in vessels <3mm [10]. CBA was associated with a lower six-month angiographic restenosis rate (27% vs

47% p<0.05) and fewer bailout procedures. The CAPAS study (single centre CBA and PTA in small coronary arteries) also demonstrated a lower restenosis rate at three months (25% vs 41.5%; p=0.009) and improved event-free survival at one year (72.8% vs 61%; p=0.047) in patients randomly assigned to CBA (n= 248) [11].

Muramatsu *et al* compared CBA with PTA for ostial coronary artery stenosis and found improved technical success (94% vs 84.6%) and a lower short-term restenosis rate at 5.3 months (43% vs 53%) for CBA [12]. Kondo and colleagues undertook a matched comparison of CBA and PTA for the treatment of non-ostial coronary artery stenosis and and demonstrated lower restenosis at four months (23% vs 42%) for CBA [13].

Nakamura looked at the impact of deep vessel wall injury on acute response and remodelling of coronary artery segments after CBA [14]. They suggest that deep vessel wall injury tends to occur in small diameter arteries and that such lesions show favourable response after CBA.

However, in the cutting balloon global randomised trial (1238 lesions), Mauri *et al* found no significant difference in angiographically-determined restenosis rates between CBA and PTA (31.4% vs 30.4%) at six months [15]. At 270 days, the rates for CBA vs PTA for myocardial infarction were 4.7% vs 2.4%, for death were 1.3% vs 0.3%, and for major adverse cardiac events were 13.6% vs 15.1%. There were five coronary perforations in the CBA group and none in the PTA group. They suggested reserving the use of cutting balloons for difficult lesions resistant to conventional balloons and in-stent restenosis.

Adamian compared the results of CBA vs PTA vs rotational atherectomy vs stent for the treatment of in-stent restenosis [16]. CBA was associated with better clinical and angiographic outcomes (restenosis rates 20% for CBA, 35.9% for rota, and 41.4% for stent) and was suggested as an option for treating these difficult lesions. Albiero reported the results of the RESCUT multicentre prospective randomised trial comparing CBA with PTA for in-stent restenosis in 428 patients [17]. At seven-month angiographic follow-up there was no difference in the rate or pattern of recurrent restenosis or incidence of major cardiac events between groups.

Clearly, there is no evidence to support the use of cutting balloons in routine coronary angioplasty and there is no definitive consensus on their selective use. However, there may be a role for cutting balloons in the treatment of focal lesions resistant to conventional angioplasty, such as heavily calcified lesions, ostial coronary lesions and in-stent restenosis. CBA will have to stand comparison with other new technologies, including brachytherapy, and the increasing use of drug-eluting stents may further impact on its coronary applications.

Extrapolation of the selective use of cutting balloons from the coronary circulation to other areas has led to their use in a diversity of clinical sites as previously listed.

Perhaps the most positive literature relating to non-coronary CBA lies in the treatment of haemodialysis fistula stenoses which are notoriously resistant to dilatation by standard balloons. Their use in this area is considered further in Chapter 28.

Lower limb arteries

There are only a few articles concerning the application of CBA to the lower limb circulation and there is no published literature relating to use of CBA in either *de novo* or recurrent iliac disease. Available publications at present relate mostly to situations which are normally considered resistant to conventional balloons, such as bypass graft stenoses.

A number of factors affect the patency of arterial bypass grafts in the leg and these include graft material, anastomotic site, quality of inflow and run-off etc. Five-year patency of infrainguinal vein grafts up to 80% is reported in some series, but this reduces to around 50% for prosthetic grafts above the knee and even less below the knee. Anastomotic stenosis due to neointimal hyperplasia is a frequent cause of delayed graft failure and may result in graft occlusion if left untreated. The short-term risk of graft occlusion in the presence of a critical stenosis is reported to be nearly 80%.

Vein patch revision and jump grafting are surgical alternatives to percutaneous interventional techniques. The results of PTA for graft stenoses have been disappointing in comparison with dilatation of native arterial narrowing. Such lesions are often resistant to dilatation with conventional balloons and primary technical success is compromised by elastic recoil. This is reflected in poor one-year patency rates of the order of 44-53%. Whittemore *et al* described the use of PTA in 54 stenoses in 30 patients with infrainguinal vein bypass grafts [18]. They identified three-year patency of 59% where a single PTA was required compared to only 6% where repeat PTAs were performed. Attempts to remedy this situation have resulted in the application of both atherectomy catheters and cutting balloons.

Engelke and colleagues reported the feasibility and safety of cutting balloon angioplasty in terms of immediate success and long-term graft patency for lower limb arterial bypass graft salvage [19]. CBA was technically successful in 15 of 16 (15 patients) lesions of which seven were PTFE (five femoropopliteal, one aortobifem, one cross-over), three were composite (common femoral to below knee), four were reversed vein (femoropopliteal), and one external iliac to femoral stent-graft. Five patients presented with acute limb ischaemia due to graft occlusion and were treated initially with thrombolysis which revealed significant anastomotic stenosis and ten were detected on duplex scan surveillance. Conventional balloon angioplasty was performed unsuccessfully in six vein graft stenoses, followed immediately by CBA and in ten lesions, CBA was performed as the primary procedure. In all cases CBA was followed by conventional balloon angioplasty. A mean anastomotic stenosis of 75% was reduced to 8% after CBA and PTA. There were no significant complications in this series. The cumulative one-year primary patency rate was 76%, which compares favourably with results of conventional PTA and is similar to the results obtained when atherectomy is used in the treatment of graft stenoses. The authors conclude by admitting that this is a small series and further work is required to determine the long-term effectiveness of CBA in the treatment of bypass graft stenosis in comparison with other new endovascular techniques.

Kasirajan *et al* treated 19 patients with infrainguinal vein bypass grafts of which ten were above knee and nine were below knee [20]. Mean velocity pre-procedure was 373cm/sec and at one month post-procedure was 144cm/sec. One patient developed recurrent stenosis at a mean of 11.4 months follow-up. There were no other complications or recurrent graft thrombosis. This study concluded that their results are superior to conventional PTA for the treatment of graft stenoses and comparable to open surgical revision.

Although these results are encouraging in the treatment of bypass graft stenoses, they offer a combined total of only 34 patients treated and so far no trial has been published randomising such patients prospectively to CBA compared with other endovascular technologies or surgery.

The literature is similarly thin when CBA is used for *de novo* disease in the lower limb. Ansel *et al* reported their experience using CBA in popliteal and infrapopliteal disease [21]. CBA performed in 93 popliteal or infrapopliteal vessels in 73 limbs were identified for this retrospective study. Eighty-two percent were *de novo* lesions and the other 18% were in-stent restenotic lesions. Post-CBA angiographic result was deemed inadequate in 20%, all of whom underwent stent placement. There were no dilatation-related complications. Only clinical follow-up was available at a mean of 12 months, with a limb salvage rate of 89.5% in survivors (17% mortality) who were at least Rutherford class four pre-procedure. No data relating to restenosis rates at the intervention site are available from this study and no definition of criteria used to determine the indications for CBA are offered.

Rabbi *et al* report the use of CBA in 11 out of a total of 45 patients undergoing femoropopliteal angioplasty over a one-year period in their institution [22]. Selection for CBA was based on a target vessel diameter of <4mm and absence of autologous vein for bypass. Technical success was achieved in ten of 11 cases and there were no cases of vessel perforation, dissection, or adjunctive surgical revascularisation. Two patients suffered periprocedural thrombosis following incomplete graft lysis. At a mean follow-up of only three months, seven of the remaining eight CBA sites were patent with one asymptomatic restenosis.

Engelke *et al* utilised CBA in five patients for peripheral arterial stenoses resistant to conventional angioplasty [23]. All had short focal stenoses (one post-irradiation external iliac lesion, one iliac in-stent restenosis, one intragraft axillobifemoral stenosis, two anastomotic stenoses of aortobifemoral grafts). Initial conventional PTA with high inflation pressures failed to produce angiographically acceptable results or abolish pressure gradients in all cases and was immediately followed by CBA using the 6mm diameter device. PTA was performed after CBA in four cases using the same balloon diameter as had been used prior to CBA. Technical success was achieved in all cases after CBA and this correlated with good clinical and colour duplex follow-up results at a mean of 6.4 months. The authors point out that although atherectomy may confer another alternative for the treatment of resistant lesions caused by neointimal hyperplasia, their use is limited by their relatively large diameter and rigidity.

It will be clear from the above data that there is a paucity of evidence concerning the role of CBA in lower limb arteries. There are as yet no randomised trials of any sort comparing the effectiveness of CBA with conventional PTA for *de novo* lower limb disease nor in comparison with other newer endovascular techniques or surgery for the treatment of resistant lesions. At least one randomised controlled trial is in progess for femoropopliteal TASC A lesions, but has not yet been published [24]. The cutting balloon currently remains a niche product for use in the lower limb which may have a limited role in treating focal lesions, especially when caused by neointimal hyperplasia. This role is supported by the small-scale observational studies published to date, but larger scale randomised studies will be required if CBA is to define a permanent place in the endovascular armamentarium available for the treatment of peripheral vascular disease.

Summary

- The application of cutting balloons in the lower limb circulation is limited by the available range of diameters from 2-8mm and particularly by their short length.

- Their mode of action produces microincisions in the stenotic lesion which disrupt the fibro-elastic continuity of diseased intima or neointimal hyperplasia.

- This produces greater plaque disruption and less vessel wall stretching than conventional angioplasty.

- Elastic recoil is minimised and the reduction in barotrauma in theory should reduce the proliferative vessel wall response, which results in restenosis, but translation into better long-term patency has not yet been proved.

- Cutting balloons can be used easily and safely with few reported complications.

- There is no level I evidence to support the use of cutting balloons in lower limb vascular disease.

- Limited observational studies suggest that cutting balloons may be of value in treating resistant lesions such as bypass graft stenoses, although this application has not been tested against alternative endovascular or surgical techniques.

References

1. Dormandy JA, Rutherford RB. Management of peripheral arterial disease. TransAtlantic Inter-Society Consensus (TASC). *J Vasc Surg* 2000; 31: S1-S296.

2. Rutherford RB, Durham J. Percutaneous balloon angioplasty for arteriosclerosis obliterans: long-term results. In: *Techniques in Vascular Surgery*. Yao JST, Pearde WH, Eds. Philadelphia: Saunders, 1992: 329-45.

3. Bolia A. Subintimal angioplasty in lower limb ischaemia. *J Cardiovasc Surg* (Torino) 2005; 46(4): 385-94.

4. Schillinger M, Exner M, Mlekusch W, *et al*. Vascular inflammation and percutaneous transluminal angioplasty of the femoropopliteal artery: association with restenosis *Radiology* 2002; 225: 21-6.

5. Okura H, Hayase M, Shimodozono S, *et al*. Mechanisms of acute lumen gain following cutting balloon angioplasty in calcified and non-calcified lesions: an intravascular ultrasound study. *Catheter Cardiovasc Interv* 2002; 57: 429-36.

6. Lary BG. Coronary artery incision and dilatation. *Arch Surg* 1980; 115: 1478-80.

7. Inoue T, Sakai Y, Hoshi K, *et al*. Lower expression of neutrophil adhesion molecule indicates less vessel wall injury and might explain lower restenosis rates after cutting balloon angioplasty. *Circulation* 1998; 97: 2511-8.

8. Barath P, Fishbein MC, Vari S, *et al*. Cutting balloon: a novel approach to percutaneous angioplasty. *Am J Cardiol* 1991; 68: 1249-52.

9. Ajani AE, Kim HS, Castagna M, *et al*. Clinical utility of the cutting balloon. *J Invasive Cardiol* 2001; 13: 554-7.

10. Ergene O, Seyithanoglu BY, Tastan A, *et al*. Comparison of angiographic and clinical outcome after cutting balloon and conventional balloon angioplasty in vessels smaller than 3mm in diameter: a randomised trial. *J Invasive Cardiol* 1998: 10: 70-5.

11. Izumi M, Nakaoka Y, Otsuji S. Predictors of restenosis after cutting balloon angioplasty and plain old balloon angioplasty in small coronary arteries: results of the CAPAS study. *Circulation* 1999; 100: 1305.

12. Muramatsu T, Tsukahara R, Ho M, *et al*. Efficacy of cutting balloon angioplasty for lesions at the ostium of the coronary arteries. *J Invasive Cardiol* 1999; 11: 201-6.

13. Kondo T, Kawaguchi K, Awaji Y, *et al*. Immediate and chronic results of cutting balloon angioplasty: a matched comparison with conventional angioplasty. *Clin Cardiol* 1997; 20: 459-63.

14. Nakamura M, Yock PG, Kataoka T, *et al*. Impact of deep vessel wall injury on acute response and remodelling of coronary artery segments after cutting balloon angioplasty. *Am J Cardiol* 2003; 91: 6-11.

15. Mauri L, Bonan R, Weiner BH, *et al*. Cutting balloon angioplasty for restenosis: results of the Cutting Balloon Global Randomised Trial. *Am J Cardiol* 2002; 90: 1079-83.

16. Adamian M, Marisco F, Di Mario C. Cutting balloon for the treatment of in-stent restenosis: a matched comparison with conventional angioplasty and atherectomy. *Circulation* 1999; 100: I-305.

17. Albiero R, Nishida T, Karvouni E, *et al*. Cutting balloon angioplasty for the treatment of in-stent restenosis. *Catheter Cardiovasc Interv* 2000; 50: 452-4.

18. Whittemore AD, Donaldson MC, Polack JF, *et al*. Limitations of balloon angioplasty for vein graft stenosis. *J Vasc Surg* 1991; 14: 340-5.

19. Engelke C, Morgan RA, Belli AM. Cutting balloon percutaneous transluminal angioplasty for salvage of lower limb arterial bypass grafts: feasibility. *Radiology* 2002; 223: 106-14.

20. Kasirajan K, Schneider PA. Early outcome of 'cutting' balloon angioplasty for infrainguinal vein graft stenosis. *J Vasc Surg* 2002; 39: 702-3.

21. Ansel GM, Sample NS, Botti JC Jr, *et al*. Cutting balloon angioplasty of the popliteal and infrapopliteal vessels for symptomatic limb ischaemia. *Catheter Cardiovasc Interv* 2004; 61: 1-4.

22. Rabbi JF, Kiran RP, Gersten G, *et al*. Early results with infrainguinal cutting balloon angioplasty limits distal dissection. *Ann Vasc Surg* 2004; 18: 640-3.

23. Engelke C, Sandhu C, Morgan RA, *et al*. Using 6mm cutting balloon angioplasty in patients with resistant peripheral arterial stenosis: preliminary results. *Am J Roentgenol* 2002; 179: 619-23.

24. Cejna M. Cutting balloon: review on principles and background of use in peripheral arteries. *Cardiovasc Interv Radiol* 2005; 28: 400-8.

Chapter 22

The endovascular treatment of popliteal aneurysms: current evidence and future predictions

Ian Loftus BSc MB ChB FRCS MD, Consultant Vascular Surgeon
St. George's Vascular Institute, St. George's Hospital, London, UK

Introduction

The most common site for peripheral aneurysms is the popliteal artery (Figure 1). Whilst often asymptomatic and detected coincidentally, they have a high cumulative risk of complications, in particular thrombosis or distal embolisation (Figure 2) [1]. Rarely, popliteal aneurysms can present with progressive ischaemia due to chronic embolisation, or rupture.

Conventionally, popliteal aneurysms are repaired by bypass surgery with proximal and distal aneurysm ligation. The results of conventional surgery are well documented, and both graft patency and limb salvage rates are very high. Furthermore, concerns about peri-operative morbidity and mortality have not been recognised in most of the published series. The potential advantages of a minimally invasive approach are, therefore, not as attractive as for endovascular aortic aneurysm repair.

Currently, there are few data to support the use of endovascular stent grafts in the treatment of popliteal aneurysms. The reported patency rates are poor, probably because the stent must be positioned across the knee joint. At the present time, popliteal stent grafts should probably be reserved for selected patients who are deemed unfit for surgery, and for

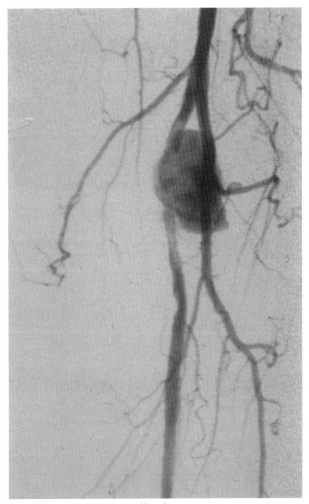

Figure 1. Localised popliteal aneurysm.

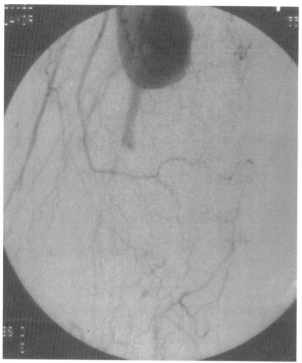

Figure 2. Embolisation from a popliteal artery aneurysm, completely occluding distal run-off.

entry into clinical trials. Improvements in stent design and the aggressive use of antiplatelet agents or anticoagulation may improve long-term patency results.

Technique of endovascular repair

Stent grafts

The main concern regarding the deployment of stent grafts in the popliteal artery is the position across the knee joint. This excludes the use of balloon expandable stents, which are prone to deformity from external pressure. Stents, therefore, must be self-expandable, and there are several such devices suitable for deployment in the popliteal artery.

The Viabahn and Hemobahn devices are self-expandable, flexible nitinol-supported PTFE grafts (WL Gore & Associates, Flagstaff, USA). The Viabahn stent is said to allow more accurate

deployment than the Hemobahn device, commencing distally rather than proximally. It is available in a smaller diameter range than the Hemobahn, from 6-8mm compared to 6-13mm, but a greater range of lengths from 2.5-15cm, rather than 5-15cm.

Similarly, the Fluency device comprises a nitinol stent, though this is encapsulated between two layers of PTFE (CR Bard, Karlsruhe, Germany). Designed for used in the tracheobronchial tree, the Fluency device comes in a range of diameters from 6-10mm, and three lengths (40, 60 and 80mm).

The Wallgraft device is a braided polyester graft bonded to a stainless steel Wallstent with a thin layer of polycarbonate urethane (Boston Scientific Corp., Galway, Ireland). It is available in a wide range of diameters, from 6-14mm, and four different lengths (20, 30, 50 and 70mm).

Imaging and device selection

The aim of initial imaging is to assess the size of the aneurysm, and the calibre and quality of the vessel proximally and distally. This can be achieved adequately by the use of duplex ultrasound. However, if considering endovascular repair, more detailed anatomical information is required for accurate measurements and device selection. It is important to assess the run-off vessels and the relationship of the aneurysm to the popliteal bifurcation. MR and CT angiography may well supersede the need for conventional angiography.

When selecting a device, the stent must be oversized by 1mm both proximally and distally. If the landing zones proximally and distally are not the same calibre, two or more different size devices may be required. The smaller device should be deployed first to prevent an endoleak, and there must be at least a 20mm overlap between devices to prevent dislocation. Clearly, there must be a suitable landing zone above and below the aneurysm, preferably with at least 20mm of normal calibre popliteal artery between the aneurysm and the bifurcation.

Technique of deployment

Under local anaesthetic, and using either a surgical cut down or percutaneous puncture, a selective catheter and guidewire are advanced from the common femoral artery down the ipsilateral superficial femoral artery. Angiography is performed to accurately delineate the popliteal anatomy, usually using a road-map facility. Heparin should be administered, along with intra-arterial glyceryl trinitrate to prevent arterial spasm.

The guidewire is then advanced through the aneurysm and positioned several centimetres below, over which is positioned the stent graft. After deployment, balloon dilatation of the device should be considered, using a balloon of similar calibre to the stent graft. Completion angiography should be performed to ensure accurate deployment with no endoleak. Generally, an arterial closure device should be used if the procedure has been performed percutanously.

All patients should be discharged on antiplatelet therapy, although the optimal treatment regime has not been determined. It may be that a combination of agents should be used. Follow-up should include regular duplex ultrasound (Figure 3), although again

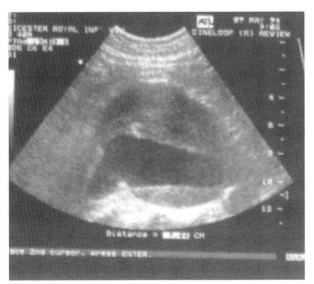

Figure 3. Popliteal aneurysms treated by stent graft require interval duplex ultrasound surveillence, although the optimal timing of scans has not been clarified.

the best protocol for interval scans is yet to be determined.

Current evidence

Elective surgical repair of popliteal aneurysms, by exclusion and bypass, is a safe and durable technique. Similarly, it is reasonable to manage smaller aneurysms by close follow-up including ultrasound surveillance. Many surgeons consider a diameter of greater than 2cm as an indication for repair [2]. In the presence of significant comorbidity, some recommend sequential ultrasound for aneurysms below 3cm in diameter [3].

The primary goals of treatment are exclusion of the aneurysm from the circulation, with effective revascularisation and prevention of distal embolisation. Conventional surgery involves bypass using autologous vein or prosthetic graft, and ligation of the aneurysm proximally and distally. Alternatively, the aneurysm may be excluded by aneurysmorraphy and interposition bypass graft. Excellent long-term patency and limb salvage rates are achievable, although this is dependent on the quality of the distal run-off vessels and whether surgery is performed in the elective or emergency setting.

The long-term graft patency and limb salvage rates from conventional surgery have been documented to be as high as 96% and 100%. In one study of 51 aneurysm repairs in 39 patients, with mean follow-up of greater than four years, the overall primary patency, secondary patency, limb salvage and actuarial survival rates were 95.5%, 100%, 98% and 98% at one year, and 85.1%, 96.9%, 98% and 83.8% at five years [4]. There were no deaths or serious cardiac complications in the 30-day postoperative period. Interestingly, in this series, there were no differences between the aneurysms repaired electively and those that were treated in an emergency setting. However, in this series, less than 30% of the group presented acutely.

Martelli and co-workers presented a cohort in which over 70% of aneurysm repairs were performed in the emergency setting [5]. In a series of 38 patients with 42 aneurysms, the secondary patency rate at

Table 1. Overview of the literature regarding the endovascular treatment of popliteal aneurysms using commercially available stent grafts.

Author	No of aneurysms	No of emergencies	Follow-up (mean months)	Occlusions
Mercade [8]	6	0	6	1
Kudelko [9]	1	0	10	0
Bürger [10]	1	1	6	0
Beregi [11]	3	0	24	0
Müller-Hülsbeck [12]	6	6	4	4
Henry [13]	10	Unknown	Unknown	5
Ihlberg [14]	1	0	5	0
Howell [15]	13	0	12	4
Gerasimidis [16]	9	0	14	4
Tielliu [18]	57	5	24	12
Antonello [20]	15	0	46	1

three years approached 80%, with estimated ten-year limb salvage rates of 96%, and six-year overall survival of 82.6%. The authors determined that poor run-off and continued smoking affected the long-term patency rate. Despite the preponderance of emergency procedures, these graft patency and limb salvage rates exceed those published for occlusive disease.

In a further study of 52 operations in 41 patients, overall five-year secondary patency and limb salvage rates were 87%, but in the sub-group of asymptomatic patients, the equivalent patency and limb salvage rates were 100% [6]. Of the four deaths in this series, all occurred in patients with symptomatic aneurysms.

Other studies have suggested that vein bypass grafts produce better long-term patency results than prosthetic grafts, although still presenting excellent long-term durability. In a study of 70 bypass procedures over an 11-year period, Blanco et al achieved early primary and secondary patency rates of 96% and 97%, with a peri-operative mortality of 2.8% [7]. The ten-year patency of vein grafts was 86%. While the patency rate for prosthetic grafts fell below 80%, the number of patients was too small to make any firm conclusions regarding graft material.

There are obvious potential advantages of a minimally invasive endovascular technique for the exclusion of popliteal aneurysms over conventional surgery. However, current evidence would suggest that the potential advantages fail to outweigh the disadvantages. Endovascular stent graft placement requires a smaller incision, less blood loss and shorter hospital stay, but evidence is mounting that short and long-term patency rates are unacceptably poor. There are a paucity of trial data, and most of the retrospective studies are of selected patients with suitable anatomy, and predominantly asymptomatic aneurysms [8-15] (Table 1). It is precisely this group of patients in whom conventional surgery achieves the best results [6].

A particular problem with the technique of endovascular popliteal aneurysm exclusion is the positioning of a stent graft across the knee joint. Repetitive stress in this area leads to kinking and fracture of the stent graft, with high rates of occlusion.

Early experience with endovascular repair suggested that the technique was feasible but the results were not promising. In a study of nine cases, six of which were elective, four thromboses occurred in the first 14 months of follow-up [16]. Overall, the

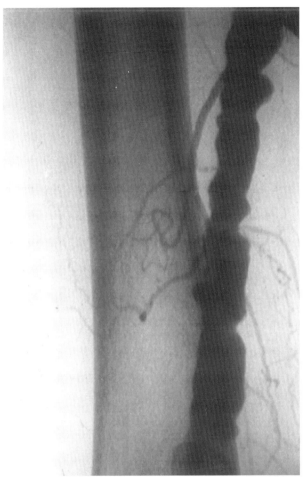

Figure 4. Diffuse aneurysmal disease is very difficult to treat using endovascular techniques, and reflects the systemic nature of the disease process.

primary and secondary patencies at 12 months were only 47% and 75% respectively. A variety of the commercially available stent grafts were used in this early study.

In Howell's series, 13 popliteal aneurysms were treated with Wallgraft prostheses[15]. This was a very select group, excluding all cases in which the stent graft would have crossed the knee joint. Technical success was achieved in all cases, with one endoleak demonstrated which sealed at one month, but no other procedural complications. In all, 19 devices were used. At one year, the primary and secondary patency rates were 69% and 92% respectively.

In a further study, using the Hemobahn stent graft, technical success was achieved in all of 23 cases,

although 24% required further vascular interventions at the same sitting [17]. Five stents occluded in the six months following deployment. The same group have recently published a larger cohort, now consisting of 67 aneurysms in 57 patients, the most recent of whom have been treated with the Viabahn device [18]. It should be noted that ten patients were excluded, mainly because they were deemed anatomically unsuitable for stenting. Of these, seven underwent conventional surgery. Of the remaining 57 cases, only five were patients presenting acutely, 68% required more than one stent, and 12% required ancillary procedures, including five cases that required proximal interposition grafts. During a mean 23-month follow-up, 12 grafts occluded (21%), of which nine underwent thrombectomy or thrombolysis, but only four remained patent. Other complications included stent migration and endoleak. In all, 13 of the 57 cases (22%) developed stent-related complications other than occlusion. These included eight stent migrations, three of which were associated with endoleaks that required further intervention. There were two stent breakages, one patient who demonstrated continued aneurysm enlargement and two stent stenoses requiring treatment.

A concern specific to endovascular repair is the risk of further dilatation above and below the position of the stent graft. There is good evidence now to show that localised aneurysmal disease is a manifestation of a systemic dilating process [19]. While this has not prevented the widespread use of endovascular techniques for aortic aneurysm repair, most surgeons aim to achieve significant over-sizing of the aortic graft with suprarenal fixation, minimising the risk of stent graft displacement related to subsequent neck dilatation. This is not as simple in the popliteal artery. Often the aneurysm is not focal, rather part of a generally ectatic vessel (Figure 4). The use of longer stents in the popliteal artery may predispose to increased risk of stent graft occlusion. Also, it is clear that the forces exerted on the stent graft in the popliteal artery are quite different to those in the aorta, associated with bending of the knee joint.

There has only been one published randomised trial of open repair versus endovascular treatment for popliteal artery aneurysm [20]. This was a small trial, of 30 selected patients with suitable anatomy and asymptomatic aneurysms, who were randomised to operative or endovascular repair. There were no complications or occlusions in the operative group, and only one occlusion in the stent group. However, the authors admitted that the trial was grossly underpowered, and the conclusions drawn from this study are very limited. Further, it is not clear how many patients were excluded from the study. Interestingly however, the stent graft deployment did take three times as long as the operative technique, the longest taking almost five hours.

Future predictions

While the endovascular treatment of popliteal aneurysms is feasible, with a low peri-procedure mortality and morbidity, the durability of the technique is currently questionable. All of the useful data are from retrospective studies, mostly from selective and asymptomatic patients. There are currently no trial data to recommend the use of this technique; the only published randomised trial is too underpowered to make any useful contribution to the discussion. In contrast, conventional bypass surgery and aneurysm exclusion is safe and durable, with excellent long-term patency and limb salvage rates. Endovascular stent graft treatment of popliteal aneurysms should currently be reserved for a select group of patients with suitable anatomy and with a high operative risk, or for patients being entered into further clinical trials. For other patients, the results of conventional surgery will be hard to improve upon, although developments in device design, and the role of antiplatelet therapy or anticoagulation may improve long-term durability.

Summary

◆   Endovascular repair of popliteal aneurysms is a safe technique with few early complications.

◆   Long-term durability appears to be dubious, with stent graft occlusion rates possibly as high as 20%.

◆   There may be a significant risk of stent graft migration and endoleak associated with endovascular repair.

◆   The morbidity and mortality associated with conventional surgery are low.

◆   The long-term graft patency and limb salvage from conventional surgery are excellent, approaching 100% in some series.

◆   There have been no useful randomised trials of conventional surgery versus stenting.

◆   Endovascular repair should currently be reserved for a few, selected patients in whom conventional surgery is deemed too risky, and for patients entered into clinical trials.

References

1. Galland RB, Magee TR. Management of popliteal aneurysm. *Br J Surg* 2002; 89: 1382-5.

2. Lowell RC, Gloviczki P, Hallett JW Jr, *et al*. Popliteal artery aneurysms: the risk of non-operative management. *Ann Vasc Surg* 1994; 8: 14-23.

3. Galland RB. Popliteal aneurysms: controversies in their management. *Am J Surg* 2005; 190: 314-8.

4. Aulivola B, Hamdan AD, Hile CN, *et al*. Popliteal aneurysms: a comparison of outcomes in elective versus emergent repair. *J Vasc Surg* 2004; 39: 1171-7.

5. Martelli E, Ippoliti A, Ventoruzzo G, *et al*. Popliteal artery aneurysms: factors associated with thromboembolism and graft failure. *Int Angiol* 2004; 23: 54-65.

6. Mahmood A, Salaman R, Sintler M, Smith SR, Simms MH, Vohra RK. Surgery of popliteal aneurysms: a 12-year experience. *J Vasc Surg* 2003; 37: 586-93.

7. Blanco E, Serrano-Hernando FJ, Monux G, *et al*. Operative repair of popliteal aneurysms: effect of factors related to the bypass procedure on outcome. *Ann Vasc Surg* 2004; 18: 86-92.

8. Mercade JP. Stent graft for popliteal aneurysms: six cases with Cragg Endo-Pro System 1 Mintec. *J Cardiovasc Surg* 1996; 37(suppl 1): 41-4.

9. Kudelko PE 2nd, Alfaro-Franco C, Dietrich EB, Krajcer Z. Successful endoluminal repair of a popliteal artery aneurysm using the Wallgraft endoprosthesis. *J Endovasc Surg* 1998; 5: 373-7.

10. Bürger T, Meyer F, Tautenhahn J, Halloul Z, Fahlke J. Initial experience with percutaneous endovascular repair of popliteal artery lesions using a new PTFE stent-graft. *J Endovasc Surg* 1998; 5: 365-72.

11. Beregi JP, Prat A, Willoteaux S, Vasseur MA, Boularand V, Desmoucelle F. Covered stents in the treatment of peripheral artery aneurysms: procedural results and mid-term follow-up. *Cardiovasc Intervent Radiol* 1999; 22: 13-9.

12. Müller-Hülsbeck S, Link J, Schwartzenberg H, Walluscheck KP, Heller M. Percutaneous endoluminal stent and stent graft placement for the treatment of femoropopliteal aneurysms: early experience. *Cardiovasc Intervent Radiol* 1999; 22: 96-102.

13. Henry M, Amor M, Henry I, *et al*. Percutaneous endovascular treatment of peripheral aneurysms. *J Cardiovasc Surg* 2000; 41: 871-83.

14. Ihlberg LH, Roth WD, Alback NA, Kantonen IK, Lepantalo M. Successful percutaneous endovascular treatment of a ruptured popliteal artery aneurysm. *J Vasc Surg* 2000; 31: 794-7.

15. Howell M, Krajcer Z, Diethrich EB, *et al*. Wallgraft endoprosthesis for the percutaneous treatment of femoral and popliteal artery aneurysms. *J Endovasc Ther* 2002; 9: 76-81.

16. Gerasimidis T, Sfyroeras G, Papazoglou K, Trellopoulos G, Ntinas A, Karamanos D. Endovascular treatment of popliteal artery aneurysms. *Eur J Vasc Endovasc Surg* 2003; 26: 506-11.

17. Tielliu IF, Verhoeven EL, Prins TR, Post WJ, Hulsebos RG, van den Dungen JJ. Treatment of popliteal artery aneurysms with the Hemobahn stent-graft. *J Endovasc Ther* 2003; 10: 111-6.

18. Tielliu IF, Verhoeven EL, Zeebregts CJ, Prins TR, Span MM, van den Dungen JJ. Endovascular treatment of popliteal artery aneurysms: results of a prospective cohort study. *J Vasc Surg* 2005; 41: 561-7.

19. Loftus IM, McCarthy MJ, Lloyd A, Naylor AR, Bell PRF, Thompson MM. Prevalence of true vein graft aneurysms: implications for aneurysm pathogenesis. *J Vasc Surg* 1999; 29: 403-8.

20. Antonello M, Frigatti P, Battocchio P, *et al*. Open repair versus endovascular treatment for asymptomatic popliteal artery aneurysms: results of a prospective randomised study. *J Vasc Surg* 2005; 42: 185-93.

Chapter 23

Radiofrequency ablation for varicose veins: current evidence and practice

Sriram Subramonia MB BS MS FRCS, Specialist Registrar, General Surgery
Grantham and District Hospital, Grantham, UK
Tim Lees MB ChB FRCS MD, Consultant Vascular Surgeon
Northern Vascular Centre, Freeman Hospital, Newcastle upon Tyne, UK

Introduction

Ablation of the great saphenous vein (GSV) using radiofrequency energy is a minimally invasive alternative to conventional surgery for the treatment of great saphenous incompetence. Over the past few years evidence from randomised trials and large case series have confirmed its safety and efficacy and gradually led to its increased acceptance among vascular surgeons. In the earlier accompanying edition of this book, *Endovascular Intervention: Current Controversies*, we discussed the principles underlying the procedure, the technique, the selection of patients suitable for the procedure, and the early results reported in the literature. In this book, after a brief overview of the technique and equipment, we will focus on mid-term and long-term outcomes, factors influencing failure and the risk of deep vein thrombosis (DVT).

Technique

Radiofrequency ablation (RFA) involves a continuous feedback-controlled heating of the great saphenous vein to 85°C, using radiofrequency energy to cause endothelial destruction, contraction of vein wall collagen and thickening of the vein wall to produce a complete and durable fibrotic seal of the lumen. The technique is now increasingly performed under tumescent anaesthesia alone. Following introduction of the catheter, the tissue immediately surrounding the great saphenous vein in the thigh is infiltrated, under duplex ultrasound guidance, with normal saline, which may be combined with local anaesthetic (20ml of 1% lidocaine with 1:200,000 adrenaline diluted in 500ml of 0.9% saline). Tumescent infiltration with a solution containing adrenaline produces a temporary blanching of the skin over the treated vein (Figure 1). The volume infiltrated is variable and is determined by satisfactory compression of the vein lumen, as judged by duplex ultrasonography. An extra bolus of the infiltrate is usually required at the proximal part of the thigh, due to the greater volume of subcutaneous tissue and a larger vein dimension in this region than in the rest of the limb. The advantages of tumescent infiltration include avoidance of general anaesthesia, the ability to anaesthetise large areas of the body without producing toxic plasma levels of the anaesthetic, reduced postoperative pain and recovery time, a reduced risk of skin burns and paraesthesia from thermal nerve damage, and the ability to treat large calibre veins. Large veins (more than 12mm diameter), initially considered unsuitable for treatment with RFA, can now be safely treated to achieve results similar to that for smaller veins. Veins up to 24mm in

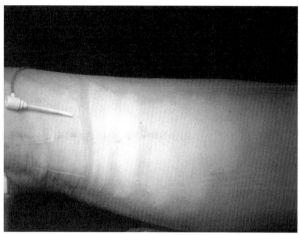

Figure 1. Temporary blanching of the skin following tumescent infiltration.

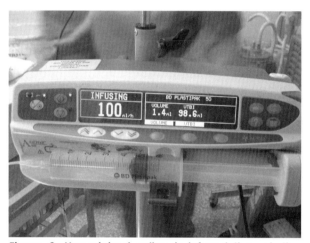

Figure 2. Heparinised saline is infused through the central lumen of the catheter via a syringe pump at 100ml/hour.

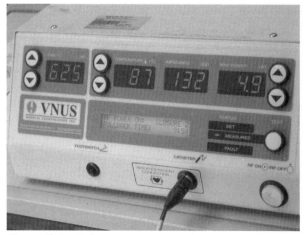

Figure 3. Radiofrequency generator.

diameter have been treated effectively [1]. Heparinised saline is infused continuously into the catheter via a central lumen to avoid thrombus formation on the electrodes. The authors use a syringe pump to deliver the heparinised saline at a rate of 100ml per hour (Figure 2). Additional stab avulsions, if required, can be performed during the same sitting under local anaesthesia.

Instrument design

The VNUS Closure® system (VNUS Medical Technologies, California, USA), comprising a bipolar radiofrequency energy generator (Figure 3) and catheters with collapsible electrodes, has several built-in mechanisms to ensure optimum control during the procedure. The generator sets the target temperature and power limits automatically, and adjusts the delivered power 50 times per second for optimal heating. The speed of catheter withdrawal can be adjusted according to the pullback timer display. The contact with the vein wall is continuously monitored via impedance display and the vein wall temperature is continuously measured by a micro-thermocouple at the tip of the catheter. Newer catheters have a light handle for ease of use, a reinforced shaft for better bend control and an integrated catheter cable for ease of set up.

Current evidence

At the beginning of this century, enthusiasm for the procedure was sustained by evidence from small case series reporting early results. Randomised trials [2-4] and large non-comparative studies [5-7] have now confirmed the safety, efficacy and clinical benefits of the procedure. Mid-term and long-term outcomes appear to confirm the durability of the procedure, [1, 4, 8, 9] with overall results comparable to conventional surgery.

GSV occlusion rate

The treated GSV remains occluded under duplex ultrasonography in 88-100% of cases at the end of one week of the procedure [3, 5, 6, 10]. In a large series involving 1006 patients and 1222 limbs, 84.9% (of

119 limbs) and 87.2% (of 117 limbs) of the GSV remained occluded at four and five years respectively [1].

Anatomical failure and clinical failure

The incidence of duplex-confirmed segmental or total reflux in the treated GSV, or groin reflux, despite a completely occluded GSV, was seen in 12% at three years [1, 8] and 16.2% at five years [1]. Most of these anatomical failures were noted early in follow-up and reflux-free rates tended to remain fairly constant over the follow-up period after the first year. Anatomical failure, however, does not necessarily indicate clinical failure and most patients demonstrated continued symptomatic benefit over the follow-up, despite duplex-demonstrable reflux [1]. A partially occluded GSV (less than 5cm open segment) did not influence the overall outcome with regard to symptoms or visible varicose veins, but a greater than 5cm non-occluded segment in the treated GSV increased the risk of recurrence [8]. Catheter withdrawal speed (optimum 2-3cm/min) and body mass index (BMI) were identified as risk factors for anatomical failure by logistic regression [1]. The latter finding is somewhat disappointing, because conventional surgery is technically more difficult and more prone to failure in patients with a high BMI. Recurrent varicosities of any degree were observed in 11.8%, 21.4% and 27.4% at three, four and five years respectively [1, 8, 9]. Improvement in pre-operative symptoms or its complete resolution were seen in over 90% of patients following RFA and sustained over the follow-up period [3, 5, 9, 11]. Moreover, 70-80% of the limbs with duplex evidence of recurrent reflux after RFA remained symptom-free for up to five years after treatment [1]. Patient satisfaction following the procedure ranged from 94% to 100% [2, 5, 10, 12]. Improvement in CEAP clinical class (Clinical, Etiology, Anatomical distribution, Pathophysiological condition) was sustained over a five-year period in over two-thirds of patients [1].

Neovascularisation

Neovascularisation induced by groin dissection increases the risk of recurrence after varicose vein surgery [13, 14]. RFA, by avoiding groin dissection and maintaining antegrade flow in the superficial epigastric vein to the GSV, has the potential to reduce the chances of neovascularisation. Although some studies have indicated that this is likely to be true [11, 15], the absence of a standard definition for neovascularisation and operator-dependent variability in the performance of duplex scans have caused difficulty in the interpretation of this relationship from different studies.

Randomised controlled trials

In *Endovascular Intervention: Current Controversies*, we reported the early results from two randomised controlled trials that compared RFA with conventional surgery that showed early clinical benefits following RFA in terms of postoperative pain, quality of life and return to activity and work [2, 3]. The latter (85 patients recruited) has now reported intermediate results with a two-year follow-up of 65 patients [4]. Recurrence and neovascularisation rates and improvement in CEAP clinical class were similar in both groups at two years. Patients who underwent RFA showed significantly improved quality of life scores compared to those who underwent conventional surgery that persisted throughout the follow-up period.

Complications

The majority of postoperative complications are transient and self-limiting. These include bruising, haematoma, purpura, phlebitis, infection at the access site and oedema. The incidence of skin burns (0.5%) and heat-induced paraesthesia (2% at four years) have decreased since the introduction of tumescent anaesthesia [9]. Necrotising fasciitis has been reported following tumescent anaesthesia for liposuction and GSV stripping [16].

Recent studies have highlighted the risk of DVT following endovenous ablation techniques [17, 18]. The cumulative incidence of DVT and pulmonary embolism after RFA has been estimated to be 2.1% and 0.2% respectively [17]. Experienced centres have reported a lower incidence [3]. The potential risk of DVT and pulmonary embolism cannot, however, be ignored and also has implications for informed consent. A 16% (12 of 73 extremities) incidence of DVT was observed in one study during early duplex scanning following RFA [18]. Undiagnosed hypercoagulable states, endothelial damage from the catheter or electrodes and propagation of thrombus from the GSV have been postulated as possible causes. We believe that commencing ablation too close to the saphenofemoral junction is possibly the most important risk factor for development of postoperative DVT. Accurate positioning of the catheter tip distal to the superficial epigastric vein prior to commencing ablation, early mobilisation following the procedure, and thromboprophylaxis in those at high risk of developing DVT, are important preventive measures. Duplex scanning within the first week of RFA will help early detection and prevention of propagation of thrombus.

Cost

RFA is significantly more expensive than conventional surgery due to the use of the generator, the catheter, intra-operative duplex imaging and possibly longer operating time. However, an earlier return to work and shorter sick leave together with improved clinical benefits in terms of pain and quality of life may offset this increased cost and prove beneficial to the individual and to society at large. Only a cost-effective analysis of the two forms of treatment within the context of an adequately powered randomised trial will help to find out if this is indeed the case.

RFA and small saphenous vein (SSV) incompetence

RFA has been used to treat SSV in some centres. The technique is similar to the treatment of GSV and tumescent anaesthesia has helped to reduce the risk of nerve injury. Insufficient numbers and limited follow-up preclude an evaluation of the long-term outcome, but results are unlikely to be significantly different from that for GSV incompetence.

Summary

◆ Radiofrequency ablation is a safe and effective minimally invasive procedure for treating great saphenous vein incompetence.

◆ It offers significant early benefits over conventional surgery in terms of postoperative pain, return to activity and quality of life.

◆ Clinical and haemodynamic outcomes after five years are comparable to conventional surgery.

◆ Tumuscent anaesthesia is now widely used and has helped to treat larger calibre veins and reduce the risk of heat-induced paraesthesia and skin burns.

◆ Non-occlusion of treated great saphenous vein for greater than 5cm increases the risk of recurrence.

◆ Catheter withdrawal speed and body mass index are risk factors for anatomical failure.

◆ The potential risk of deep vein thrombosis and pulmonary embolism is always present, but published incidence from most centres is low and acceptable for current practice.

References

1. Merchant RF, Pichot O. Long-term outcomes of endovenous radiofrequency obliteration of saphenous reflux as a treatment for superficial venous insufficiency. *J Vasc Surg* 2005; 42(3): 502-9.

2. Rautio-Tero O-A, Perälä-Jukka, Ohtonen-Pasi, *et al.* Endovenous obliteration versus conventional stripping operation in the treatment of primary varicose veins: a randomized controlled trial with comparison of the costs. *J Vasc Surg* 2002; 35(5): 958-65.

3. Lurie F, Creton D, Eklof B, *et al.* Prospective randomized study of endovenous radiofrequency obliteration (closure procedure) versus ligation and stripping in a selected patient population (EVOLVeS Study). *J Vasc Surg* 2003; 38(2): 207-14.

4. Lurie F, Creton D, Eklof B, *et al.* Prospective randomised study of endovenous radiofrequency obliteration (closure) versus ligation and vein stripping (EVOLVeS): two-year follow-up. *Eur J Vasc Endovasc Surg* 2005; 29(1): 67-73.

5. Weiss RA, Weiss MA. Controlled radiofrequency endovenous occlusion using a unique radiofrequency catheter under duplex guidance to eliminate saphenous varicose vein reflux: a 2-year follow-up. *Dermatol Surg* 2002; 28(1): 38-42.

6. Merchant RF, DePalma RG, Kabnick LS. Endovascular obliteration of saphenous reflux: a multicenter study. *J Vasc Surg* 2002; 35(6): 1190-6.

7. National Institute for Health and Clinical Excellence (NICE). Radiofrequency ablation of varicose veins. Interventional Procedure Guidance 8. http://www.nice.org.uk/pdf/ip/IPG008 guidance.pdf. Sep 2003. Accessed Jan 25, 2006.

8. Nicolini P, ClosureGroup. Treatment of primary varicose veins by endovenous obliteration with the VNUS closure system: results of a prospective multicentre study. *Eur J Vasc Endovasc Surg* 2005; 29(4): 433-9.

9. Merchant RF, Pichot O, Myers KA. Four-year follow-up on endovascular radiofrequency obliteration of great saphenous reflux. *Dermatol Surg* 2005; 31(2): 129-34.

10. Wagner WH, Levin PM, Cossman DV, *et al.* Early experience with radiofrequency ablation of the greater saphenous vein. *Ann Vasc Surg* 2004; 18(1): 42-7.

11. Pichot O, Kabnick LS, Creton D, *et al.* Duplex ultrasound scan findings two years after great saphenous vein radiofrequency endovenous obliteration. *J Vasc Surg* 2004; 39(1): 189-95.

12. Goldman MP, Amiry S. Closure of the greater saphenous vein with endoluminal radiofrequency thermal heating of the vein wall in combination with ambulatory phlebectomy: 50 patients with more than 6-month follow-up. *Dermatol Surg* 2002; 28(1):2 9-31.

13. Jones L, Braithwaite BD, Selwyn D, *et al.* Neovascularisation is the principal cause of varicose vein recurrence: results of a randomised trial of stripping the long saphenous vein. *Eur J Vasc Endovasc Surg* 1996; 12(4): 442-5.

14. Winterborn RJ., Foy C, Earnshaw JJ. Causes of varicose vein recurrence: late results of a randomized controlled trial of stripping the long saphenous vein. *J Vasc Surg* 2004; 40(4): 634-9.

15. Fassiadis N, Kianifard B, Holdstock JM, *et al.* Ultrasound changes at the saphenofemoral junction and in the long saphenous vein during the first year after VNUS closure. *Int Angiol* 2002; 21(3): 272-4.

16. Hubmer M, Koch H, Haas F, *et al.* Necrotizing fasciitis after ambulatory phlebectomy performed with use of tumescent anesthesia. *J Vasc Surg* 2004; 39(1): 263-5.

17. Mozes G, Kalra M, Carmo M, *et al.* Extension of saphenous thrombus into the femoral vein: a potential complication of new endovenous ablation techniques. *J Vasc Surg* 2005; 41(1): 130-5.

18. Hingorani AP, Ascher E, Markevich N, *et al.* Deep venous thrombosis after radiofrequency ablation of greater saphenous vein: a word of caution. *J Vasc Surg* 2004; 40: 500-4.

Chapter 24

Endovenous laser therapy for varicose veins: current evidence and recommendations

Michael J Gough ChM FRCS, Consultant Vascular Surgeon

The General Infirmary at Leeds, Leeds, UK

Introduction

Truncal varicosities due to superficial venous incompetence are common (Edinburgh Vein Study: 32% of women, 40% of men [1]) and in 2001 cost the National Health Service £20-£25 million in performing around 40,000 operations.

Most (60-70%) primary varicose veins are the result of saphenofemoral (SFJ) and great saphenous vein (GSV) reflux with 10-20% being due to saphenopopliteal (SPJ) and small saphenous (SSV) incompetence. The remainder arise as a result of perforator incompetence, or, in a few cases, from pelvic veins.

Successful treatment should abolish reflux and during surgery this is achieved by ligation of the SFJ or SPJ and GSV stripping. The case for SSV stripping is controversial because of the risk of nerve injury. However, its equivalent is easily, and safely, achieved by endovenous laser therapy.

Although varicose vein surgery may be considered a simple procedure for benign disease (only about 5% of patients suffer complications from this condition [2]), it consumes a significant proportion of the healthcare budget with additional indirect costs for community nursing services, particularly if complications occur, and absence from work. Thus, it is not surprising that there is considerable interest in the newer minimally invasive techniques for treating varicose veins.

This chapter will examine the evidence for the safety and efficacy of endovenous laser ablation (EVLA) of the great or small saphenous veins in treating superficial venous incompetence. Aspects of training in this procedure will also be considered.

Laser ablation of the GSV was described by Navarro and Min in 2001 [3], who called the procedure EVLT. Although this term has become synonymous with the technique it is a registered trademark (EVLT®) for a specific laser kit (Diomed Inc, Andover, MA). Thus, the generic name of the procedure should be EVLA, since the procedure can be performed with other manufacturer's equipment.

When do varicose veins require treatment?

In recent years, funders of healthcare in parts of the UK have implemented criteria to identify patients in whom varicose vein surgery can be performed, sometimes limiting intervention to patients who have developed complications such as thrombophlebitis,

guidewire can also be difficult to pass, particularly if the GSV/SSV is tortuous. A Terumo hydrophilic guidewire may overcome this difficulty. Problems may also be encountered if venous spasm occurs. This often reverses with patience, but, if there is sufficient guidewire in the vein, the catheter can be partly introduced and the wire withdrawn. The catheter may then advance with controlled pressure. Finally, 12.5mg papaverine in 5ml saline can be instilled into the vein via the sheath to promote venous dilatation.

Tumescent anaesthesia

Up to 200ml of 0.1% lignocaine is infiltrated along the length of the GSV/SSV under ultrasound guidance. This very important step provides anaesthesia, compression of the vein around the catheter, and a mechanism for absorption of heat when the laser is fired. If this is not done thoroughly, the patient will experience discomfort and the risks of nerve injury or skin burns are increased.

Laser ablation

The laser fibre is inserted as far as the tip of the catheter, following which the latter is withdrawn 2cm so that the fibre protrudes beyond the catheter. The laser is fired during stepwise withdrawal (12 watts energy, 810nm diode laser; one-second pulses, one-second intervals allowing withdrawal by 2mm). During treatment manual pressure is exerted over the GSV/SSV.

Following laser removal, the exit wound is closed with a suture strip and a non-stretch compression bandage applied over a length of sponge positioned over the treated vein. This remains *in situ* for one week, followed by a class II compression stocking for a further week. Patients mobilise immediately, are encouraged to resume normal activity as soon as possible and are discharged 20-30 minutes following the procedure. Usual treatment times are around 35 minutes/vein. Bilateral GSV/SSV ablation can be performed at a single visit.

Post-EVLA analgesia

Patients generally experience little pain in the first few days after EVLA and rarely require analgesia. However, 10-15% develop discomfort two to three days later due to 'phlebitis' of the GSV/SSV. The frequency and severity of this is reduced by the routine prescribing of diclofenac 50mg tds for the first three days.

Patient suitability

Suitability for EVLA is determined by ultrasound demonstration of the sites of venous incompetence and assessment of GSV/SSV tortuosity. Ideally, this is done with a portable ultrasound at the first outpatient visit. Although uncommon, a very tortuous GSV or SSV may be a relative contraindication due to difficulties in advancing the guidewire. In most patients, these veins are reasonably straight with varicosities confined to their tributaries.

In some patients, anterior thigh and lateral knee varicosities arise from an incompetent anterior saphenous vein (ASV) which usually joins the GSV just distal to the saphenofemoral junction. The anatomy of this vein is variable and it is important to determine its precise course. For successful treatment, at least 10cm of the proximal vein should be ablated. The anatomical variations of the ASV and their suitability for EVLA are shown in Figure 1.

Finally, some patients with recurrent varicose veins may be suitable for laser treatment if the GSV or SSV were not stripped at the time of their previous surgery. In addition, foam sclerotherapy can be administered via the sheath, prior to insertion of the laser fibre, if there is significant neovascularisation refilling the truncal vein.

In a pilot study, the suitability for EVLA was assessed in 591 consecutive patients with truncal varicosities. Of 515, 365 (71%) with primary varicose veins and 34/76 (45%) with recurrent varicosities were offered laser therapy.

perforation (extravasation of blood and post-ablation bruising), damage to perivenous nerves and arteries, and skin burns. Although some of these events were observed in an animal model [9], the protective effect of perivenous tumescent anaesthesia was not assessed. In order to assess the risk of irreversible nerve damage, which occurs at temperatures above 45°C, we measured perivenous temperatures 3mm, 5mm, and 10mm from the GSV during laser fibre withdrawal, after administration of tumescent anaesthesia. The median temperature 3mm from the vein was 34.5°C (maximum 43.3°C), making nerve injury unlikely during EVLA. In contrast, a radiofrequency ablation catheter generates a constant temperature of 85°C with the catheter being withdrawn much more slowly. This is likely to generate higher perivenous temperatures and may account for the higher incidence of nerve injuries and skin burns reported with this technique.

Portable or static ultrasound?

Although superior imaging will be obtained from a static ultrasound machine in a radiology department or vascular laboratory, performing EVLA in either will compromise the work of that department. Furthermore, the image quality of currently available portable ultrasound equipment is sufficient to allow the safe performance of EVLA.

Who should perform ultrasound imaging?

To provide the most cost-effective service, the clinician undertaking EVLA should be competent in performing the required ultrasound imaging. For surgeons acquiring these skills there is the additional advantage of applying them in the outpatient clinic to assess patient suitability for EVLA. Currently, training programmes in vascular ultrasound are not freely available, but are clearly needed. Thus, many surgeons are self taught or have spent time with a specialist ultrasonographer/vascular technician to develop their skills. Alternatively, an ultrasonographer or radiologist can provide ultrasound imaging. The latter could also undertake EVLA given their expertise in interventional procedures. Under this circumstance

patients must undergo initial assessment by a vascular surgeon who can assess their symptoms and counsel them in respect of the risks and benefits of the various therapeutic options.

Where should EVLA be performed?

For maximum cost-effectiveness, EVLA can be performed as an outpatient procedure in a clean treatment room, and does not require the use of an operating theatre or a day-case surgery unit, although the latter may provide a waiting room and changing facilities. Another alternative, particularly if portable ultrasound is not available, is to undertake EVLA in the radiology department. The drawbacks to this have been alluded to above.

EVLA technique

Patient position

For GSV ablation, the patient lies supine on a tilting table with the leg to be treated slightly flexed at the knee and hip with the latter externally rotated. The patient lies prone for SSV treatment.

Cannulation of the GSV or SSV

After preparing the skin with povidine iodine, a sterile, disposable drape is placed beneath it. The table is tilted into the Trendelenberg position. Under ultrasound guidance, the GSV/SSV is cannulated percutaneously, after anaesthetising the overlying skin (1% lignocaine) just above or below the knee (mid-calf for SSV) and a guidewire passed beyond the SFJ or SPJ. A 5 French catheter is passed over the guidewire and the tip positioned (ultrasound control) 0.5-1cm distal to the junction. Visualisation of a jet of saline flushed through the catheter may aid identification of the tip. The table is then placed in the horizontal position.

If percutaneous cannulation proves difficult (superficial vein, spasm or haematoma after an initial attempt), the vein can be delivered through a small stab incision with a vein hook. Occasionally, the

varicose eczema, lipodermatosclerosis or ulceration. Inevitably, many potential patients will find this approach unacceptable and much of the difficulty in identifying patients for intervention, if cosmetic surgery is to be denied, centres on the rather loose association between varicose veins and symptoms.

Whilst common symptoms include aching, heaviness, pruritis, and oedema, the Edinburgh Vein Study found that almost half of all women complained of aching legs irrespective of the presence of varicose veins and that there was a poor correlation between symptoms and the existence of truncal varices [4]. Conversely, asymptomatic superficial venous reflux occurs in up to 39% of the population [5]. Thus, many surgeons offer varicose vein treatment to those patients who wish to proceed with it, provided that they are aware of potential complications.

The ideal management for varicose veins

Successful management depends upon accurate identification of the site or sites of superficial venous reflux and its subsequent abolition. The chosen intervention should relieve symptoms, improve cosmesis, and be associated with low complication and recurrence rates. Therapies that allow a rapid return to normal activity and reduce treatment costs are clearly advantageous. These are attributes that may be achieved by the three minimally invasive treatment methods, endovenous laser therapy, radiofrequency ablation and foam sclerotherapy.

Endovenous laser ablation of the great or small saphenous vein

Equipment

The principal requirements for EVLA are a laser power source, single-use laser fibres, an ultrasound machine (portable or static), a tilting couch or theatre recovery trolley, a procedure pack and a number of disposable items including 200ml 0.1% lignocaine with adrenaline (190ml N/Saline and 10ml 2% lignocaine and 1:200,000 adrenaline) for tumescent

anaesthesia. A vein hook and mosquito forceps are useful if there is difficulty cannulating the GSV or SSV and a Terumo hydrophilic guidewire in the event of difficulty in passing the wire.

Which laser power source?

The choice of 810nm or 940nm diode lasers for EVLA is based on the absorption peak of haemoglobin to red/infrared light (800-1000nm). It was originally believed that heat generated by the laser produced steam bubbles from blood that caused thermal damage to the endothelium and sub-endothelial layer, resulting in focal coagulative necrosis and shrinkage, and leading to thrombotic occlusion of the vein [6]. Histological studies at three and six months indicate failure of endothelial regeneration and progressive damage to the muscle layers of the vein wall, resulting in further shrinkage [7].

Although this mechanism of venous injury has been widely accepted, it is not entirely logical. Following catheterisation, venous spasm often occurs. Further, administration of the tumescent perivenous anaesthesia compresses the vein, as does manual pressure over the vein during laser withdrawal. Direct contact between the laser and vein wall therefore seems a more likely explanation for the injury which results in permanent ablation, since recanalisation should be relatively common following a simple thrombotic occlusion.

In practical terms, there seems to be no difference in the safety and efficacy of either the 810nm or 940nm diode laser for EVLA. In contrast, a single report describes the use of a 1064nm Nd:YAG laser for EVLA. The laser energy delivered in this study was ten-fold greater than that in other EVLA studies and resulted in a high incidence of temporary paraesthesia and thermal injury (36% and 5% respectively), making it unsuitable for clinical use [8].

Is laser therapy safe?

In animal studies, the average laser tip temperature was 729°C. Such high temperatures could have a number of potential adverse effects, including vein

Chapter 24

Endovenous laser therapy for varicose veins: current evidence and recommendations

Michael J Gough ChM FRCS, Consultant Vascular Surgeon

The General Infirmary at Leeds, Leeds, UK

Introduction

Truncal varicosities due to superficial venous incompetence are common (Edinburgh Vein Study: 32% of women, 40% of men [1]) and in 2001 cost the National Health Service £20-£25 million in performing around 40,000 operations.

Most (60-70%) primary varicose veins are the result of saphenofemoral (SFJ) and great saphenous vein (GSV) reflux with 10-20% being due to saphenopopliteal (SPJ) and small saphenous (SSV) incompetence. The remainder arise as a result of perforator incompetence, or, in a few cases, from pelvic veins.

Successful treatment should abolish reflux and during surgery this is achieved by ligation of the SFJ or SPJ and GSV stripping. The case for SSV stripping is controversial because of the risk of nerve injury. However, its equivalent is easily, and safely, achieved by endovenous laser therapy.

Although varicose vein surgery may be considered a simple procedure for benign disease (only about 5% of patients suffer complications from this condition [2]), it consumes a significant proportion of the healthcare budget with additional indirect costs for community nursing services, particularly if complications occur, and absence from work. Thus, it is not surprising that there is considerable interest in the newer minimally invasive techniques for treating varicose veins.

This chapter will examine the evidence for the safety and efficacy of endovenous laser ablation (EVLA) of the great or small saphenous veins in treating superficial venous incompetence. Aspects of training in this procedure will also be considered.

Laser ablation of the GSV was described by Navarro and Min in 2001 [3], who called the procedure EVLT. Although this term has become synonymous with the technique it is a registered trademark (EVLT®) for a specific laser kit (Diomed Inc, Andover, MA). Thus, the generic name of the procedure should be EVLA, since the procedure can be performed with other manufacturer's equipment.

When do varicose veins require treatment?

In recent years, funders of healthcare in parts of the UK have implemented criteria to identify patients in whom varicose vein surgery can be performed, sometimes limiting intervention to patients who have developed complications such as thrombophlebitis,

Table 1. Results for endovenous laser ablation of the great saphenous vein.

Author	Year	Limbs	FU	% success	Paraesthesia	Burns	DVT
Navarro et al [3]	2001	40	4.2	100	0	0	0
Min et al [11]	2001	90	6	97	1	0	0
Min et al [15]	2003	499	17	98.2	0	0	0
Proebstle et al [12]	2003	104	12	90.4	0	0	0
Oh et al [14]	2003	15	3	100	0	0	0
Sadick et al [36]	2004	30	24	96.8	0	0	0
Perkowski et al [13]	2004	203	0.5	97.0	0	0	0
Theivacumar et al [37]	2005	502	6	92*	3	0	1

* 100% occlusion when ≥60 joules/cm used

to three years [15]. GSV occlusion rates were 98% at one month and 93% at two years (n=121). Eight of nine patients whose GSV was patent at two years were successfully retreated and no further recurrences occurred in 40 patients followed-up for three years. In a recent review article, the same author cited further follow-up data describing 98% occlusion at up to five years with 99.8% success in 500 patients treated with ≥70 joules/cm [17].

Although there are no published randomised trials comparing EVLA with conventional surgery, preliminary results of such a study were presented at the annual meeting of the Vascular Society of Great Britain & Ireland in 2005 [16]. This showed that abolition of reflux and improvements in symptom scores three months after either EVLA or surgery were identical. However, the time taken to return to normal activity and to paid employment was significantly lower in EVLA patients. Long-term follow-up on these patients is continuing.

SSV occlusion

Since EVLA was initially developed for abolishing GSV reflux, there are few studies describing its use for SPJ and SSV incompetence. Further, the risk of

thermal damage to the common peroneal nerve and its branches meant that this concept was pursued with caution. Following the results of our temperature studies described earlier we have ablated 45 SSV. All received ≥60 joules/cm, resulting in 100% occlusion rates. Three patients experienced transient paraesthesia or numbness in the distribution of the sural nerve, despite cannulating the SSV at or above the mid-point of the calf, where the nerve normally joins the vein. Two other reports describe success rates of 95% and 97% [12, 13] for SSV ablation in a total of 78 limbs with a median follow-up of three months. These results are encouraging given that conventional SPJ ligation is associated with recurrence rates of up to 50%, often as the result of inadequate surgery [18].

Treatment of residual varicosities

Conventional surgery aims at eliminating superficial venous reflux (SFJ ligation and stripping GSV or SPJ ligation ± SSV stripping) and removing the varicosities (multiple phlebectomies). In contrast, EVLA only achieves the primary aim of eliminating reflux. In most centres patients are reviewed after 6-12 weeks and varicosities that have not disappeared spontaneously following abolition of reflux are treated by injection sclerotherapy. In our series sclerotherapy has been

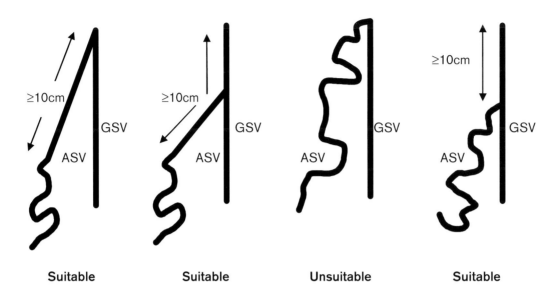

Figure 1. Anatomy and suitability of the anterior saphenous vein (ASV) for EVLA.

Results for GSV ablation

Laser energy

Navarro and Min [3], who initially described the procedure, employed an 810nm-diode laser and this has arguably been more widely used than 940nm-diode lasers. In early reports, Min and his colleagues used laser powers varying from 10-14 watts delivered as intermittent pulses (12 watts, one-second pulses, one-second intervals, stepwise withdrawal, four pulses/cm) or continuous laser (14 watts) with continuous withdrawal (2mm/sec). These techniques delivered around 50 joules/cm treated vein.

Recently we have assessed a number of factors that might influence the success of EVLA, including GSV diameter, the length of vein ablated, total laser dose, joules of energy delivered/cm vein and body mass index. In 476 consecutive GSV procedures, the vein was occluded or non-visible (duplex ultrasound) throughout the treated length in 432 (91%) at six-month follow-up. Occlusion rates were not influenced by body mass index, which might affect the efficacy of post-treatment compression, GSV diameter or the total laser dose after correction for differences in the length of vein ablated. However, there was a significant difference in the median energy delivery to occluded (61.2 [50.4-68.4] joules/cm) and partially occluded or patent veins (43.2 [36.0-55.2] joules/cm), p<0.01. Further, successful ablation was achieved in all veins that received ≥60 joules/cm. This equates to ≥5 pulses/cm using the protocol described earlier.

GSV occlusion

Observational studies report GSV closure rates of 94-100% (assessed by duplex ultrasound), with relief of symptoms and improvement in the appearance of superficial varicosities (Table 1). In most studies, follow-up was one year or less [3, 10-16]. Nevertheless, Min *et al* have provided some data to support the longer-term efficacy of EVLA, describing the outcome in almost 500 patients who had been assessed at up

required in 45% and 12.5% of GSV and SSV patients respectively. Although the results of primary sclerotherapy for truncal varicosities have been disappointing, long-term efficacy is likely when truncal reflux has been abolished.

Alternative approaches to the management of residual varicosities include multiple phlebectomies, either at the time of EVLA, or at 6-12 weeks or early sclerotherapy. None of these options seem particularly attractive, since with the latter up to 95% of patients require sclerotherapy whilst the former negates much of the benefit of a minimally invasive procedure.

Patient-related outcomes

The potential advantages of EVLA compared to surgery are shown in Table 2. Data from our randomised trial, and from a prospective audit of other patients treated with laser ablation, confirm that it is associated with the same reduction in venous symptom scores (Aberdeen Venous Symptom Score)

as surgery, but with a more rapid return to normal activity and a reduced complication rate. These results are summarised in Table 3. Furthermore, 93% of patients would chose EVLA again.

Potential complications

Phlebitis and superficial thrombophlebitis

Symptomatic 'phlebitis' in the ablated vein is the commonest adverse event following EVLA and appears more frequent in patients treated with 14 watts laser power compared to 12 watts. Its severity can be minimised by the prescription of a non-steroidal anti-inflammatory agent for 72 hours following the procedure, although compliance with this advice is variable.

Rarely, patients develop superficial thrombophlebitis in the tributaries of the ablated vein secondary to stasis. This risk is reduced when adequate post-treatment compression is applied as described above.

Table 2. Potential advantages and cost factors for EVLA and surgery.

Potential advantages	Cost factors for EVLA	Cost factors for surgery
Outpatient procedure	Equipment £50,000 (laser power source + US)	Surgical instruments
Avoid general anaesthesia	Disposables/case £275 (laser fibre £225)	Disposables
'No scars'	1 'surgeon'	2 surgeons 1 anaesthetist/1 ODA
Reduced risk of complications	1-2 nurses	2 nurses (minimum)
More rapid recovery	Waiting room	Day unit/IP bed
Potential reduction in direct and indirect costs	Treatment room	Operating theatre Recovery room and staff

Table 3. Patient outcomes following EVLA or surgery (medians±IQR).

	GSV EVLA~ n=66	SSV EVLA n=48	Surgery~ n=33
Abolition of reflux	91% *	100%	88%
Time to normal activity (days)	3.5 (0-8)	0 (0-4)	14 (3-28)
Return to work (days)	4 (2-10)	Not recorded	17 (5-32)
Analgesia requirement (days)	2 (1-7)	3 (0-14)	3 (2-8)
Sclerotherapy	45%	12.5%	-
Aberdeen Venous Symptom Score	13.83 (10.21-2.3) v	14.2 (11.2 - 19.5) v	14 (9.3-18.2) v
	6.05 (2.70-11.64)	4.8 (3.3-6.8)	5.3 (1.4-7.4)
Complications			
Phlebitis	12% #	4%	-
Nerve 'injury'	3.8%	6%	15%
DVT/PE	0.29%	0	0
Wound problems	-	-	6.7%
Other	-	-	1 ARDS
Would choose EVLT again	93%	98%	-

~ patients from randomised trial

* includes patients treated prior to establishing requirement of ≥60 joules/cm

includes patients treated prior to routine prescription of diclofenac (50mg tds x 72hr)

Time to normal activity: p=0.016 GSV EVLA v surgery

Return to work: p=0.011

Aberdeen Venous Symptom Score: p=0.001, pre- v post-treatment for all groups

Bruising

Minor bruising along the line of the treated vein is uncommon and is much less severe than the bruising associated with GSV stripping, after which haematoma and wound infection are relatively common (up to 10%).

Skin burns

Although skin burns were reported in the study using the 1064nm Nd:YAG laser [8], and have been described after radiofrequency ablation, this complication has not been observed after EVLA (Table 1), presumably because of the protective effect of the tumescent infiltration.

Nerve injury

Surgical treatment of varicose veins results in permanent neurological deficits in 5-7% of patients [19]. Although numbness or paraesthesia in the distribution of the saphenous or sural nerves may occur following EVLA, it is uncommon (Table 3) and resolves within three months.

Min has proposed that variations in the laser energy throughout the length of the treated vein might be beneficial in avoiding complications when the vein for ablation is particularly superficial or close to nerves or arteries. Thus, for the proximal 10-15cm of the GSV he suggests up to 140 joules/cm, 70 joules/cm for the mid-portion of the vein, and around 50 joules/cm for the below-knee GSV or the SSV close to the saphenopopliteal junction [17].

Vascular injury

A single vascular complication, an arteriovenous fistula between the SSV and the superficial sural artery in the popliteal fossa after SSV ablation, has been described after EVLA [20]. This risk should be avoided by thorough infiltration of relatively large volumes of tumescent anaesthesia around the SSV to separate it from adjacent structures. Further, it is possible that the reported injury was traumatic from the spinal needle used for tumescence rather than thermal. Although Min's protocol for reducing the laser energy when close to the saphenopopliteal junction might avoid this type of complication, it may compromise effective ablation of the proximal SSV.

DVT and pulmonary embolism

Following conventional surgery, this risk is no greater than for comparable surgery and the incidence of pulmonary embolism is 0.2-0.5% [21]. In our series of >700 GSV EVLA procedures, a single patient (0.14%) has suffered a non-fatal pulmonary embolus. However, there has been debate about the risk of thrombo-embolic complications following EVLA and radiofrequency ablation, due to propagation of thrombus from the GSV into the common femoral vein. A recent report by Puggioni et al [22] found evidence of this on early post-procedure ultrasound scans in 3/54 (5.6%) EVLA patients. Although none had occlusive thrombus in the common femoral vein, all were anticoagulated and a temporary IVC filter was deployed in one. None suffered a pulmonary embolus and the thrombus had lysed on subsequent scans.

Although this is a potentially important finding, all patients underwent concomitant phlebectomies and all received a general or spinal/epidural anaesthetic. Thus, procedures inevitably took longer and immediate ambulation was prevented. This could explain the discrepancy between this and other observational series. Technical factors might also be relevant when considering the risk of thrombus propagation and again large volumes of tumescent anaesthesia that empty the proximal GSV should diminish this risk.

In another study involving rigorous duplex examination ten days after radiofrequency ablation, 16% of patients had evidence of a DVT [23], with 11/12 due to extension of thrombus from the GSV. These procedures were also performed under general anaesthesia in conjunction with phlebectomies. In addition, during radiofrequency ablation the catheter is *in situ* for much longer, thus encouraging the development of catheter-related thrombus. Although early thrombus resolution occurred following anticoagulation, the authors recommend that early duplex scans should be performed following radiofrequency ablation. The issue of the thrombo-embolic risk associated with this technique, and perhaps EVLA, remains controversial and good prospective data are required.

Complications and litigation

Although a relatively minor procedure, varicose vein surgery is the commonest reason for litigation in general/vascular surgery in the UK, accounting for 17% of settled claims, including the highest Medical Defence Union settlement for these specialties between 1990-1998. Further, the NHS Litigation Authority (NHSLA) has paid almost £5.5 million in compensation to varicose vein patients since 1995. Most claims result from a failure to warn patients of the risk of sensory nerve injury, which highlights the importance of obtaining fully informed consent. More serious nerve injuries also occurred with 12 cases of foot drop after saphenopopliteal ligation being recorded on the NHSLA database. Ligation or injury to either the femoral vein or artery may also occur and are impossible to defend. That EVLA avoids these complications is of considerable importance.

Risk of recurrence

It has been suggested that recurrent reflux, and subsequently recurrent varicose veins, may occur because of recanalisation of the GSV or SSV and because the GSV tributaries in the groin are likely to remain patent since ligation of these may be pivotal in reducing recurrence rates [24]. In our own series of >700 GSV ablations, the vein is occluded up to the level of the SFJ, provided that ablation is commenced within 1cm of the junction, thus protecting these veins from the effects of SFJ reflux. Further, recanalisation only occurs following thrombotic occlusion of the truncal vein. The importance of tumescent anaesthesia, manual compression and elevation of the limbs during EVLA has already been stressed. Provided that these principles are adhered to, the treated vein should be empty during the procedure and occlusion will be the result of vein wall injury rather than thrombosis. That this is the case is supported by our own observation that the ablated vein becomes invisible on sequential post-procedure ultrasound scanning.

Neovascularisation is a major cause of recurrent reflux and further varicosities following surgery. Chandler *et al* have suggested that avoiding surgical disruption of the SFJ or SPJ may reduce this risk following EVLA [25]. In our series, neovascularisation was evident in 3.7% of 109 limbs specifically scanned for this purpose at 12 months. In contrast, Dwerryhouse *et* *al* found evidence of neovascularisation in 52% of post-surgery patients by two years [26]. Although far from conclusive, this data would suggest that neovascularisation may be less likely after EVLA.

Training in minimally invasive techniques for varicose veins

Effective performance of EVLA requires three essential skills. These are the clinical assessment of venous patients and a full knowledge of all potential therapeutic options, the ability to perform a reliable venous ultrasound assessment, and the technical ability to perform the procedure. Traditionally, vascular surgeons are only trained in the first skill. To gain expertise in ultrasound, time can be spent in the vascular laboratory or radiology department, although there is clearly a need for short but intensive 'hands-on' training courses. For surgical trainees, the acquisition of such skills should become part of the training curriculum. Once the ultrasound skills have been acquired, the ability to perform EVLA can be easily learnt in the skills laboratory using available models and in the clinical setting. Alternatively, an EVLA service could be run jointly by a surgeon and an interventional radiologist. Although the latter might argue that they are capable of running a service on their own, this would be difficult with current NHS referral practices and would require a period of training in clinical assessment.

EVLA compared to radiofrequency ablation, foam sclerotherapy and surgery

Such a comparison is not the specific purpose of this chapter, although it is a question that inevitably arises. Briefly, occlusion rates seem to be slightly lower for radiofrequency ablation (85-100% [27-31]), although there are no comparative studies. Some of the reported difference between EVLA and radiofrequency ablation are summarised in Table 4. Of some importance is the much greater cost of radiofrequency ablation catheters.

One of the difficulties in assessing the reported outcomes for radiofrequency ablation is the variety of techniques employed. Thus, it has been performed using general, loco-regional or local anaesthesia, with or without tumescent anaesthesia, and frequently in combination with multiple phlebectomies. These variations may influence both its efficacy and the prevalence of complications.

Sclerotherapy of varicose veins is associated with high recurrence rates in patients with saphenofemoral or saphenopopliteal incompetence [32]. However, greater success has been reported for foam sclerotherapy, which allows a smaller quantity of sclerosant to cover a greater surface area and to displace blood from the vein when used for GSV incompetence. GSV occlusion rates of 81-90% have

Table 4. Comparison of EVLA and RFA.

	EVLA	RFA
Anaesthetic	Local	General, regional, local (inconsistent approach)
Treatment for varicosities	Delayed sclerotherapy (early sclerotherapy) (phlebectomy)	Phlebectomy (sclerotherapy)
GSV diameter	Any size	≤12mm
Patient suitability	>70%	30-58%
Success	94-100%	85-100%
Mode of action	? steam bubbles ? direct vein wall injury	Endothelial and collagen damage, venoconstriction
Paraesthesia	Up to 7.8%	13-16%
Thrombophlebitis	Up to 12%	Up to 20%
DVT	Up to 5.6% if under GA	Up to 16%
Skin burns	None	Up to 20% in early studies
Costs	Less expensive OP procedure, LA	RFA catheter ≥2x laser fibre ±GA, operating theatre etc RCT = more expensive than surgery

been reported [33, 34], the lowest rate being at three-year follow-up. Thus, although foam sclerotherapy is associated with minimal cost, early occlusion rates are lower and its durability is unproven. In addition, a few serious adverse events have been reported with this technique including DVT, anaphylaxis, visual disturbance, stroke and cardiac events.

The initial success of EVLA and surgery in abolishing reflux appears similar, although there is fairly good evidence to suggest that the risk of serious complications and of more minor morbidity is lower with laser ablation. In addition, return to normal activity and employment are more rapid after EVLA. For health providers, EVLA performed under local anaesthesia in an outpatient setting is almost certainly less expensive than conventional surgery. The outstanding issue that remains is that of the long-term results for EVLA and this has been discussed earlier.

Conclusions

The results of EVLA were the subject of a recent systematic review [35], which concluded that although EVLA seems beneficial, its effectiveness and safety cannot be judged without comparative data from randomised clinical trials. Our recently completed study (GSV EVLA versus conventional surgery) confirms that laser therapy is as effective as surgery in eliminating reflux, improving symptoms and enhancing cosmesis, but with the advantage that it avoids general anaesthesia, is associated with fewer complications, a rapid convalescence, and potentially, a lower risk of recurrent varicosities.

A large multicentre randomised trial against surgery would provide the best evidence about treatment efficacy. From experience, it is difficult to recruit patients to such a trial, since many opt for EVLA.

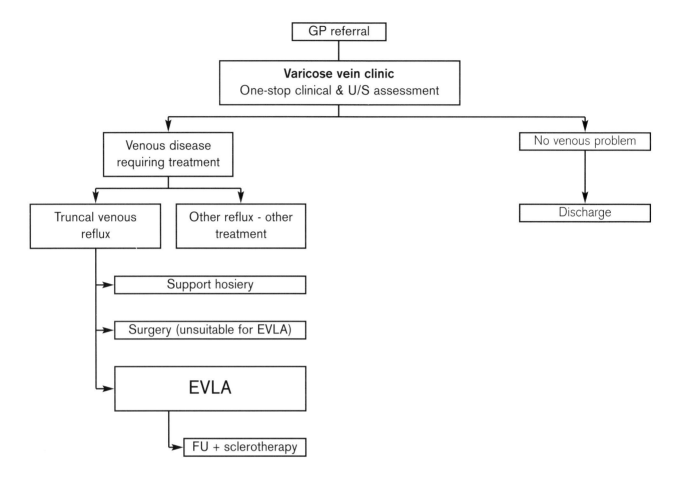

Figure 2. Algorithm for the management of new referrals with varicose veins.

Further, such a study should include long-term follow-up for five or more years. This is likely to be incomplete.

If it is accepted that the choice of treatment for varicose veins will be increasingly driven by patient choice, then management algorithms are required. Thus, our current recommendations for the management of patients with varicose veins are shown in Figure 2.

On the assumption that minimally invasive treatment will replace conventional surgery for patients in whom it is appropriate, there remains the difficulty of selecting the most appropriate method of those currently available. Whilst it might be argued that EVLA has some advantages over radiofrequency ablation in terms of cost and complication rates, there is no clear evidence that either is superior. A randomised trial might answer this question although, without corporate sponsorship, the cost of equipping centres to undertake both procedures makes this unlikely. Further, since any differences between the techniques may be small, a large multicentre study is likely to be required. Finally, the information derived from such a trial may not be attractive to the relevant manufacturers and thus, funding may not be forthcoming!

For foam sclerotherapy, there is certainly an advantage in terms of cost, although its durability is unlikely to match that of EVLA or radiofrequency ablation and its efficacy may be lower in patients with larger diameter veins. Further, serious complications have been reported following foam sclerotherapy, which although rare, may mitigate against its routine use for a largely benign and often cosmetic intervention.

Summary

◆ 71% primary and 45% recurrent varicose veins are suitable for EVLA.

◆ Equally effective for GSV and SSV reflux.

◆ 60-70 joules laser energy per cm vein results in optimum occlusion rates.

◆ Symptom and cosmetic improvement is equivalent to surgery.

◆ More rapid return to normal activity and employment than after surgery.

◆ Fewer complications than surgery, particularly for nerve injury and wound problems.

◆ Popular with patients.

◆ Further evidence regarding long-term efficacy is required for all minimally invasive therapies.

References

1. Evans C, Fowkes FG, Ruckley CV, *et al*. Prevalence of varicose veins and chronic venous insufficiency in men and women in the general population: Edinburgh Vein Study. *J Epidemiol Community Health* 1999; 53: 149-53.

2. Tibbs DJ. *Varicose Veins and Related Disorders*, 1st ed. Oxford: Butterworth-Heinemann Ltd, 1992.

3. Navarro L, Min RJ, Bone C. Endovenous laser: a new minimally invasive method of treatment for varicose veins - preliminary observations using an 810nm diode laser. *Dermatol Surg* 2001; 27(2): 117-22.

4. Bradbury A, Evans CJ, Allan P, *et al*. The relationship between lower limb symptoms and superficial and deep venous reflux on duplex ultrasonography: The Edinburgh Vein Study. *J Vasc Surg* 2000; 32: 921-31.

5. Labropoulos N, Delis KT, Nicolaides AN. Venous reflux in symptom-free vascular surgeons. *J Vasc Surg* 1995; 22: 150-4.

6. Proebstle TM, Sandhofer M, Kargl A, *et al*. Thermal damage of the inner vein wall during endovenous laser treatment; key role of energy absorption by intravascular blood. *Dermatol Surg* 2002; 28: 596-600.

7. Bush RG, Shamma HN, Hammond KA. 940-nm laser for treatment of saphenous insufficiency: histological analysis and long-term follow-up. *Photomed Laser Surg* 2005; 23: 15-9.

8. Chang CJ, Chua JJ. Endovenous laser photocoagulation (EVLP) for varicose veins. *Lasers Surg Med* 2002; 31(4): 257-62.

9. Weiss RA. Comparison of endovenous radiofrequency versus 810nm diode laser occlusion of large veins in an animal model. *Dermatol Surg* 2002; 28(1): 56-61.

10. Bush RG. Regarding "Endovenous treatment of the greater saphenous vein with a 940-nm diode laser: thrombolytic occlusion after endoluminal thermal damage by laser-generated steam bubbles". *J Vasc Surg* 2003; 37(1): 242.

11. Min RJ, Zimmet SE, Isaacs MN, *et al*. Endovenous laser treatment of the incompetent greater saphenous vein. *J Vasc Interv Radiol* 2001; 12(10): 1167-71.

12. Proebstle TM, Gul D, Kargl A, *et al*. Endovenous laser treatment of the lesser saphenous vein with a 940-nm diode laser: early results. *Dermatol Surg* 2003; 29(4): 357-61.

13. Perkowski P, Ravi R, Gowda RC, *et al*. Endovenous laser ablation of the saphenous vein for treatment of venous insufficiency and varicose veins: early results from a large single-center experience. *J Endovasc Ther* 2004; 11: 32-8.

14. Oh CK, Jung DS, Jang HS, *et al*. Endovenous laser surgery of the greater saphenous vein with a 980nm diode laser. *Dermatol Surg* 2003; 29: 1135-40.

15. Min RJ, Khilnani N, Zimmet SE. Endovenous laser treatment of saphenous vein reflux: long-term results. *J Vasc Interv Radiol* 2003; 14: 991-6.

16. Beale RJ, Thievacumar N, Mavor AID, *et al*. Endovenous laser treatment (EVLT) or surgery for varicose veins? A randomised controlled trial in patients with sapheno-femoral and long saphenous incompetence. Presented to the Vascular Society of Great Britain and Ireland, Nov 2005.

17. Min RJ, Khilnani NM. Endovenous laser ablation of varicose veins. *J Cardiovasc Surg* 2005; 46: 395-405.

18. van Rij AM, Jiang P, Solomon C, Christie RA, Hill GB. Recurrence after varicose vein surgery: a prospective long-term clinical study with duplex ultrasound scanning and air plethysmography. *J Vasc Surg* 2003; 38: 935-43.

19. Holme JB, Skajaa K, Holme K. Incidence of lesions of the saphenous nerve after partial or complete stripping of the long saphenous vein. *Acta Chir Scand* 1990; 156: 145-8.

20. Tiperman PE. Arteriovenous fistula after endovenous laser treatment of the short saphenous vein. *J Vasc Interv Rad* 2004; 15: 625-7.

21. Critchley G, Handa A, Maw A, *et al*. Complications of varicose vein surgery. *Ann R Coll Surg Eng* 1997; 79: 105-10.

22. Puggioni A, Kalra M, Carmo M, *et al*. Endovenous laser therapy and radiofrequency ablation of the great saphenous vein: analysis of early efficacy and complications. *J Vasc Surg* 2005; 42: 488-93.

23. Hingorani A, Ascher E, Markevich N, *et al*. Deep venous thrombosis after radiofrequency ablation of greater saphenous vein: a word of caution. *J Vasc Surg* 2004; 40: 500-4.

24. Browse NL, Burnand KG, Irvine AT, *et al*. *Diseases of The Veins*. 2nd ed. London: Arnold, 1999.

25. Chandler JG, Pichot O, Sessa C, *et al*. Defining the role of extended saphenofemoral junction ligation: a prospective comparative study. *J Vasc Surg* 2000; 32: 941-53.

26. Dwerryhouse S, Davies B, Harradine K, *et al*. Stripping the long saphenous vein reduces the rate of re-operation for recurrent varicose veins: five-year results of a randomised trial. *J Vasc Surg* 1999; 29: 589-92.

27. Rautio T, Ohinmaa A, Perala J, Ohtonen P, Heikkinen T, Wiik H, *et al*. Endovenous obliteration versus conventional stripping operation in the treatment of primary varicose veins: a randomized controlled trial with comparison of the costs. *J Vasc Surg* 2002; 35: 958-65.

28. Sybrandy JE, Wittens CH. Initial experiences in endovenous treatment of saphenous vein reflux. *J Vasc Surg* 2002; 36: 1207-12.

29. Merchant RF, DePalma RG, Kabnick LS. Endovascular obliteration of saphenous reflux: a multicenter study. *J Vasc Surg* 2002; 35: 1190-96.

30. Manfrini S, Gasbarro V, Danielsson G, Norgren L, Chandler JG, Lennox AF, *et al*. Endovenous management of saphenous vein reflux. Endovenous Reflux Management Study Group. *J Vasc Surg* 2000; 32: 330-42.

31. Lurie F, Creton D, Eklof B, Kabnick LS, Kistner RL, Pichot O, *et al*. Prospective randomized study of endovenous radiofrequency obliteration (Closure procedure) versus ligation and stripping in a selected patient population (EVOLVeS Study). *J Vasc Surg* 2003; 38: 207-14.

32. Jakobsen BH. The value of different forms of treatment for varicose veins. *Br J Surg* 1979; 66: 182-4.

33. Tessari L, Cavezzi A, Frullini A. Preliminary experience with a new sclerosing foam in the treatment of varicose veins. *Dermatol Surg* 2001; 27: 58-60.

34. Cabrera J, Cabrera J, Garcia-Olmedo MA. Treatment of varicose long saphenous veins with sclerosant in microfoam form: long-term outcomes. *Phlebology* 2000; 15: 19-23.

35. Mundy L, Merlin TL, Fitridge RA, Hiller JE. Systematic review of endovenous laser treatment for varicose veins. *Br J Surg* 2005; 92(10): 1189-94.

36. Sadick NS, Wasser S. Combined endovascular laser with ambulatory phlebectomy for the treatment of superficial venous incompetence. *J Cosmet Laser Ther* 2004; 6: 44-9.

37. Theivacumar N, Beale RJ, Mavor AID, *et al*. Factors influencing the effectiveness of endovenous laser treatment for varicose veins due to sapheno-femoral and long saphenous reflux. Presented to the Vascular Society of Great Britain and Ireland, Nov 2005.

Chapter 25

Foam sclerotherapy for varicose veins: current evidence and recommendations

Philip Coleridge Smith DM FRCS, Reader in Surgery

UCL Medical School, London, UK

Introduction

Surgery for varicose veins is widely used in the UK for the management of symptomatic varicose veins, but this is a far from perfect treatment. Although regarded as an effective method of management, recent publications show that recurrence may be expected in 25-50% of patients at five years [1-4]. Patients require on average two weeks away from work following treatment to allow postoperative bruising and discomfort to subside. Surgery leaves scars and may result in damage to adjacent structures, including nerves, lymphatics, major arteries and veins [5]. Deep vein thrombosis and pulmonary embolism may also follow surgical treatment for varicose veins [6, 7]. These problems have led to the development of a number of new treatments for varicose veins, including radiofrequency obliteration (RF obliteration) [8], endovenous laser treatment (EVLT) [9] and ultrasound-guided foam sclerotherapy (UGFS).

Sclerotherapy has been used to treat varicose veins for 150 years. A detailed review of the history of this subject has been published recently [10]. One of the first descriptions of a method of sclerotherapy that resembles the techniques used today was published in a monograph by Dr. R Thornhill in 1929 [11]. The apparatus used to make the injections included a syringe which had been modified to include a small glass window between the syringe and the needle. This was used to aspirate blood from the vein to be injected in order to confirm that the tip of the needle was in the lumen of the vein. Thornhill used a solution of quinine and urethane to treat veins.

Fegan devised his own injection-compression technique, which involved firm bandaging of the lower limb following injection of a sclerosant [12]. This method along with strategies described by other European authors has been widely used for more than half a century. In the UK and other northern European countries, sclerotherapy is substantially less popular than in southern European countries such as France, Spain and Italy. The reasons for this are not entirely clear, but there was a diminishing of interest in sclerotherapy in the UK following the publication of a randomised study between sclerotherapy and surgery published by Hobbs [13]. This showed that the outcome of surgical treatment after ten years was substantially better than for conventional sclerotherapy. Many took this to mean that sclerotherapy was not a very useful treatment in the management of varicose veins and its use declined in the UK and northern European countries.

Ultrasound-guided sclerotherapy

In the 1980s, ultrasound was introduced for the diagnosis of venous disease of the lower limb. In France, where enthusiasm for the use of sclerotherapy had remained strong, this led Schadeck and Vin to improve the efficacy of their treatment by using ultrasound imaging to guide the placing of injections into incompetent saphenous trunks [14, 15]. This method of treatment was found to achieve obliteration of the saphenous trunks in a substantial proportion of patients, resulting in long-term relief from varices. As with conventional sclerotherapy, the problem of recanalisation of veins was encountered in up to one quarter of patients at one year [16]. Proponents of sclerotherapy argue that, even if recurrence occurs, the resulting varices and incompetent saphenous trunk are easily managed by further sessions of sclerotherapy.

Foam sclerotherapy

In 1944, Orbach described the 'air block' technique. A small volume of air is included in the syringe with the sclerosant. The air is injected ahead of the sclerosant in order to prevent blood diluting the sclerosant and reducing its efficacy. In 1950, he published a further paper describing the use of a foam which he created by vigorously shaking a syringe containing air and sclerosant to produce a froth [17]. He modestly records that this method was also suggested by Foote [18]. Fegan refers to the use of sodium tetradecyl sulphate (STS) as a foam in the management of vulval varices of pregnancy in his book on sclerotherapy, originally published in 1967 [19].

The next significant advance came in 1993 when Cabrera suggested that foam could be created using carbon dioxide mixed with polidocanol, a detergent sclerosant [20]. Cabrera published a further article in 1997, describing his experience in 261 limbs with long saphenous varices and eight patients with vascular malformations [21]. He had used sclerotherapy with foam, guiding his injections by ultrasound imaging. Some of the varicose veins reached 20mm in diameter. He considered that foam greatly extended the range of vein sizes which could be managed by sclerotherapy. He felt that the increased efficacy of

foam was attributable to it displacing blood from the treated vein and increasing the contact time between the sclerosant and the vein. He used a 'microfoam', consisting of very small bubbles, created by the use of a small rapidly rotating brush.

Preparation of sclerosant foam

Several authors have described methods of preparing 'home-made' foam, which may be used for ultrasound-guided sclerotherapy. Monfreux described a method utilising a glass syringe to produced small quantities of polidocanol foam, which he used to treat a series of patients with truncal varicose veins [22]. Sadoun described a method of preparing foam using a plastic syringe, avoiding the need for reusable glass syringes [23]. Subsequently, Tessari has described a method of preparing foam using two disposable syringes and a three-way tap [24]. This method can be used to produce large quantities of foam, suitable for treating saphenous trunks and large varices. Frullini has added his own method of producing foam to this increasing list [25], based on that of Flückinger [26].

The most widely used method is that of Tessari, which is readily achieved using materials available in most clinics (Figure 1). Two syringes are connected using a three-way tap. These can be either 2ml or 5ml syringes or a combination. A mixture of sclerosant and

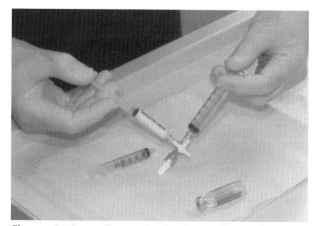

Figure 1. Tessari's method of creating sclerosant foam. A mixture of sclerosant (3% Fibrovein) and air is oscillated between two syringes connected by a three-way tap.

air is drawn into one syringe at a ratio of one part of sclerosant to three or four parts of air. The sclerosant can be STS 1-3% (Fibrovein®, STD Pharmaceuticals, Hereford, UK) or polidocanol 0.5-3% (Sclerovein®, Resinag AG, Zurich, Switzerland). Low concentrations of polidocanol (0.5%) make better foam when mixed 1:1 with air. The mixture is oscillated vigorously between the two syringes about 10 or 20 times. The tap can be turned slightly to reduce the aperture and increase the smoothness of the foam. The foam produced in this way is stable for about two minutes, so it should be injected immediately it has been created.

Applications of foam sclerotherapy

Sclerosant foam can be injected instead of liquid sclerosant, in the management of varicose veins and reticular varices not associated with truncal saphenous incompetence. The advantage of using foam in these veins is that more varices appear to be treated per injection and lower volumes of sclerosant are required. Since veins injected with foam have

blood displaced from them and develop spasm, it is usually obvious which veins have been treated without the need for ultrasound imaging.

In 1999, Henriet reported his results in 10,000 patients with reticular varices and telangiectases of the lower limb treated between the years 1995-8 [27]. He found that the outcome of foam treatment in small varices was excellent and that reduced volumes and concentrations of sclerosant could be employed compared to liquid sclerosants. Benigni reported the findings of a pilot study comparing liquid and foam sclerosants. He measured the outcome using a visual analogue scale to describe the improvement in appearance. He found that foam resulted in a 20% improved appearance compared to liquid sclerosant [28].

Treatment of saphenous trunks

Foam sclerotherapy, as described by Cabrera, was intended to be used to treat saphenous trunks as an alternative to surgery (Figure 2). This requires

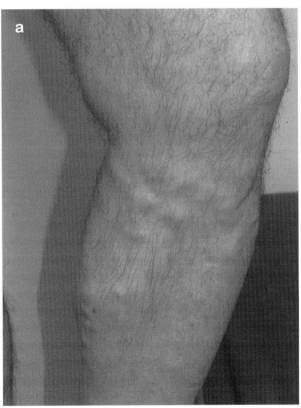
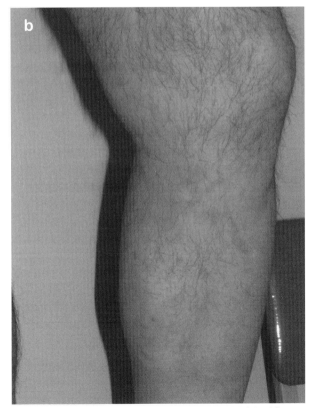

Figure 2. a) Varices arising from incompetence of the SFJ and GSV. b) Two weeks after ultrasound-guided foam sclerotherapy of the saphenous trunk.

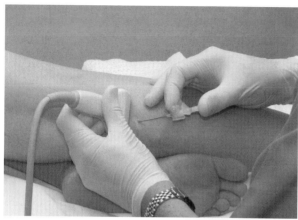

Figure 3. Ultrasound-guided cannulation of the SSV during UGFS of varices, arising from the SSV. The patient is lying in the left lateral position.

ultrasound-guided injecting (UGFS), since the saphenous trunks cannot be readily treated safely and effectively without imaging control (Figure 3). Cabrera described cannulation of the affected saphenous trunk, followed by injection of foam until the vein was completely filled along with its tributaries. Any unfilled tributaries were managed by injection using a butterfly needle. Other strategies are possible and it is common practice in France to inject the saphenous trunk using a needle and syringe. The complete length of the incompetent vein and tributaries is managed by several injections carried out over a number of sessions. Direct needle injection has the advantage of simplicity, but in some anatomical regions, such as the popliteal fossa, a number of large arteries may lie adjacent to the small saphenous vein. Inadvertent intra-arterial injection causes disastrous results.

A wide range of maximum suggested volumes have been reported. Cabrera injected up to 100ml of his foam, whereas other authors have averaged 1-2ml in a single session. A recent consensus document suggested that 6-8ml of foam per session is the maximum appropriate amount [33].

It is conventional to apply compression following foam sclerotherapy. Some authors use stockings alone [20, 32] and others use bandages [29]. As with earlier practices in sclerotherapy, immediate ambulation and return to work are encouraged. There is little need for time away from work.

Any vein suitable for injection may be treated by foam sclerotherapy. In contrast to techniques requiring the passage of a catheter, such as RF closure or EVLT, UGFS can be used to manage primary and recurrent varices arising in saphenous tributaries or trunks. The treatment is limited only by the skill of the sclerotherapist to inject the vein.

Outcomes

Cabrera has published a clinical series of 500 lower limbs treated by foam sclerotherapy. He reported that, after three or more years, 81% of treated great saphenous trunks remained occluded and 97% of superficial varices had disappeared. This required one session of sclerotherapy in 86% of patients, two in 11% and three sessions in 3% of patients. No DVT or pulmonary embolism was encountered in this series Subsequently, a number of authors have published clinical series based on this technique, including Frullini and Cavezzi, who reported a series of 453 patients [30], and Barrett who reported a series of 100 limbs [31]. Cavezzi has subsequently published a detailed analysis of the efficacy of foam sclerotherapy in 194 patients, reporting a good outcome in 93% of patients [32]. In fact, this technique has become widely used in southern Europe, Australia, New Zealand, South America and the USA [33]. However, few surgeons in the UK use this method, perhaps because of limited evidence of efficacy. One series has been recently reported from the UK involving 60 patients comparing surgical treatment with foam sclerotherapy combined with saphenofemoral ligation [34].

No randomised study of foam sclerotherapy in comparison to surgery has yet been published, although a multicentre European study has been conducted and the results presented at a scientific meeting [35]. This randomised controlled trial included two separate studies. The first study involved surgeons, who randomised patients to saphenous stripping or UGFS. The second study involved sclerotherapists, who randomised patients to ultrasound-guided sclerotherapy conducted using either foam or liquid sclerosant. A total of 654 patients were treated during this study. Up to four sessions of ultrasound-guided foam sclerotherapy were allowed over a three-month period, in order to obliterate the saphenous trunks. After 12 months, the surgeons had eliminated truncal saphenous reflux in 130 of 176 patients (74%) by UGFS and in 84/94 (88%) by surgery. In comparison, sclerotherapists had eliminated reflux in 239 of 254 patients (91%) by UGFS and 104/125 (83%) by liquid sclerotherapy. Post-treatment pain was assessed by a visual analogue scale, which showed that surgery was much more painful than UGFS during the first week. Normal activities were resumed after a median of 13 days in the surgery group and two days in the UGFS group. Deep vein thrombosis was seen in ten patients treated by UGFS and one patient treated by liquid sclerotherapy.

Personal experience

The author's experience of the use of ultrasound-guided foam sclerotherapy is based on an analysis of all patients treated for varicose veins, during the period January 2002 to August 2005. A total of 808 patients (666 women, 142 men) were managed by ultrasound-guided foam sclerotherapy for truncal saphenous incompetence. In all, 1411 limbs were affected by varices (CEAP C1 n=212, 15%, CEAP C2 n=1154, 82%). Treatments were selected according to the preference of the patients and upon the advice of the author. This was not a randomised study. Patients often requested foam sclerotherapy, since they considered that surgery was excessively invasive, and many of them had previous experience of surgical treatment. Nearly one third treated for GSV reflux had had previous surgical treatment. Patients were investigated by clinical examination and duplex ultrasonography by the author. Those with isolated saphenous varices and reticular varices are not included in this analysis. All treatments were carried out in a consulting room, without sedation or general anaesthesia. The techniques were based on those published by Cabrera, in which ultrasound-guided cannulation of the great saphenous vein (GSV) or small saphenous vein (SSV) was used to deliver foam to the saphenous trunk. Direct needle injection of foam was used to manage superficial varices.

The sclerosants used to prepare the foam were, either polidocanol (POL - Sclerovein®, Resinag AG, Zurich, Switzerland), or purified sodium tetradecyl sulphate (STS - Fibrovein®, STD Pharmaceuticals Ltd, Hereford, UK). POL was used as a 1% solution to create the foam to treat saphenous trunks and STS was used as either a 1% or 3% solution for saphenous trunks. The author's practice changed during the clinical series, with the use of greater volumes of foam and stronger solutions to minimise the likelihood of recurrence. Foam was prepared in a ratio of 0.5ml of sclerosant to 1.5ml of air, in keeping with the practice reported in previous publications [30].

Compression bandaging was applied to limbs where saphenous trunks and varices had been injected. Pehahaft cohesive bandage (Pehahaft®, Hartmann, Germany) was used most often with Velband (Velband®, Johnson & Johnson Medical, Ascot, Berkshire, UK) cotton wool padding applied over the saphenous trunks to increase compression. This results in a thin bandage which fits beneath most clothes and shoes. A class 2 medical compression stocking was measured and applied to secure the bandage (Credelast®, Credenhill, Ilkeston, Derbyshire, UK). Initially, bandaging was left in place for three to five days, but later in the series this was increased to 10-14 days to minimise the incidence of thrombophlebitis.

Treatment sessions were carried out at intervals of two weeks. Duplex ultrasonography was used to check the treated veins for completeness of occlusion and additional segments of saphenous trunk and associated varices were treated as required.

All patients were invited to return for review after six months following completion of treatment. Those who did not attend were sent further appointments. Despite this, not all patients attended for follow-up.

Not all venous disease detected on clinical and ultrasound examination underwent ultrasound-guided foam sclerotherapy. Some patients considered that only one limb required treatment. In all, 1109 limbs were managed by foam sclerotherapy. In these limbs, duplex ultrasonography showed that the main cause was GSV or SSV reflux. GSV reflux alone was present in 766 limbs (69%), SSV reflux alone in 223 limbs (20%) and combined GSV and SSV reflux in 120 (11%). A surprisingly high proportion of patients had undergone previous surgery for varicose veins in

Outcome of treatment of GSV

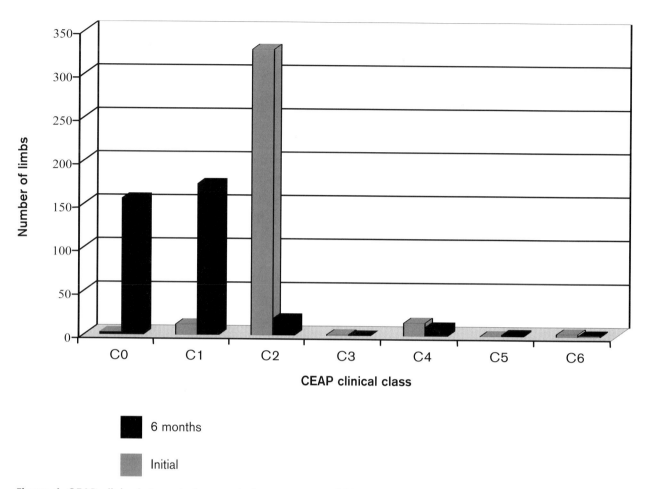

Figure 4. CEAP clinical stage before and at an average of 11 months after UGFS carried out to the GSV.

the vessel being treated (n=267, 30% of GSVs and n=60, 17% of SSVs). The median diameter of the GSVs treated was 5mm (IQR 4-6mm) and for the SSVs 5mm (IQR 4-6mm). In this series, four limbs were treated in which post-thrombotic damage was found, leading to deep vein incompetence in association with GSV or SSV reflux.

Thrombophlebitis occurred in a small number of patients (5%) and was managed by analgesia, compression and aspiration of thrombus. Calf vein thrombosis was confined to isolated gastrocnemius veins or to part of the posterior tibial vein (ten cases). All resolved with compression, by stocking or bandage, and exercise without use of anticoagulants. In one case, a short occlusive thrombus arose in the

common femoral vein two weeks following treatment of the GSV. The mechanism appeared to be due to direct extension of thrombus from the GSV into the femoral vein. This case was managed by anticoagulation using low molecular weight heparin and warfarin continued for six months. The occluded femoral vein recanalised within four weeks and at six months of follow-up, no residual scarring or valve damage could be demonstrated on duplex ultrasonography. In two further cases, thrombus extended from the SFJ and SPJ (one case each) into the femoral and popliteal vein. The thrombus was noted to be firmly adherent to the vein wall and of limited extent. This was managed by compression stockings and exercise whilst the extent of the thrombus was monitored by duplex ultrasonography.

In these cases, the thrombus resolved without further intervention. No major systemic complication, such as anaphylaxis, stroke or transient ischaemic attack occurred in this series. A number of patients (14, 2% of all patients treated) reported visual disturbance following treatment. Patients with a previous history of migraine were especially at risk of this problem. In all but one case, the only effect was to produce a scotoma with flashing lights or a ground glass appearance in part of the visual field, which resolved within one hour.

A total of 457 limbs have been reviewed at six months or more, following treatment (average 11 months, range 6-46 months). Figure 4 shows the CEAP clinical class before and after sclerotherapy in the limbs where the GSV was treated. A substantial improvement in clinical venous disease was obtained. Duplex examination of the GSVs showed occlusion had been obtained in 322 of 364 (88%). In the SSVs, occlusion was present in 118 of 143 (83%). The median diameter of the GSVs and SSVs fell from 5mm before treatment to GSV: 2 mm and SSV: 1mm at follow-up of six months or more.

The only residual adverse events still present at six months or more of follow-up were skin pigmentation (115 of 457 limbs) and palpable lumps (21 limbs). The skin pigmentation was almost always of a minor extent and continued to fade with the passage of time. In those patients reviewed one year or more following treatment, skin pigmentation was present in 11 of 115 limbs. Small palpable lumps were sometimes detectable in the calf and comprised residual elements of treated veins. These could be identified by ultrasound imaging, but were not otherwise visible. In contrast to surgery, no scars, neurological damage or lymphatic injuries were encountered.

Safety of foam sclerotherapy

Complications arising from foam sclerotherapy are those which may also arise from and have been previously described in connection with conventional liquid sclerotherapy. Problems may arise locally at the site of injection, in the same limb or systemically.

Local complications include extravasation of sclerosant foam associated with skin necrosis. This is more commonly seen with STS than with polidocanol foam, which is much less likely to cause problems if it leaks from a vein during treatment. Thrombophlebitis occurs reasonably frequently following sclerotherapy, but is readily managed by aspiration of thrombus. Frullini reported two cases of skin necrosis and seven of thrombophlebitis in a series of 196 patients treated by foam sclerotherapy.

Deep vein thrombosis may occur following surgery or sclerotherapy for varicose veins. Gastrocnemius veins in the calf are at risk of exposure to sclerosant foam injected into superficial varices. Frullini also reported one case of gastrocnemius thrombosis and a further case of popliteal vein thrombosis in his series of 196 patients.

Systemic complications, which have been described following both liquid and foam sclerotherapy, include visual disturbance and chest symptoms such as coughing. These occur in about 1-2% of patients. Visual disturbance often occurs in patients with a previous history of migraine associated with a visual aura. They develop a scotoma following treatment, which resolves completely within 30-60 minutes. There is some evidence that this may be attributable to the passage of bubbles via a patent foramen ovale (PFO, which is in any case present in 20% of people). There is a rapidly expanding literature on the association of PFO and migraine in the general population [36]. However, the fact that visual disturbance, and other neurological symptoms, are well known following injection of liquid sclerosants, suggests that this may be a simplistic explanation. A case of 'stroke' following foam sclerotherapy has been reported [37]. Right-sided weakness occurred following a session of foam sclerotherapy. However, there was no identifiable lesion on MR imaging and the patient made a complete recovery. He was found to have a large patent foramen ovale.

Severe allergic reactions to sclerosants are rare but not unknown. These represent the most severe adverse reaction to treatment. Anyone performing sclerotherapy of any type should be suitably equipped to deal with such an event.

A large number of patients are treated by foam sclerotherapy throughout the world on a daily basis and the extent of the recorded complications is very low. In the author's opinion, this treatment carries a low risk of serious adverse reactions. The cause of visual disturbance caused by sclerotherapy remains unknown. It would be desirable to understand this phenomenon better. It appears to be strongly related to a history of migraine and resolves without sequelae.

Conclusions

Foam sclerotherapy offers an alternative to surgical intervention for patients with varicose veins. It can be conducted on an outpatient basis and is far less complex than endovenous laser therapy or radiofrequency ablation of saphenous veins. It can also be used in primary or recurrent truncal incompetence as well as in tributaries and small varices. The recurrence rate following this treatment has yet to be established in comparison to surgery. Ultrasound imaging studies suggest that 85-90% of veins treated in this way remain occluded after three years. This is comparable to endovenous laser therapy and radiofrequency ablation and similar to rates of neovascularisation reported following surgery. This technique promises to be a useful addition to the methods currently in use for managing superficial venous incompetence.

Summary

- Ultrasound-guided foam sclerotherapy has become widely used in the management of superficial venous incompetence in many countries.

- Treatment is directed towards incompetent saphenous trunks which are injected under ultrasound control.

- This treatment is painless and can be used in an outpatient setting.

- No complex or special equipment is required other than an ultrasound machine.

- The cost of management of varicose veins performed in this way is low in comparison to surgical interventions.

- Patients can normally continue their usual work following treatment.

- The complications of this treatment include local skin necrosis, due to the sclerosant, thrombophlebitis and deep vein thrombosis. Transient visual disturbance and chest problems may also arise.

- In contrast to surgery, peripheral nerves are not at risk during this treatment.

- Primary and recurrent veins can be treated whether arising from saphenous trunks or tributaries.

- Data from clinical series suggest that after three years 85-90% of saphenous trunks treated by UGFS remain occluded.

References

1. van Rij AM, Jiang P, Solomon C, Christie RA, Hill GB. Recurrence after varicose vein surgery: a prospective long-term clinical study with duplex ultrasound scanning and air plethysmography. *J Vasc Surg* 2003; 38: 935-43.

2. Winterborn RJ, Foy C, Earnshaw JJ. Causes of varicose vein recurrence: late results of a randomized controlled trial of stripping the long saphenous vein. *J Vasc Surg* 2004; 40: 634-9.

3. Fischer R, Linde N, Duff C, Jeanneret C, Chandler JG, Seeber P. Late recurrent saphenofemoral junction reflux after ligation and stripping of the greater saphenous vein. *J Vasc Surg* 2001; 34: 236-40.

4. Perrin MR, Guex JJ, Ruckley CV, dePalma RG, Royle JP, Eklof B, Nicolini P, Jantet G. Recurrent varices after surgery (REVAS), a consensus document. REVAS group. *Cardiovasc Surg* 2000; 8: 233-45.

5. Campbell WB, France F, Goodwin HM; Research and Audit Committee of the Vascular Surgical Society of Great Britain and Ireland. Medicolegal claims in vascular surgery. *Ann R Coll Surg Engl* 2002; 84: 181-4.

6. van Rij AM, Chai J, Hill GB, Christie RA. Incidence of deep vein thrombosis after varicose vein surgery. *Br J Surg* 2004; 91: 1582-5.

7. Srilekha A, Karunanithy N, Corbett CRR. Informed consent: what do we tell patients about the risk of fatal pulmonary embolism after varicose vein surgery? *Phlebology* 2005; 20: 175-6.

8. Merchant RF, Pichot O; Closure Study Group. Long-term outcomes of endovenous radiofrequency obliteration of saphenous reflux as a treatment for superficial venous insufficiency. *J Vasc Surg* 2005; 42: 502-9.

9. Mundy L, Merlin TL, Fitridge RA, Hiller JE. Systematic review of endovenous laser treatment for varicose veins. *Br J Surg* 2005; 92: 1189-94.

10. Wollmann JC. The history of sclerosing foams. *Dermatol Surg* 2004; 30: 694-703.

11. Thornhill R. *Varicose veins and their treatment by 'empty vein' injection.* London: Balliere, Tindall & Cox, 1929: 64.

12. Fegan WG. Injection with compression as a treatment for varicose veins. *Proc R Soc Med* 1965; 58: 874-6.

13. Hobbs JT. Surgery or sclerotherapy for varicose veins: 10-year results of a random trial. In: *Superficial and deep venous diseases of the lower limbs.* Tesi M, Dormandy JA, Eds. Turin: Panminerva Medica, Sept 1984: 243-8.

14. Schadeck M, Allaert F. Echotomographie de la sclérose. *Phlébologie* 1991; 44: 111-30.

15. Vin F Echo-sclérothérapie de la veine saphène externe. *Phlébologie* 1991; 44: 79-84.

16. Kanter A, Thibault P. Saphenofemoral incompetence treated by ultrasound-guided sclerotherapy. *Dermatol Surg* 1996; 22: 648-52.

17. Orbach EJ. The thrombogenic activity of foam of a synthetic anionic detergent (sodium tetradecyl sulfate NNR). *Angiology* 1950; 1: 237-43.

18. Foote RR. *Varicose veins.* London: Butterworth & Co., 1949: 1-225.

19. Fegan G. *Varicose veins: compression sclerotherapy.* London: Heinemann Medical, 1967: 1-114.

20. Cabrera Garido JR, Cabrera Garcia Olmedo JR, Garcia Olmedo Dominguez. Nuevo meodo de esclerosis en las varices tronculares. *Pathologia Vasculares* 1993; 1: 55-72.

21. Cabrera Garrido JR, Cabrera Garcia-Olmedo JR, Garcia-Olmedo Dominguez MA. Elargissement des limites de la schlérothérapie: noveaux produits sclérosants. *Phlébologie* 1997; 50: 181-8.

22. Monfreux A. Traitement sclérosant des troncs saphèniens et leurs collatérales de gros calibre par le méthode mus. *Phlébologie* 1997; 50: 351-3

23. Sadoun S, Benigni JP. The treatment of varicosities and telangiectases with TDS and Lauromacrogol foam XIII World Congress of Flebology, 1998, Abstract Book: 327.

24. Tessari L. Nouvelle technique d'obtention de la scléro-mousse. *Phlébologie* 2000; 53: 129.

25. Frullini A. New technique in producing sclerosing foam in a disposable syringe. *Dermatol Surg* 2000; 26: 705-6.

26. Flückinger P. Nicht-operative retrograde Varizenverödung mit Varsylschaum. *Schweizer Med Wochenschrift* 1956; 86: 1368-70.

27. Henriet JP. Expérience durant trois années de la mousse de polidocanol dans le traitement des varices réticulaires et des varicosités. *Phlebologie* 1999; 52: 277-82.

28. Benigni JP, Sadoun S, Thirion V, Sica M, Demagny A, Chahim M. Télangiectasies et varices réticulaires traitement par la mousse d'aetoxisclérol à 0.25% présentation d'une étude pilote. *Phlebologie* 1999; 52: 283-90.

29. Yamaki T, Nozaki M, Iwasaka S. Comparative study of duplex-guided foam sclerotherapy and duplex-guided liquid sclerotherapy for the treatment of superficial venous insufficiency. *Dermatol Surg* 2004; 30: 718-22

30. Frullini A, Cavezzi A. Sclerosing foam in the treatment of varicose veins and telangiectases: history and analysis of safety and complications. *Dermatol Surg* 2002; 28: 11-5.

31. Barrett JM, Allen B, Ockelford A, Goldman MP. Microfoam ultrasound-guided sclerotherapy of varicose veins in 100 legs. *Dermatol Surg* 2004; 30: 6-12.

32. Cavezzi A, Frullini A, Ricci S, Tessari L. Treatment of varicose veins by foam sclerotherapy: two clinical series. *Phlebology* 2002; 17: 13-8.

33. Breu FX, Guggenbichler S. European Consensus Meeting on Foam Sclerotherapy, April, 4-6, 2003, Tegernsee, Germany. *Dermatol Surg* 2004; 30: 709-17.

34. Bountouroglou DG, Azzam M, Kakkos SK, Pathmarajah M, Young P, Geroulakos G. Ultrasound-guided foam sclerotherapy combined with sapheno-femoral ligation compared to surgical treatment of varicose veins: early results of a randomised controlled trial. *Eur J Vasc Endovasc Surg* 2006; 31(1): 93-100.

35. International Union of Phlebology, Chapter Meeting, San Diego, USA, Sept 2003.

36. Holmes DR Jr. Strokes and holes and headaches: are they a package deal? *Lancet* 2004; 364: 1840-2.

37. Forlee MV, Grouden M, Moore DJ, Shanik G. Stroke after varicose vein foam injection sclerotherapy. *J Vasc Surg* 2006; 43: 162-4.

Chapter 26

Conventional surgery for varicose veins: current evidence and predictions for the future

Mo Adiseshiah MA MS FRCS FRCP, Consultant Vascular & Endovascular Surgeon
University College Hospital, London, UK

Introduction

Many modern therapies for the treatment of varicose veins represent variants of ancient traditional remedies. As one considers alternatives to conventional surgery, the long tradition of scientific evaluation of the subject should be revisited. The reader is referred to the leading reference text [1], which reviews the scientific evidence on this subject.

In summary, varicose veins were recognised as a pathological phenomenon in 1550 BC [2], and after William Harvey's [3] ground-breaking research on the circulation, first Trendelenberg [4] in 1891, and then Homans [5] in 1916 described the operation of saphenofemoral vein junction disconnection, which remains the gold standard to the present day. Earlier in 1905, Keller [6] described the technique of stripping the great saphenous vein (GSV), and thus the stage was set for one of the most enduring surgical procedures: saphenofemoral flush disconnection and great saphenous vein stripping. The technique of avulsion and excision of individual varicosities was popularised by Lofgren [7], who used incisions in Langer's lines, and Chester [8], who used stab incisions and vein hooks to produce more acceptable cosmetic results. Infrageniculate communicating vein ablation has been developed using open and endoscopic sub-fascial (sub-fascial perforator surgery or SPS) approaches [9, 10, 11], as well as by the use of blunt metal phlebotomes inserted just deep to the deep fascia [12], followed by division of all perforating vessels in this anatomical plane.

The introduction of sclerosant results in venospasm, sterile inflammatory change in the vein wall, thrombus formation and ultimately, vein sclerosis in some of the treated veins. Lindser [13] developed injection sclerotherapy in its present form in 1916. Since then, several variants on the theme have been described including the current popular technique of ultrasound-guided foam sclerotherapy (UGFS) in which treatment of the whole varicose system is the aim. This form of sclerotherapy is the subject of Chapter 25 in this book.

An alternative to flush saphenofemoral or saphenopopliteal junction ligation coupled with surgical stripping of the GSV or small saphenous vein (SSV) is the development of devices employing radiofrequency (RF) or laser energy (LA) to ablate these truncal veins and obviate the need to perform a flush junctional ligation and stripping procedure. The evidence for these technologies is evaluated in Chapters 23 and 24, and attempts to compare the newer treatments with classic surgery are undertaken there.

Clinical aspects

As ever, the clinical diagnosis and assessment for treatment must underwrite all approaches to therapy. The following are the usually accepted goals of treatment:

- relief of symptoms - aching, swelling;
- treatment of complications - lipodermato-sclerosis, venous ulceration, superficial thrombophlebitis, vein haemorrhage;
- prevention of complications above;
- prevention of recurrence;
- improvement of appearance of legs.

At the present time of proposed rationing within the NHS, it is important to justify the massive expenditure necessary for the treatment of varicose veins. There is ample evidence of benefit for intervention for the latter four factors above. With respect to the first factor (relief of symptoms), a recent randomised controlled trial of conventional surgery versus conservative treatment for uncomplicated varicose veins showed that there was a significant quality of life benefit for surgery within the first two years [14]. Clearly the history and physical examination concentrating on the five factors mentioned above is the starting point. A past history of treatment of varices, deep vein thrombosis and a family history are also sought. On examination, the distribution of varices and the presence of a saphena varix is noted. The traditional Trendelenberg tourniquet test has been superseded by the use of duplex/Doppler ultrasound scanning of the lower limb and pelvic veins. Using this technology, saphenofemoral, saphenopopliteal and perforator vein incompetence are diagnosed, and the surface marking of the saphenopopliteal junction and other perforators is carried out. Finally, deep venous thrombosis and deep venous incompetence, if present, can be demonstrated using this technology.

In a reasonably fit subject, with the full clinical and duplex scanning, it is possible in most cases to select patients for interventional therapies after obtaining fully informed consent. In patients unfit for intervention, or in whom the results of intervention are unlikely to be of benefit, or in those unwilling to accept intervention, alternative approaches are necessary.

The use of graduated compression elastic stockings, four-layer bandaging for ulcers, elevation of the foot of the bed and ambulation are recommended.

Current evidence

Intervention strategies for treatment of varicose veins

There is ample evidence [15, 16] that saphenofemoral junction and saphenopopliteal junction disconnection, coupled with ablation of the respective truncal veins, is the basis for successful treatment of varicose veins when these junctions are incompetent. In addition, either communicator/perforator vein ablation [11] and/or phlebectomies [8] of varicose complexes are essential as well as the ablation of the truncal veins and their communication with the deep system to achieve maximum success rates.

A fundamental realisation based upon published evidence is that attention to only part of the pathology, i.e. only truncal disease ablation when there is accompanying perforator disease will undoubtedly result in residual veins after surgery or in recurrence [17], and vice versa [18].

The first task is to establish the most effective and most patient-acceptable technique for ablation of the GSV and SSV. Further, the presence or absence of junctional tributaries after intervention should be addressed. For the GSV, the four current techniques are open surgery and stripping (OS) - usually to the level of the knee, radiofrequency ablation (RF), laser ablation (LA), or ultrasound-guided foam sclerotherapy (UGFS). Traditional surgery gives immediate and late failure rates for GSV ablation and loss of reflux of 1% and 23% respectively [19]. The immediate results of optimally administered LA are comparable with OS, but the late results of junctional and GSV reflux are awaited. Currently, the results of RF are less good with 81% immediate and 75% late freedom from junctional and GSV reflux [20]. This may be because the optimum dose of energy is at present unknown. Cases of deep vein thrombosis with RF have been reported by some workers [21], probably because of higher energy delivery given with less precision. On the other hand, the dose of energy with LA has been better researched [22], and better results are obtained as a result. Recent randomised controlled trials of OS versus LA have shown greater patient satisfaction with LA. This is because it is less invasive and less traumatic to the patient [23].

At present, the standard treatment for SSV and junctional incompetence is OS. The operation is accompanied by a high recurrence rate and a significant incidence of nerve injury [24]. The proximity of the sural nerve and the branches of the sciatic nerve at the saphenopopliteal junction are the cause of this intra-operative nerve damage. Anecdotal reports [25] of LA of the SSV are emerging, but there is no registry or randomised controlled trial of LA, RF and OS.

Attention to the main trunks of the GSV and SSV system and ignoring perforators and other varicose complexes leads to recurrence and unsatisfactory patient outcomes. The need for additional surgery is high and unacceptable to the patient [26].

OS is indicated when there is recurrence of saphenofemoral and saphenopopliteal reflux. If there is accompanying truncal reflux in the GSV and / or the SSV, LA or RF may be used if the fibre will pass, and UGFS may have a role in such circumstances. Even after successful LA, RF or UGFS, if saphenofemoral junction reflux persists, OS is necessary. The presence of significant calf perforating veins is a challenge for OS, RF and LA. UGFS is an attractive option in these circumstances, but for reasons stated in the complications section, some caution should be exercised with this form of therapy. Sub-fascial perforator surgery can only be undertaken at present by OS, although there is an option for a minimally invasive endoscopic approach.

Sub-fascial perforator surgery (SPS)

Symptomatic truncal incompetence is invariably accompanied by varicose complexes, and in a significant number, with perforator disease. In a registry of 632 patients [27], perforator disease was present in 62%. Thus this transfascial incompetence is substantial. The role of this phenomenon in severity

of CEAP classification and recurrence of varicose veins has been disputed. However, in a systematic review of 20 published studies involving 1140 limbs using sub-fascial endoscopic perforator surgery (SEPS) with or without truncal ablation, 88% of ulcers healed in the short term, and 13% recurred at a mean of 21 months [28]. SPS surgery may be performed by employing the open or endoscopic methods. A randomised controlled trial in which 39 patients were randomly allocated to one or other method showed equivalence of these methods [29].

An additional factor is the presence of deep venous incompetence (DVI). In a series of 51 CEAP 5 and 6 Class patients who underwent SEPS, 76% were found to have DVI on duplex scanning [30]. Seventy-four percent of venous ulcers healed in this group within six months, with 13% ulcer recurrence at five years.

To date there is no level I evidence to compare outcomes after SEPS versus stab avulsions with pre-operative marking of calf perforators.

Analgesia; local, regional and general anaesthesia

The use of local, regional or general anaesthesia must be determined with the patient's best interests in mind. The 'office procedure' should be undertaken only when extensive avulsions are not part of the procedure. With proper monitoring of the patient, preferably by an anaesthetist, LA, RF or OS may be undertaken with infiltration anaesthesia, including tumescent anaesthesia in a properly equipped room. In this situation, the patient can literally walk in and walk out after the intervention. However, if there are residual veins or recurrence at the postoperative visit, the original decision to perform the intervention as an office procedure must be called into question. Such cases are better treated in a minor procedure room with regional or general anaesthesia administered by an anaesthetist.

Complications

The complications of LA, RF and UGFS have been dealt with in the preceding chapters. The complications following OS (Table 1) include injury to the femoral

Table 1. Complications following open surgery, radiofrequency and laser ablation, SPS and foam sclerotherapy.

	OS	RF	LA	SPS	UGFS
Nerve damage	+++	++	+	++	
Wound infection	++			+++	
Lymphocoele	++				
DVT	+	+	+/-	+	+
Cough/scotoma/stroke					++
Phlebitis	+	++	+/-		++
Skin pigmentation					+++
Skin burn		++	+/-		

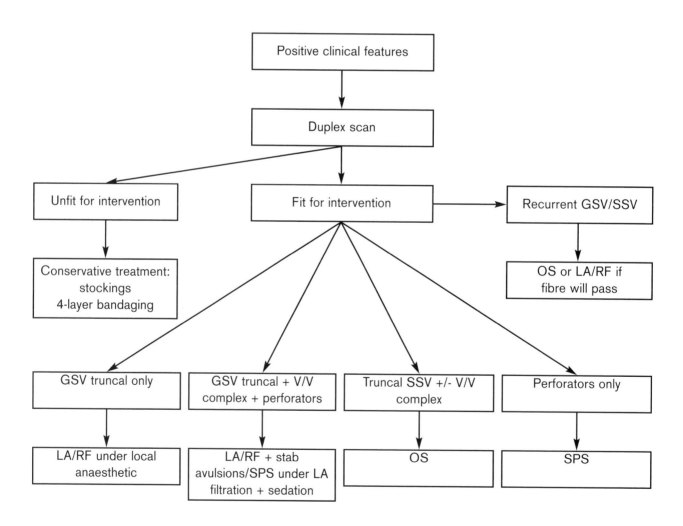

Figure 1. Suggested algorithm for the assessment and treatment of varicose veins.

artery and vein in the groin dissection, and to the popliteal vein and artery in the SSV/popliteal disconnection. Nerve damage of up to 5% of all cases is the commonest occurrence and constitutes the largest area for litigation. The saphenous, sural and common peroneal nerves are most often traumatised.

Wound complications, especially wound infection and lymphocoele occur in 2-10% of groin wounds and OS wounds for SPS.

Predictions for the future

For primary varicose veins with no perforator disease and few varicose complexes, it is likely that LA under local anaesthetic will replace OS. An alternative is RF with careful attention paid to delivery of energy. Provided the patient is fully informed regarding its complications, and agrees to treatment, UGFS will be employed as the least invasive of all the current treatments.

When significant perforator disease is demonstrated on duplex scanning, SPS and/or stab avulsions should be performed. If only stab avulsions are to be performed, the perforators should be marked pre-operatively and avulsed. Anaesthesia and analgesia should be administered by local tumescence/infiltration and sedation as necessary by an anaesthetist. SPS is best performed with a combination of infiltration of local anaesthetic and a short general anaesthetic.

The treatment of venous ulcers is likely to be addressed by a combination of LA and SPS if there is significant perforator disease in addition to truncal incompetence. If the former predominates, the procedure will require local anaesthetic infiltration and general anaesthetic. If the problem is due to mainly truncal disease, LA of the whole trunk with proper administration of tumescent LA will suffice.

A suggested algorithm for the assessment and treatment of varicose veins is presented in Figure 1.

Summary

◆ A full and careful clinical and duplex Doppler evaluation should be undertaken, and patients properly selected for interventional therapy.

◆ LA and RF are less traumatic and better tolerated alternatives to OS for saphenofemoral and GSV incompetence.

◆ UGFS is a cheap, effective alternative. The risks of scotomata, stroke, cough and migraine are of concern, and the problem of skin pigmentation and phlebitis in the short term may be a deterrent for the patient.

◆ In early cases, LA or RF under local anaesthetic may be used as an 'office procedure' when no other procedure is indicated.

◆ In the presence of accompanying perforator disease and varicose complexes, LA and RF must be accompanied by avulsions and/or SPS. It is not good practice to do half the job, i.e. only avulsions/SPS or only SSV ablation when both are indicated. Save the patient a second procedure.

◆ At the present time, saphenopopliteal and SSV reflux should be treated by OS to minimise the risk of nerve damage, until more experience and better data from the use of LA and RF become available. Recurrent saphenopopliteal and saphenofemoral junction recurrence should be treated by OS.

References

1. Browse NL, Burnand KG, Irvine AT, Wilson NM. *Diseases of the veins*. Oxford: Arnold Hodder HEADLINE group, Oxford University Press, 1999.

2. Major RH. *A History of Medicine*. Oxford: Blackwell, 1954: Vol I.

3. Harvey W. *Exercitatio Anatomica de Motu Cordis at Sanguini in Animalibus*. Frankfurt: W Fitzer, 1628.

4. Trendelenberg F. Uber die Unterbindung der Vena Saphena magna bie unterschenkel varicen. *Beitr Clin Chir* 1891; 7: 195.

5. Homans J. Operative treatment of varicose veins and ulcers. *Surg Gynaecol Obstet* 1916; 22: 143-58.

6. Keller. A new method of extirpating the internal saphenous and similar veins in varicose conditions. *NYJ Med* 1905; 82: 385.

7. Lofgren KA. Management of varicose veins: Mayo Clinic experience. In: *Venous Problems*. Bergan JJ, Yao JST, Eds. Chicago IL: Year Book Medical Publishers, 1978.

8. Chester JF, Taylor RS. Hookers and French strippers: a technique for varicose vein surgery. *Br J Surg* 1990; 77: 560-1.

9. Linton RR. The communicating veins of the lower leg and the operative technique for their ligation. *Ann Surg* 1938; 107: 582-93.

10. Royle JP. Operative treatment of varicose veins. *Hosp Update* 1984; 941-9

11. Bentley RJ. The obliteration of the perforating veins of the leg. *Br J Surg* 1972; 59: 199.

12. Albanese AR. New instruments of varicose vein surgery. *J Cardiovasc Surg* 1969; 3: 194-9.

13. Lindser P. Die Behandlung der Krampfadern mit intravarikosen Kochsalzinjektionen. *Dermatol Wochenschr* 1925; 81: 1345-51.

14. Michaels JA, Brazier JE, Campbell WB, Macintyre JB, *et al*. Randomised clinical trial comparing surgery with conservative treatment for uncomplicated varicose veins. *Br J Surg* 2006; 93; 175-81.

15. Sarin S, Scurr JH, Coleridge-Smith P. Assessment of stripping the long saphenous vein in the treatment of primary varicose veins. *Br J Surg* 1992; 79: 889-93.

16. Winterborn R, Foy C, Earnshaw J. Causes of varicose vein recurrence: late results of a randomized controlled trial of stripping the long saphenous vein. *J Vasc Surg* 2004; 40: 634-9.

17. Massel TB. Problem of adequate therapy for varicose veins: new procedure. *West J Surg* 1950; 58: 112-5.

18. Corbett CR, McIrvine AJ, Aston NO, Jamieson CW, *et al*. The use of varicography to identify the sources of incompetence in recurrent varicose veins. *Ann R Coll Surg Eng* 1984; 66: 412-5.

19. Van Rij AM, Jiang P, Solomon C, Christie RA Hill GB. Recurrence after varicose vein surgery: a prospective long-term clinical study with duplex ultrasound scanning and air plethysmography. *J Vasc Surg* 2003; 38: 935-43.

20. Nicolini P. Treatment of primary varicose veins by endovenous closure with VNUS closure system: results of a prospective multicentre study. *Eur J Vasc Endovasc Surg* 2005; 29: 433-9.

21. Hingorani AP, Ascher F, Markevich N, *et al*. Deep vein thrombosis after radiofrequency ablation of greater saphenous vein: a word of caution. *J Vasc Surg* 2004; 40: 500-4.

22. Theivacumar N, Beale R, Mavor R, Gough MJ. Factors influencing the effectiveness of Endovenous Laser Treatment (EVLT) for varicose veins due to saphenofemoral (SF) and long saphenous (LSV) reflux. The Vascular Society Year Book, 2005: 40.

23. Beale R, Theivacumar N, Mavor AID, Gough MJ. Endovenous laser treatment (EVLT) or surgery for varicose veins? A randomized controlled trial in patients with saphenofemoral and long saphenous incompetence. The Vascular Society Year Book, 2005: 77.

24. Winterborn RJ, Campbell WB, Heather BP, Earnshaw JJ. The mangement of short saphenous veins: a survey of the members of the Vascular Surgical Society of Great Britain and Ireland. *Eur J Vasc Endovasc Surg* 2004; 28: 400-3.

25. Watson AB, Bani-Hani M, Madaresi K, Greenstein D. Early experience of endovenous laser ablation of the short saphenous vein. The Vascular Society Year Book, 2005: 85.

26. Min RJ, Khilnani N, Zimmet N. Endovascular laser treatment of saphenous reflux: long-term results. *J Vasc Intervent Radiol* 2003; 14: 991-6.

27. Jeanneret C, Fischer R, Chandler JG, Galeazzi RL, *et al*. Great saphrenous vein stripping with liberal use of subfascial endoscopic perforator vein surgery (SEPS). *Ann Vasc Surg* 2003; 17: 539-49.

28. Tenbrook JA Jr, Infrati MD, O'donnell TF Jr, Wolf MP, *et al*. Systematic review of outcomes after surgical management of venous disease incorporating subfascial endoscopic perforator surgery. *J Vasc Surg* 2004; 39: 583-9.

29. Sybrandy JE, van Gent WB, Pierik EH, Wittens CH. Endoscopic versus open subfascial division of incompetent perforating veins in the treatment of venous leg ulceration: long-term follow-up. *J Vasc Surg* 2001; 33: 1028-32.

30. Infrati MD, Pare GJ, O'Donnell TF, *et al*. Is the nihilistic approach to surgical reduction of superficial and perforator vein incompetence for venous ulcer justified ? *J Vasc Surg* 2002; 36: 1167-74.

Chapter 27

Management of major trauma: is there a role for endovascular therapy?

Tony Nicholson MSc FRCR, Consultant Vascular Radiologist

Leeds Teaching Hospitals NHS Trust, The General Infirmary at Leeds, Leeds, UK

Introduction

The means of controlling haemorrhage by endovascular treatment was first described in 1972 [1]. Since then there have been developments in technology and techniques that have seen endovascular methods applied to all areas where there has been vascular injury. Yet the surgeon and open surgery are still considered the mainstay of haemostasis and repair. The current 2006 edition of *The Advanced Trauma Life Support Manual for Doctors* [2], a bible for trauma teams everywhere, does not consider endovascular therapy at all. Radiologists are usually brought late into the treatment algorithm, usually when surgery has failed. The development of trauma teams in hospitals reflects this. Traditionally, haemodynamically unstable patients have been taken straight to theatre rather than undergo any CT or angiography to localise and potentially treat haemorrhage. Yet appropriately sited multislice CT, combined with endovascular approaches to haemostasis and blood flow restoration, provide the control, speed and specificity to fulfil all the requirements learnt from hard lessons in the historical development of vascular repair.

Initial diagnosis of vascular trauma

Before any treatment can be given, bleeding has to be recognised and preferably its source identified. Sometimes the source of bleeding is clinically obvious such as in a ruptured abdominal aortic aneurysm. In trauma patients, who may have multiple injuries, bleeding may be initially suspected or its source uncertain. Ultrasound is said to be the diagnostic imaging procedure of choice in the resuscitation room [3]. It certainly has a role, and should have consigned peritoneal lavage to the medical history books. However, its role is limited due to the resuscitation room environment, patient factors and inherent deficiencies. CT has emerged as the modality of choice in imaging the acute abdomen and has fewer limitations than ultrasound [4], diagnostic peritoneal lavage [5] or laparoscopy [6, 7]. In a large multicentre analysis of 938 patients, 11% of liver and 12% of splenic injuries on CT had no free fluid and hence may be missed by diagnostic peritoneal lavage or ultrasound [7]. Multislice CT will not only show haematoma but will often show contrast extravasation or a jet that immediately identifies the source of bleeding [8-12] (Figure 1). It is vital that trauma centres have easy access to multislice CT, which must be sited close to resuscitation facilities. Arrangements also need to be made for an endovascular team to be on standby. If not, some severely unstable patients

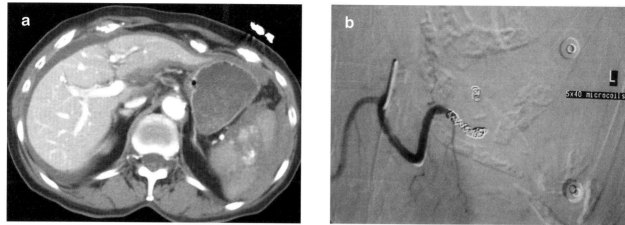

Figure 5. a) This grade 4 injury to the spleen in a haemodynamically unstable 80-year-old lady was shown at CT to be actively bleeding. **b)** Angiography confirmed this and also demonstrated multiple small traumatic aneurysms. Coil embolisation of the splenic artery beyond the dorsal pancreatic artery reduced the pulse pressure enough to stop bleeding and preserve viable splenic tissue by short gastric perfusion.

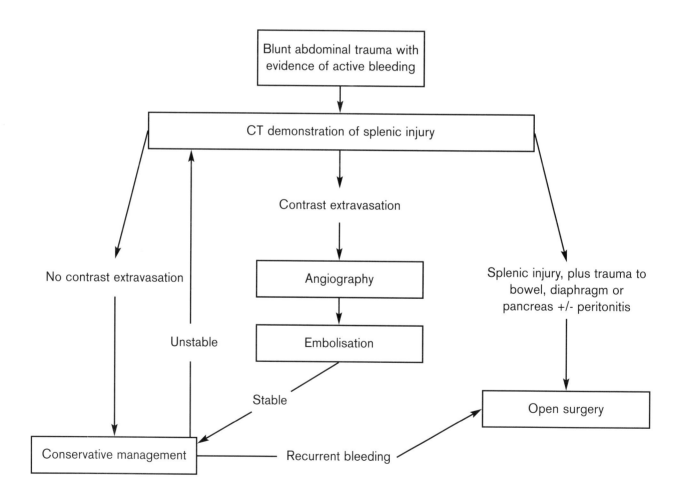

Figure 6. Algorithm for dealing with splenic injury in blunt abdominal trauma (adapted from Sclafani [48]).

Chapter 27

Management of major trauma:
is there a role for endovascular therapy?

Tony Nicholson MSc FRCR, Consultant Vascular Radiologist
Leeds Teaching Hospitals NHS Trust, The General Infirmary at Leeds, Leeds, UK

Part VI

Miscellaneous

Introduction

The means of controlling haemorrhage by endovascular treatment was first described in 1972 [1]. Since then there have been developments in technology and techniques that have seen endovascular methods applied to all areas where there has been vascular injury. Yet the surgeon and open surgery are still considered the mainstay of haemostasis and repair. The current 2006 edition of *The Advanced Trauma Life Support Manual for Doctors* [2], a bible for trauma teams everywhere, does not consider endovascular therapy at all. Radiologists are usually brought late into the treatment algorithm, usually when surgery has failed. The development of trauma teams in hospitals reflects this. Traditionally, haemodynamically unstable patients have been taken straight to theatre rather than undergo any CT or angiography to localise and potentially treat haemorrhage. Yet appropriately sited multislice CT, combined with endovascular approaches to haemostasis and blood flow restoration, provide the control, speed and specificity to fulfil all the requirements learnt from hard lessons in the historical development of vascular repair.

Initial diagnosis of vascular trauma

Before any treatment can be given, bleeding has to be recognised and preferably its source identified. Sometimes the source of bleeding is clinically obvious such as in a ruptured abdominal aortic aneurysm. In trauma patients, who may have multiple injuries, bleeding may be initially suspected or its source uncertain. Ultrasound is said to be the diagnostic imaging procedure of choice in the resuscitation room [3]. It certainly has a role, and should have consigned peritoneal lavage to the medical history books. However, its role is limited due to the resuscitation room environment, patient factors and inherent deficiencies. CT has emerged as the modality of choice in imaging the acute abdomen and has fewer limitations than ultrasound [4], diagnostic peritoneal lavage [5] or laparoscopy [6, 7]. In a large multicentre analysis of 938 patients, 11% of liver and 12% of splenic injuries on CT had no free fluid and hence may be missed by diagnostic peritoneal lavage or ultrasound [7]. Multislice CT will not only show haematoma but will often show contrast extravasation or a jet that immediately identifies the source of bleeding [8-12] (Figure 1). It is vital that trauma centres have easy access to multislice CT, which must be sited close to resuscitation facilities. Arrangements also need to be made for an endovascular team to be on standby. If not, some severely unstable patients

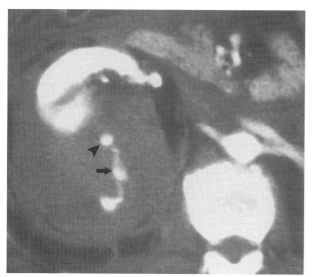

Figure 1. Contrast jet from the mid-pole of the right kidney following a road traffic accident. Such contrast jets signify active bleeding and should be an indication for intervention.

may have to go straight to theatre without angiography. If, however, an endovascular team is available, angiography can be invaluable in all traumatised patients with vascular injury, allowing confirmation of active bleeding and absolutely accurate localisation of the bleeding site. This is not only useful for the surgeon, allowing accurate planning if surgery is necessary, but also allows distinction of intimal disruption over spasm via the use of vasodilators and the diagnosis of false aneurysms, arteriovenous fistulae and most importantly, active bleeding suitable for endovascular palliation or therapy.

Techniques of endovascular treatment of vascular injury

There are three approaches to endovascular therapy that may be used in any traumatised organ or extremity if appropriate. These are balloon occlusion, embolisation and the use of stents or stent grafting.

Balloon occlusion

Achieving haemostasis rapidly in vascular trauma is probably the single most important life-saving manoeuvre. Mere pressure in the hands of the layperson can often save a life. There are some areas where pressure alone cannot adequately control bleeding. Such areas include the subclavian and axillary arteries, the carotid artery (particularly above the skull base), the thoracic and abdominal aorta, the mid-superficial femoral artery and the inferior vena cava. The successful use of balloon occlusion was first described in 1953 in the aorta [13]. In each of these areas the inflation of a suitable size balloon proximal to the bleeding site can achieve haemostasis, allow resuscitation and achieve a bloodless operative field [13-20].

Embolisation

The successful use of embolisation has been described in all areas of the body following vascular injury [21]. Selective arterial embolisation that does not cause ischaemia or infarction to non-haemorrhaging areas, allows surgery to be avoided or, where there are other injuries requiring open operation, haemodynamic stability. The development of delayed complications such as pseudoaneurysm or arteriovenous fistula can also be avoided. It is essential that vascular radiologists have a sound knowledge of embolic agents and devices, including their mode of delivery, together with a good appreciation of vascular anatomy if embolisation is to be performed rapidly and efficiently. The development of co-axial catheter systems as small as 2.5 French and steerable fine wires, along with microcoils, means that there is practically no area of the vascular tree that cannot be superselected and embolised. In the emergency situation where a patient is very unstable, coils are often the quickest agent to deliver and can be done so with considerable accuracy. Particles, gel foam and glue take time to prepare and can occasionally cause non-target embolisation. They are, however, very effective embolisation agents. Gelfoam in particular is very useful, especially where a specific bleeding point cannot be identified in an unstable patient due to vascular compression or spasm, but where the bleeding site can be accurately predicted from CT. This is particularly the case after pelvic trauma. In other areas like the kidney and liver, the biodegradability of Gelfoam may allow interval recanalisation [22].

Stents and stent grafts

Dotter first described the concept of endovascular stenting to provide haemostasis and vascular repair in 1969 [23]. The routine use of stents to repair arterial occlusions did not occur until the 1990s [24, 25]. Homemade stent grafts, using commercially available stents covered with polyester or vein, were first used for treating traumatic vascular injuries in the mid 1990s [26]. Commercially available stent grafts have now been used in many arteries to provide haemostasis and restoration of flow following arterial trauma [24-29].

Extremity trauma

In the extremities, arterial injury is most typically the result of penetrating trauma, either from gunshots or stab wounds. Blunt traumatic injuries also occur following road traffic accidents, particularly where there are injuries to the scapula and clavicle. Multi-slice CT not only images bony trauma under these situations but can often identify actively bleeding arteries (Figure 2). Time is a most precious commodity for patients with major extremity vascular injuries.

Haemorrhaging subclavian injuries require proximal and distal control that often necessitates thoracotomy plus an extra-thoracic approach. There are in fact 17 different open surgical approaches to the innominate and subclavian arteries described in vascular trauma [30]. Demetraides recently published a review of 79 patients admitted over a two-year period. Fifty-eight had gunshot and 21 knife injuries. Eighteen died undergoing emergency thoracotomy in the emergency room. Of the 61 who underwent thoracotomy in the operating room, 24% died and in the remaining 46, 25% developed arm ischaemia or infection necessitating amputation [31]. The cause of this high mortality and morbidity is the difficulty in both the initial and operative control of bleeding. By the time patients reach theatre they have lost a considerable circulating volume. The surgeon, if he does get the patient to theatre, operates in a field obscured by blood. Until proximal and distal clamps can be placed on the artery, it is very difficult to see what needs repairing. The absolute urgency means that repairs are often done in a hurried fashion simply to save the patient's life.

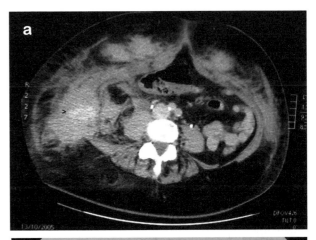

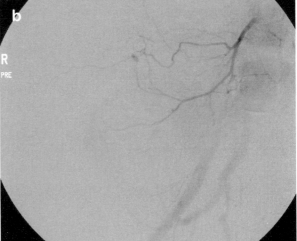

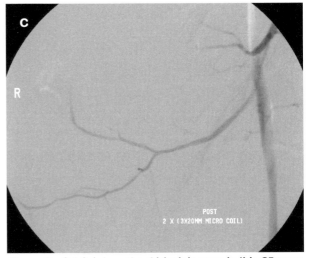

Figure 2. a) A faint contrast blush is seen in this CT scan in a patient who was haemodynamically unstable, following a road traffic accident. The increasing size of the abdomen was clinically obvious, but the CT scan points to the right 5th lumbar artery as the probable source of bleeding. b) This was confirmed at angiography. c) And dealt with by coil embolisation.

It is also often the case that the brachial plexus and thoracic duct are injured in upper extremity trauma. Though the former may well require emergency repair, it does not necessarily follow that the patient should undergo open vascular surgery at the same time as surgery to repair the damaged nerves. Surgery to both of these structures can be long and complex. It could be argued that if the stress of a second open operative procedure and control of haemorrhage can be achieved by endovascular means, then this can make operations on the brachial plexus or on the thoracic duct easier and more successful.

Balloon occlusion

Direct pressure in the superficial femoral artery or subclavian artery/axillary artery behind the clavicle or in the axilla is extremely difficult and more than 20% of patients with these injuries reach hospital with no vital signs or with imminent cardiac arrest caused by massive blood loss [31]. Balloon tamponade can be highly effective under these circumstances.

The successful use of balloon occlusion was first described in 1973 in the subclavian artery [14]. More recently, Scalea described successful control of subclavian haemorrhage in six patients with gunshot and stab injuries [15].

Embolisation

Transcatheter embolisation of small branch vessels is very safe (Figure 3), although if Gelfoam or particles are used, secure anchorage of the catheter and a slow speed of embolisation is absolutely vital if distal reflux and non-target embolisation is to be avoided.

In the lower limb, vascular injury often complicates fractures. Angiography and successful embolisation are well described in the literature, particularly in the profunda femoris artery [32-33]. It must be remembered that there is an excellent collateral circulation to the profunda femoris artery and therefore distal and proximal coil embolisation should be performed if necessary, following isolation of the bleeding point. In the calf, haemorrhage from tibial arteries is common following fractures. These often require fasciotomy.

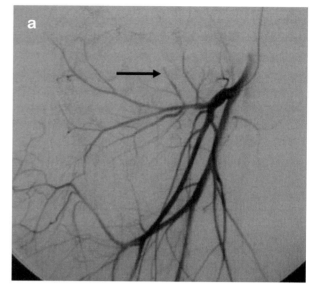

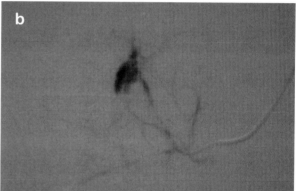

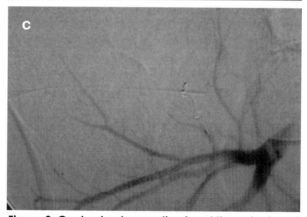

Figure 3. Contrast extravasation is not the only sign of active bleeding. Often, traumatised arteries can intermittently go into spasm due to sympathetic effects and local factors. a) In this patient who was stabbed in the buttock with a curved knife and unsuccessfully surgically explored, the clue lies in the small artery that has no branches (arrowhead), unlike the others. b) Selective catheterisation of this artery confirms it as the source of continued bleeding. c) It is successfully embolised with steel coils.

27 Management of major trauma: is there a role for endovascular therapy?

231

However, providing the patient has at least one other tibial vessel intact embolisation can be carried out with impunity.

Stents and stent grafts

Surgical repair of ischaemic extremity vascular trauma is reported to result in a 10-30% major complication rate and a 2% post-peri-operative death rate [34-36]. Where a damaged vessel is causing distal ischaemia, stents or stent grafts are indicated (Figure 4). Brandt described several patients who had intimal injuries to the subclavian, vertebral and carotid arteries, all of which were treated with stents and stent grafts [37]. None of the patients in this series had any complications and all survived long term with a follow-up of up to 52 months. Similarly, Ohki [38] described 11 patients treated by stent grafting for penetrating subclavian injuries. In this series there were no complications related to stent graft placement and stent graft function was maintained in ten of the 11 patients for a mean follow-up of 30 months. Blaszczyk [39] recently presented his experience of treating penetrating subclavian and carotid artery trauma with stent grafts in Johannesburg, South Africa. Of 37 patients successfully treated, there was one death for unrelated reasons, and five early or late stenoses treated successfully by PTA or lysis and PTA at follow-up. Although other long-term complications of subclavian stents have been reported [40, 41], overall, the results are extremely good. Stent grafts have also been used for traumatic injuries to the common carotid [42, 43] and iliac arteries [44], with similar good long-term results.

Visceral injuries

The spleen, liver and kidneys can all be damaged and bleed profusely following blunt or penetrating trauma. Such injuries may not be apparent initially, especially if the patient has head and thoracic injuries, and they are often overlooked. The patient may not initially be haemodynamically unstable. The development of ultrasound and particularly multislice CT has allowed the diagnosis of such occult injuries to be made early. There is now a positive emphasis on the need for control of haemorrhage and organ preservation, as opposed to organ removal. Indeed, such trends have gone hand in hand with developments in CT diagnosis. All too often, however, patients are taken to theatre when unstable, before any attempt at controlling haemorrhage and

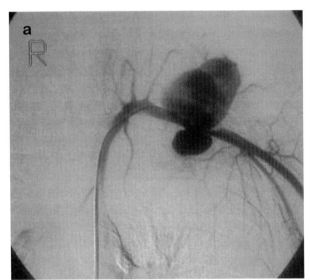
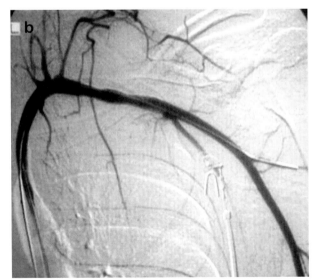

Figure 4. This patient was admitted 12 hours after a downward stabbing with a small kitchen knife. a) There was a pulsatile swelling above the left clavicle and angiography confirmed the development of a pseudoaneurysm. b) This was treated with a stent graft with a good clinical result.

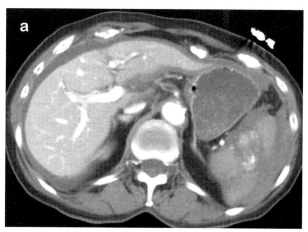
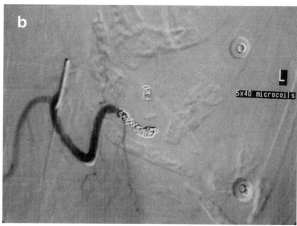

Figure 5. a) This grade 4 injury to the spleen in a haemodynamically unstable 80-year-old lady was shown at CT to be actively bleeding. b) Angiography confirmed this and also demonstrated multiple small traumatic aneurysms. Coil embolisation of the splenic artery beyond the dorsal pancreatic artery reduced the pulse pressure enough to stop bleeding and preserve viable splenic tissue by short gastric perfusion.

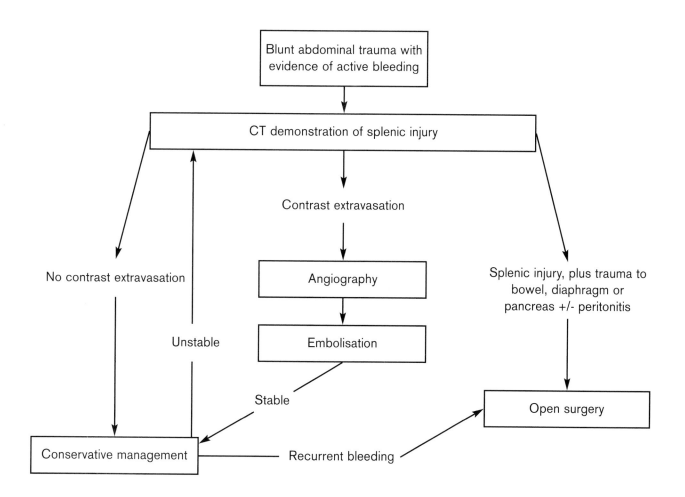

Figure 6. Algorithm for dealing with splenic injury in blunt abdominal trauma (adapted from Sclafani [48]).

preserving organs is made by endovascular means. The ATLS manual [2] calls for the immediate use of open surgery in patients with visceral damage where there is proven bleeding. Yet a recent prospective study of 100 patients with abdominal and pelvic trauma that included both haemodynamically unstable and stable patients, called for the liberal use of embolisation in abdominal and pelvic injuries [45]. In this study embolisation was quoted as being effective in 95% and safe in 94%.

The spleen is the most frequently injured solid organ. Surgical removal leads to post-splenectomy sequelae particularly in children. Prior to fast accurate multislice CT, many patients underwent splenectomy, as there was no means of assessing patients for conservative management [46]. However, a review of 524 patients suggested that CT and aggressive angiographic management reduced the failure rate of conservative management to just 6% [47, 48] (Figure 5). A useful algorithm for the diagnosis and treatment of splenic injuries has been provided by Sclafani [48], but this can be updated because of multislice CT (Figure 6). The outcomes reported in this study (Table 1) demonstrate the effectiveness of such an algorithm.

The use of endovascular therapy for controlling haemorrhage from the damaged spleen was first reported in 1981 [49]. Gelfoam embolisation can be used, but it does occlude splenic vessels distal to any collateral circulation and can result in splenic infarction. As the aim of embolisation is haemostasis with organ preservation, coils are recommended and Gelfoam should be used only to deal with refractory shock or where there is a need to control extrasplenic haemorrhage. Coil embolisation of the splenic artery in fact mimics splenic artery ligation. By reducing splenic blood flow and arterial pressure, bleeding ceases and the collateral supply from the left gastric artery, short gastric branches, dorsal pancreatic artery and pancreatic or duodenal arcades as well as omental and gastro-epiploic collaterals will all provide an alternative blood flow, maintaining the viability of the spleen. Coil sizing is important as too small a coil may migrate distally, compromising the collateral circulation. Appropriate sized coils should be placed approximately 2cm beyond the origin of the dorsal pancreatic artery proximal to the first pancreatica magna artery. Despite this, most surgeons still assert that high-grade splenic injury should be treated by prompt exploratory laparotomy [48, 50]. However, Sclafani's series demonstrated an 84% salvage with Grade IV splenic hilar injuries.

Injuries to the liver can be due either to blunt or penetrating trauma. Surgical mortality in complex injuries is in excess of 50% [51]. Again, in the experience of the author and others, modern multislice CT will often demonstrate not only the liver

Table 1. Clinical data and outcomes of blunt splenic trauma algorithm (Sclafani [48]).

	Initially observed	Initially embolised	Initially explored
Patients	90	60	22
Average Injury Severity Score	13.1	18	18
Severity of splenic Injury	2.1	2.88	2.5
Deaths	2	2	3
Haemorrhage-related	1	1	2
Head injury	1	1	1
Recurrent or persistent haemorrhage	3	1	1
Splenic or perisplenic infection	-	3	1

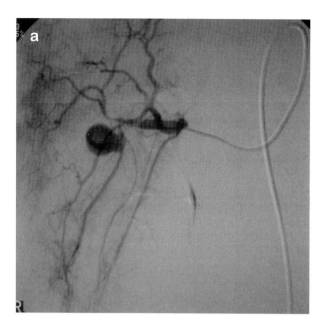

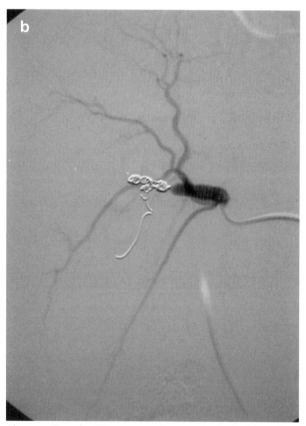

Figure 7. a) CT scan demonstrated bleeding following a stabbing. The origin was from the segment 6 hepatic artery. b) This was embolised selectively with steel coils.

laceration, but also active bleeding (Figure 7). At the same time, where there is obvious bleeding in the liver parenchyma, portal vein patency can be assessed, as bleeding is most commonly from the hepatic artery. As the portal vein provides two thirds of the liver's blood supply this is important. If the diagnosis is delayed, hepatic artery pseudoaneurysms or arteriovenous fistulae can often be diagnosed. With modern catheterisation and embolisation techniques it is possible to selectively embolise the bleeding hepatic artery whilst maintaining the majority of hepatic arterial flow. Hepatic arterial embolisation in the hands of an experienced interventional radiologist is a far better alternative to surgery with a technical success rate reported of 90%. The only reported series of complex liver injuries, where over 70% underwent embolisation, reported a remarkable 86% survival [51].

Renal injuries requiring emergency treatment are more often due to penetrating rather than blunt trauma, although the kidney is the most commonly injured retroperitoneal structure in all trauma. If intervention is required, surgical exploration can be very difficult where there is a large retroperitoneal haematoma and most patients go on to either have a heminephrectomy or total nephrectomy. In a study of 21 patients who had high-grade renal injuries on CT, eight had contrast extravasation and underwent technically and clinically successful embolisation [52]. Angiography nearly always reveals a single bleeding point (Figure 8) and this can be treated successfully by embolisation, minimising the amount of tissue and organ loss while obtaining haemostasis. Angiography and embolisation should be the procedure of choice for renal trauma where there is evidence of continuous bleeding on CT. It is vital to superselect the injured vessel in order to minimise tissue loss. If there is time Gelfoam is often better than coils, as it maximises the potential for revascularisation.

The next most commonly injured retroperitoneal structures are the lumbar arteries. These can be extremely difficult to identify and control at open surgery [53]. Though there are no cohort studies in this area, there are several case reports suggesting that selective angiography and embolisation significantly reduces morbidity and mortality in such patients [53-55] (Figure 2). Clearly, the potential for damage to the spinal cord should always be considered at

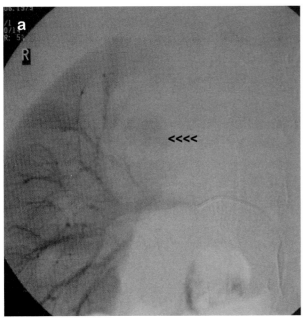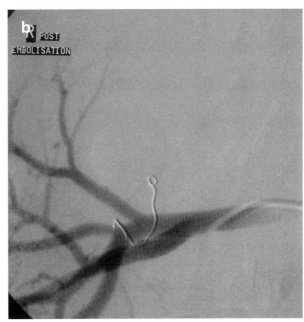

Figure 8. a) Angiography confirms a source of bleeding from the kidney in a young man who had been stabbed in the right loin (arrowheads). b) The branch was selectively catheterised and embolised preserving function in the right kidney.

angiography. Vessel branches must be identified and any potential supply to the spine isolated prior to embolisation. Gelfoam embolisation works very well, but if significant supply to the spine is seen a single coil beyond the branch artery is effective.

Pelvic injuries

Fracture and ligamentous disruption to the pelvis usually occur due to major trauma. They have a very significant association with injuries to abdominal and retroperitoneal structures and there is an increased instance of thoracic aortic and intracranial damage. For this reason, examination and imaging are vital. Plain X-rays play an important role. Ultrasound has been recommended to check for free intraperitoneal and pelvic fluid, but its usefulness is limited and multislice CT offers far more useful information [45]. It does have to be immediately available and close at hand, however, as multi-trauma patients cannot be moved far and delays cause preventable deaths in these patients. Figure 9 offers an ideal algorithm for the investigation and management of patients with pelvic injuries.

It is said that anteroposterior compression fractures that disrupt the aortic ring are most commonly associated with pelvic venous and arterial bleeding. It is also said that lateral compression fractures reduce the volume of the pelvis through rotation and that consequently haemorrhage is infrequent [2]. However, in the experience of this author and others [56], vertical shear fractures are the commonest injuries that require angiography (52%), with the rest split equally between anteroposterior and lateral compression injuries. Mortality (24-40%) and morbidity (8-15%) rates are high with these injuries [56-65]. This high mortality is partly due to comorbidities, but 60% of deaths that occur after pelvic injury are due to haemorrhage. The vast majority of patients are stabilised by pelvic traction. The literature suggests that 2-15% of patients require angiography. A technical success of 100% has been reported for embolisation in haemodynamically unstable patients with pelvic fractures (Figure 10). An analysis of seven large series containing 2403 patients with pelvic fractures suggests that 143 were unstable enough to require angiography [56]. It is by no means clear from these papers how many had external fixation and what the outcomes were in the patients who did not have angiography. One paper does suggest that those patients undergoing angiography (median severity

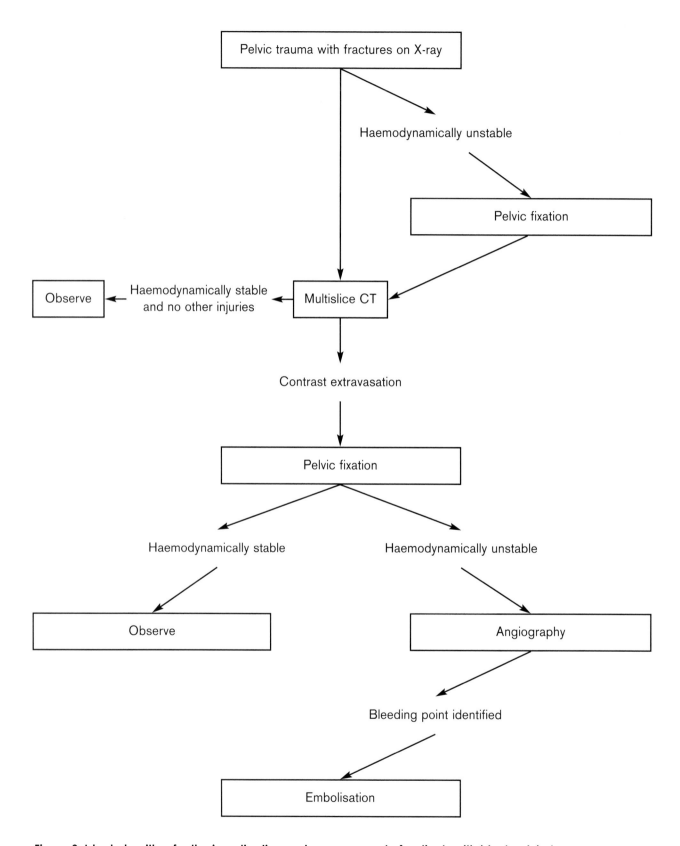

Figure 9. Ideal algorithm for the investigation and management of patients with blunt pelvic trauma.

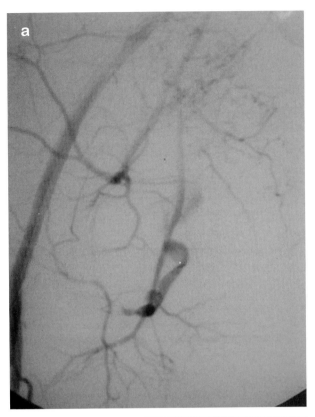

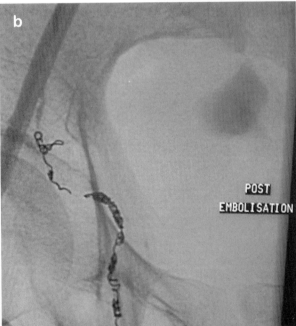

Figure 10. A contrast jet seen on a CT scan following a road traffic accident was initially ignored because of haemodynamic stability. Later, when the patient became dangerously unstable he was rushed to theatre, but the bleeding source could not be identified. The pelvis was packed and angiography requested. **a)** This showed a classic 'Corona Mortis' injury. **b)** This was easily embolised with steel coils.

score 34 [20-57]) were sicker from the outset than those that did not (median severity score 20 [9-75]). This may account in part for the high mortality of 43%, even though embolisation was successful in 98%. The point is well made that if a patient is haemodynamically unstable despite external traction, then early angiography and embolisation is vital. Delays increase mortality.

Aortic injuries

Seventeen percent of road traffic accident mortalities are due to aortic rupture [66]. The thoracic aorta may tear and rupture in a variety of accidents. The most common site for injury is in the first segment of the descending thoracic aorta at the isthmus. This is nearly always due to rapid deceleration injury caused by head-on collision. Partial tears are also common, usually in the distal arch above the isthmus, caused by shear force in side-on collisions. Traumatic dissection can rarely occur in deceleration injury at the diaphragm. Whatever the site of aortic tear, these patients nearly always have multiple injuries and are usually gravely ill. The injury is commonly missed, as the classical chest X-ray signs are not always present or are very difficult to interpret on supine chest X-rays. There are often no clinical signs at all. Modern multi-slice CT will make the diagnosis in nearly every case. Exadaktylos *et al* studied 93 consecutive trauma patients by clinical examination, AP chest radiograph and thoracic CT scanning. All patients had been involved in either high speed road traffic accidents or fallen from heights greater than five feet. The study found that over 50% of patients with normal initial chest radiographs had multiple injuries on CT, of which 8% had potentially fatal aortic transection [67]. The conclusion of this study was that all patients who had undergone major trauma to the chest should undergo routine CT scanning. A further study demonstrated 96.2% sensitivity, 99.8% specificity and 99.7% accuracy for spiral CT angiography in the diagnosis of traumatic transection [68].

Previously, surgery was the only treatment available if a traumatic thoracic aortic transection was diagnosed. However, the results of such emergency thoracic surgery are poor. Bouchart *et al* has described his unit's experience in 102 patients with traumatic dissections [69]. Five of the 102 patients were not fit for surgery due to comorbidity. A further six patients died during the operation or within 24 hours of the operation. There was a serious morbidity, resulting in permanent complications, such as stroke, in 80% of the remainder. The conclusion of this study was that endovascular stent graft insertion, though still under investigation, holds tremendous promise for non-surgical treatment of traumatic aortic dissection. The weight of evidence is now growing to support this conclusion [66-75]. Though it is true that long-term durability of endovascular repair remains to be defined, overall it is unlikely that the results will be any worse than those for surgery. In the study by Fattori et al [68], 19 patients were treated for acute traumatic transections in the proximal segment of the descending aorta. Two of these patients underwent emergency stent grafting because of suggested impending rupture. There were no complications in any of the 19 and aneurysm exclusion and shrinkage were confirmed at follow-up. All patients remained asymptomatic with a follow-up of up to 56 months.

Similarly, traumatic dissection is a recognised finding after blunt trauma to the abdominal aorta. Again, both immediate and long-term prognosis is poor and though the results of surgery are better than those for thoracic aortic transection, the avoidance of open surgery in such patients with polytrauma is highly desirable. A diagnosis can often be missed clinically and also at exploratory laparotomy [72, 74, 75]. The successful treatment of these lesions by stent grafting has been described [72, 74, 75].

Summary

◆ Endovascular repair of vascular trauma provides a minimally invasive treatment that fulfils the requirements of haemostasis, speed and asepsis, found to be essential during the long history of trauma surgery.

◆ At present they are often not considered in therapeutic algorithms and if they are, usually as a last resort.

◆ Randomised controlled trials in this field are unlikely to be ethical, possible or successful and evidence for the use of endovascular therapies will almost certainly come from a weight of cohort evidence and experience in much the same way that the evidence for surgical intervention was obtained.

◆ A great deal of that evidence already exists and the huge advantages of early whole body multi-slice CT and endovascular treatment of vascular injuries should also now be recognised.

◆ Modern multi-slice CT scanners need to be close to trauma rooms and endovascular specialists should be part of trauma teams.

References

1. Margolies MN, Ring EJ, Waltman AC. Arteriography in the management of haemorrhage from pelvic fractures. *New Engl J Med* 1972; 287: 317-21.

2. Advanced Trauma Life Support Manual for Doctors (ATLS). 6th Edition 1997. American College of Surgeons: First impression, USA

3. Britt LD, Weireter LJ, Cole FJ. Newer diagnostic modalities for vascular injuries. *Surg Clin NA* 2001; 81: 1263-79.

4. Shanmuganathan K, Mirvis SE, Sherbourne CD, Chiu WC, Rodriguez A. Hemoperitoneum as the sole indicator of abdominal visceral injuries: a potential limitation of screening abdominal US for trauma. *Radiology* 1999; 212(2): 423-30.

5. Maxwell-Armstrong C, Brooks A, Field M, Hammond J, Abercrombie J. Diagnostic peritoneal lavage analysis: should trauma guidelines be revised? *Emerg Med J* 2002; 19(6): 524-5.

6. Livingston DH, Tortella BJ, Blackwood J, Machiedo GW, Rush BF Jr. The role of laparoscopy in abdominal trauma. *J Trauma* 1992; 33(3): 471-5.

7. Ochsner MG, Knudson MM, Pachter HL, et al. Significance of minimal or no intraperitoneal fluid visible on CT scan associated with blunt liver and splenic injuries: a multicenter analysis. J Trauma 2000; 49(3): 505-10.

8. Okamoto K, Norio H, Kaneko N, Sakamoto T, Kaji T, Okada Y. Use of early-phase dynamic spiral computed tomography for the primary screening of multiple trauma. Am J Emerg Med 2002; 20: 528-34.

9. Ruchholtz S, Waydhas C, Lewan U, Piepenbrink K, Stolke D, Debatin J, Schweiberer L, Nast-Kolb D. A multidisciplinary quality management system for the early treatment of severely injured patients: implementation and results in two trauma centers. Intensive Care Medicine 2002; 28: 1395-404.

10. Willmann JK, Roos ER, Platz A. Multidetector CT: detection of active haemorrhage in patients with blunt abdominal trauma. AJR 2002; 179: 437-44.

11. Lane MJ, Katz SK, Shah RA. Active arterial contrast extravasation on helical CT of the abdomen, pelvis and chest. AJR 1998; 171: 679-85.

12. Eubanks III JW, Meier DE, Hicks BA. Significance of 'blush' on computed tomography scan in children with liver injury. J Pediatric Surg 2003; 38: 363-6.

13. Edwards WS, Salter PP, Carnaggio VA. Intraluminal aortic occlusion as a possible mechanism for controlling massive intra-abdominal haemorrhage. Surg Forum 1953; 4: 496.

14. Doty DB, Kanatahworn C, Erenhaft JL. Control of proximal subclavian artery injury with internal shunt catheter. Ann Thor Surg 1973; 15: 285.

15. Scalea TN, Scalafani SJ. Angiographically placed balloons for arterial control: a description of a technique. J Trauma 1991; 31: 1671-7.

16. Desai M, Baxter AB, Karmy-Jones R, Borsa JJ. Potentially life-saving role for temporary endovascular balloon occlusion in atypical mediastinal haematoma. AJR 2002; 178: 1180.

17. Rieger J, Linsenmaier U, Euler E. Temporary balloon occlusion as therapy for uncontrollable arterial haemorrhage in multiple trauma patients. Rofofort Schrgeb Roe Ntgenstrneun Bild Gebverfahr 1999; 170: 80-3.

18. Sensing DM. Rapid control of ruptured abdominal aortic aneurysms. Arch Surg 1981; 116: 1034.

19. Hesse FG, Kletschka HD. Rupture of abdominal aortic aneurysm; control of haemorrhage by balloon tamponade. Ann Surg 1962; 155: 320.

20. Joseph N, Levy E, Lipman S. Angioplasty-related iliac artery rupture: treatment by temporary balloon occlusion. Cardiovasc Intervent Radiol 1987; 10: 276-9.

21. Rich MN, Rhee P. An historical tour of vascular injury management. Surg Clin NA 2001; 81: 1199-1215.

22. Barth KH, Strandberg JD, White RI. Long-term follow-up of transcatheter embolisation with autologous clot, Oxycel and Gelfoam in domestic swine. Invest Radiol 1977; 12: 273-80.

23. Perodi JC, Schonolz C, Ferreira LM, et al. Endovascular treatment of traumatic arterial lesions. Ann Vasc Surg 1999; 13: 121-9.

24. Dyet JF, Cook AM, Nicholson AA. Self-expanding stents in iliac arteries. Clin Rad 1993; 48: 117-9.

25. Dyet JF, Nicholson AA, Cook AM. The use of the wallstent endoprosthesis in the treatment of malignant obstruction of the superior vena cava. Clin Rad 1993; 48: 481-5.

26. Marin ML, Veith FJ, Cynamon J, et al. Transluminal repair of penetrating vascular injury. J Vasc Interv Radiol 1994; 5: 901-5.

27. Palmaz JC. Balloon expandable intravascular stent. AJR 1988; 150: 1263-9.

28. Homma, Yukioka T, Ishimaru S. Two-year follow-up after multiple injuries treated with endovascular stent grafting of aorta and transcatheter arterial embolisation of spleen. J Trauma 2002; 52: 382-6.

29. Pfammatter T, Kunzli A, Hilfiker PR, et al. Relief of subclavian venous and brachial plexus compression syndrome caused by traumatic subclavian artery aneurysm by means of transluminal stent-grafting. J Trauma - Injury Infection & Critical Care 1998; 45: 972-4.

30. Greenough J. Operations on the innominate artery. Report of successful ligation. Arch Surg 1929; 19: 1484.

31. Demetraides D, Chahwan S, Gomez H, et al. Penetrating injuries of the subclavian and axillary arteries. J Am Coll Surg 1999; 188: 290-295.

32. Entwhistle JJ, DeNunzio M, Hinwood D. Transcatheter embolisation of pseudoaneurysm of the profunda femoris artery complicating fracture of the femoral neck. Clinical Radiology 2001; 56: 424-7.

33. Shinya H, Hirakawa A, Kitazaw Y. Application of transcatheter arterial embolisation in the treatment of profunda femoris artery injury. Japan J Clin Radiol 1997; 42: 623-5.

34. Rich NM, Baugh JH, Hughes CW. Acute arterial injuries in Vietnam: 1000 cases. Trauma 1970; 10: 359-69.

35. Perry MO, Thal ER, Shires GT. Management of arterial injuries. Ann Surg 1971; 173: 403-8.

36. Morris GC, Crech O, DeBakey ME. Acute arterial injuries in civilian practice. Am J Surg 1957; 93: 565-72.

37. Brandt MM, Kazanjian S, Wahl W. The utility of endovascular stents in the treatment of blunt arterial injuries. J Trauma 2001; 51: 901-5.

38. Ohki T, Veith FJ, Craas C. Endovascular therapy for upper extremity injury. Sem Vasc Surg 1998; 11: 106-15.

39. Blaszczyk M. Endovascular treatment of penetrating upper extremity trauma: a South African experience. Presented at IRSSA, Bloemfontein, South Africa, 2002.

40. Sitsen ME. Deformation of self-expanding stent grafts complicating endovascular aneurysm repair. J Endovasc Surg 1999; 6: 288-92.

41. Phipp LH, Scott DJ, Kessel D. Subclavian stents and stent grafts: cause for concern. J Endovasc Surg 1999; 6: 223-6.

42. Nicholson AA, Dyet JF, Galloway I. Treatment of a carotid artery pseudoaneurysm with a polyester covered nitinol stent. Clin Rad 1995; 50: 872-3.

43. Althaus SJ, Keskey TS, Harker CP. Percutaneous placement of self-expanding stents for acute traumatic arterial injury. J Trauma 1996; 41: 145-8.

44. Lyden SP, Srivastava SD, Waldman DL. Common iliac dissection after blunt trauma: endovascular repair and literature review. J Trauma 2001; 50: 339-42.

45. Velmahos GC, Toutouzas KG, Vassiliu P. A prospective study on the safety and efficacy of angiographic embolization for pelvic and visceral injuries. J Trauma - Injury Infection & Critical Care 2002; 53: 303-8.

46. Cocanour CS, Moore FA, Ware DN. Delayed complications of non-operative management of blunt adult splenic trauma. *Arch Surg* 1998; 133: 619-25.

47. Gavant M L Schurr M, Flick PA. Predicting clinical outcome of non-surgical management of blunt splenic injury: using CT to reveal abnormalities of splenic vasculature. *AJR* 1997; 168: 207-12.

48. Sclafani SJA, Schaftan GW, Scalea TM. Non-operative salvage of computed tomography diagnosed splenic injuries: utilisation of angiography for triage and embolisation for haemostasis. *J Trauma - Injury, Infection and Critical Care* 1995; 39: 818-27.

49. Scalfani SJA. The use of angiographic haemostasis in salvage of the injured spleen. *Radiology* 1981; 141: 645.

50. Smith JS, Wengrovitz MA, DeLong BS. Perspective validation of criteria including age for safe non-surgical management of the ruptured spleen. *J Trauma* 1992; 33: 363.

51. Bochicchio GV. The management of complex liver injuries. *Trauma Quarterly* 2002; 15: 55-76.

52. Hagiwara A, Sakaki S, Goto H. The role of interventional radiology in the management of blunt renal injury: a practical protocol. *J Trauma - Injury Infection & Critical Care* 2001; 51: 526-31.

53. Kajiwara M, Hanakita J, Suwa H. Coil embolization of a lacerated lumbar artery due to compression fracture. *Jap J Neurosurg* 2001; 10: 465-8.

54. Marty B, Sanchez LA, Wain RA. Endovascular treatment of a ruptured lumbar artery aneurysm: case report and review of the literature. *Ann Vasc Surg* 1998; 12: 379-83.

55. Armstrong NN, Zarvon NP, Sproat IA. Lumbar artery hemorrhage: unusual cause of shock treated by angiographic embolization. *J Trauma - Injury Infection & Critical Care* 1997; 42: 544-5.

56. Cook R, Gillespie I, Keating J. The role of angiography in the management of haemorrhage from major pelvic fractures. *J Bone Joint Surg* 2002; 84: 178-82.

57. Lane MJ. Mindelzun RE. Unenhanced CT of abdominal and pelvic haemorrhage. *Seminars in Ultrasound, CT & MR* 1999; 20: 94-107.

58. Carillo EH, Wohltmann CD, Spain DA. Common and external iliac injuries associated with pelvic fractures. *J Orthop Trauma* 1999; 13: 351-5.

59. Ben-Menachem Y, Coldwell DM, Young JWR. Haemorrhage associated with pelvic fractures: causes diagnosis and emergent management. *AJR* 1991; 157: 1005-14.

60. Agolini SF, Shah K, Jaffe J. Arterial embolization is a rapid and effective technique for controlling pelvic fracture haemorrhage. *J Trauma* 1997; 43: 395-9.

61. Evers BM, Cryer HM, Miller FB. Pelvic fracture haemorrhage, priorities in management. *Arch Surg* 1989; 124: 422-4.

62. Moreno C, Moore EE, Rosenberger A. Haemorrhage associated with major pelvic fracture: a multispecialty challenge. *J Trauma* 1986; 26: 987-94.

63. Gilliland MG, Ward RE, Flynn TC. Peritoneal lavage and angiography in the management of patients with pelvic fractures. *Am J Surg* 1982; 144: 744-7.

64. Panetta T, Scalafani SJ, Goldstein AS. Percutaneous transcatheter embolization for massive bleeding from pelvic fractures. *J Trauma* 1985; 25: 1021-9.

65. Mucha P, Farnell MB. Analysis of pelvic fracture management. *J Trauma* 1984; 24: 379-86.

66. Williams JS. Aortic rupture in vehicular trauma. *Ann Thorac Surg* 1994; 56: 726-730.

67. Exadaktylos AK, Sclaba SG, Schmid SW. Do we really need routine computer tomographic scanning in the primary evaluation of blunt chest trauma in patients with normal chest radiographs? *Trauma* 2001; 51: 1173-6.

68. Fattori R, Napoli G, Lovato L. Indications for, timing of and catheter-based treatment of traumatic injury to the aorta. *AJR* 2002; 179: 603-9.

69. Bouchart F, Bessou JP, Tabley A, *et al.* Acute traumatic rupture of the thoracic aorta and its branches - results of surgical management. *Ann Chirurg* 2001; 126: 201-11.

70. Hoffer EK, Karmy-Jones R, Bloch RD. Treatment of acute thoracic aortic injury with commercially available abdominal aortic stent grafts. *J Vasc Interv Radiol* 2002; 13: 1037-41.

71. Pickard E, Marty-Ane CH, Vernhet H, *et al.* Endovascular management of traumatic infrarenal abdominal aortic dissection. *Ann Vasc Surg* 1998; 12: 515-21.

72. Lovarto AC, Quick RC, Phillips B. Immediate endovascular repair for descending thoracic aortic transection secondary to blunt trauma. *J Endovasc Ther* 2000; 7: 16-20.

73. Hoffer E, Karmy-Jones R, Gibson K. Endovascular stent graft as a bridge to definitive repair of aortic trauma. *Emergency Radiology* 2001; 8: 233-6.

74. Voellinger DC, Saddakini S, Melton SM. Endovascular repair of traumatic infrarenal aortic transection. *Vasc Surg* 2001; 35: 385-9.

75. Borsa JJ, Hoffer EK, Karmy-Jones R. Angiographic description of blunt traumatic injuries to the thoracic aorta with specific reference to aortic endograft repair. *J Endovasc Ther* 2002; 9: 1184-91.

Chapter 28

Complications following arteriovenous fistula formation: endovascular techniques and results

Sam Chakraverty MA MRCP FRCR, Consultant Radiologist

Raj Bhat MS FRCS FRCR, Specialist Registrar in Radiology

Ninewells Hospital, Dundee, UK

Introduction

The use of surgically created arteriovenous fistulas is the preferred method of long-term haemodialysis in patients with chronic renal failure. They are more durable and avoid the long-term morbidity of tunnelled central venous catheters, which is mainly due to infection. The goal is to create the longest possible segment of superficial vein that can be used for dialysis access. The preferred fistula is, therefore, the native radiocephalic (Brescia-Cimino) fistula with the anastomosis sited peripherally. If this is not possible, alternative native fistulas can be made in the forearm (e.g. ulnar-basilic) or in the upper arm (e.g. brachiocephalic), as these are preferable to the use of synthetic grafts which have a shorter useful life expectancy [1]. Despite this, a large proportion of fistulas created in the USA are synthetic grafts. The US-based Dialysis Outcomes Quality Initative (DOQI) recommend not using data on cumulative patency rates of native fistulas as a measure of quality in an attempt to encourage their greater use! [2]. Fortunately, this is less of a problem in Europe including the UK, where native fistulas are most often used.

Fistulas do not last for ever because of the development of stenosis, due to neointimal hyperplasia in the venous segment. This process is inevitable and is due to smooth muscle cell proliferation, as a response to high pressure abnormal flow. This has effects on the efficiency of haemodialysis and puts the fistula at risk of subsequent thrombosis [3]. In each patient, appropriate vein for fistula creation is a finite resource. There is, therefore, much investment in assessment and intervention in keeping each individual fistula patent for as long as possible for a period of haemodialysis that will be lifelong, if a renal transplant is unavailable or inappropriate.

Unfortunately, while there is broad agreement that failing fistulas should be investigated and treated, there is little agreement as to the appropriate techniques that should be used and their timing. The majority of reported series in the literature are based at single centres. However, some of these detail extensive experience in large numbers of patients, such that they are reference texts and should be read by every practitioner [4]. Conversely, some multicentre trials suffer from relatively few procedures being performed at each centre. Upper arm radiocephalic native and synthetic fistulas are all mixed up in the data in some papers. Worse, some series make little distinction between fistulas that are patent at the time of intervention and those that have already thrombosed. Overall, the state of the available evidence is not as good as it should be, given the large haemodialysis patient population and the almost impossibility of losing to follow-up a group of patients who require life-saving treatment every few days.

Despite this, many European radiologists and surgeons appear to have come to roughly similar conclusions about when, and even sometimes how, to intervene on haemodialysis fistulas, presumably because they appear pragmatically to work in practice. Individual patients are likely to have multiple interventions during the lifetime of each fistula and should be aware of this. However, these can almost always be performed as an outpatient, either on a dialysis day or not. Endovascular procedures usually take less time than a dialysis session. The remainder of this chapter will attempt to answer some common controversies and questions. However, while there may be broad agreement on these, the evidence against an alternative view is never strong.

Prevention is better than cure

The better quality of the fistula created in the first place, the more likely it is to be adequate for dialysis and less likely it is to be prone to early failure. Most patients will have had multiple peripheral and central venous cannulations causing segmental stenosis or thrombosis. Unnecessary venepuncture in potential veins required for a fistula should be avoided. In practice this means using the hand veins. The subclavian venous route should be avoided for central venous access if at all possible. Duplex examination of potential veins is prudent to avoid early fistula failure and subsequent futile intervention. There should be a low threshold for contrast examination of the central veins inaccessible to duplex if problems are suspected clinically or on duplex examination.

Is any intervention worthwhile in the failing fistula?

There are two problems here: firstly, the fistula is failing and, therefore, will become increasingly difficult to use; secondly, failing fistulas are usually due to functionally significant venous stenoses which are associated with a high rate of fistula thrombosis and potential loss. Intervention delays this and may therefore prolong the useful life of the fistula. This will postpone further fistula creation or the use of central venous catheters. It would not be possible to perform a randomised trial in this patient group that included patients having insufficient dialysis treatments.

For native fistulas, the commonest intervention for venous-side stenoses is balloon angioplasty. Alternatively, surgical correction by a vein patch or interposition graft can be performed. There is no evidence overall that either treatment is superior, but surgery does use up more vein. It is, therefore, reserved in most centres for repetitive angioplasty failure.

For grafts, the same principles generally apply. Stenoses are usually present at the venous anastomosis and are amenable to endovascular treatment.

A six-month primary patency rate of 50% after intervention should be the goal [2]. This is exceeded in many reported series and centres.

Is any intervention worthwhile in the failed thrombosed fistula?

Thrombosed fistulas should have preliminary imaging of the venous drainage of the fistula performed before embarking on complex treatment. This is achievable via the clotted fistula.

Thrombosis in a native fistula should not be a frequent event in units providing the above preventative strategy. Historically, such thrombosis has been thought difficult and perhaps futile to treat. This is not the case and it is reasonable to attempt declotting of these fistulas by endovascular means [5]. A variety of combinations of mechanical, aspiration and thrombolytic means have been described and are in widespread use in many centres. Attention to detail is important and difficulties may be encountered during the procedure, but are often surmountable. Results are reasonable and again six-month primary patency rates of 50% should be the aim.

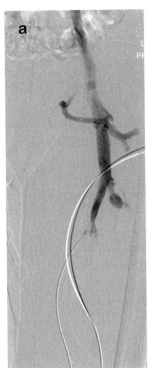
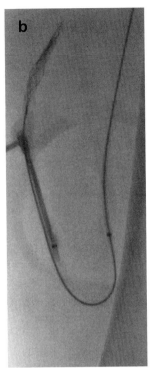
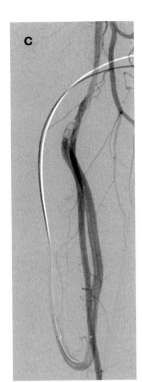
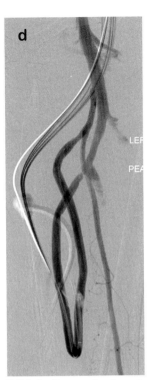

Figure 1. Some of the stages during percutaneous aspiration of an occluded loop graft fistula (femoral artery to vein) in the thigh. a) The graft has been punctured and a catheter past the venous anastomosis is confirming good outflow in the draining vein. b) A rotating basket thrombectomy device near the venous anastomosis. c) After near fistula clearance, a plug of thrombus is present at the arterial end. d) Clearance of the fistula before treatment of the venous end stenosis.

In grafts, thrombosis is more frequent and is usually due to stenosis at the venous anastomosis. Thrombectomy by endovascular or surgical means is in routine practice and many patients will have repetitive treatments. Available data does not distinguish between the two techniques, but either angioplasty or surgical revision of the venous side stenosis should be performed at the same time as thrombectomy. Again, surgical revision uses up a little more vein. There are a variety of endovascular thrombectomy devices, the newer devices having no proven superiority over older devices. Attention to detail and the sequence of intervention are important to avoid the possibility of arterial or significant pulmonary embolisation. Rethrombosis during the procedure can occur particularly before removal of the arterial 'plug', but eventual technical success is very high (Figure 1). There should be no real need for adjunctive thrombolysis in most patients with thrombosed grafts. Again six-month primary patency rates of 50% should be the aim.

The patient will have lost access for dialysis access until the fistula is working again or alternative central venous access is achieved. Good results, however, can be obtained even after several days (and even weeks for grafts). They can, therefore, be performed as semi-elective procedures, rather than as an unplanned emergency that disrupts other work. Dialysis can take place temporarily via temporary line access until fistula function can be carefully restored in a planned fashion with enough time to optimise the result.

Should interventions be performed in the non-failing fistula?

This is an area of controversy. A proportion of fistulas will be working well clinically, but will have various measurements suggesting otherwise. Many of these will have significant stenoses. Some patients with well functioning fistulas will have significant stenosis that can be detected by ultrasound without change in other parameters.

Recently reported trials from the same centre suggested that prophylactic angioplasty in these circumstances increased median graft survival and decreased the risk of other access-related morbidity [6]. However, other authors question this. In a sequential observational trial, blood flow monitoring and subsequent duplex examination and intervention increased the number of angioplasty procedures 7-fold without decreasing thrombosis rates or cumulative graft patency [7]. One study in patients with grafts even suggests waiting for thrombosis before treatment and gives similar outcomes to a programme of prophylactic angioplasty [8].

Many centres with an active duplex fistula surveillance programme adopt a pragmatic approach and wait for some supportive evidence that the fistula is starting to fail before intervening. If the fistula is clinically failing, the decision is a little easier.

The non-maturing fistula

Stenoses at the anastomosis are a common cause of non-maturation of a native fistula. These have traditionally been treated surgically by revision of the anastomosis slightly centrally, which is usually straightforward. However, these can also be treated successfully by endovascular means [9] (Figure 2). Very peripheral stenoses at the wrist are perhaps best treated surgically. Appropriate treatments for individual patients should be discussed in a multidisciplinary manner.

Diagnosis of the problem - what is the place of fistulography in 2006?

Large numbers of diagnostic fistulograms used to be performed for 'problematic' fistulas, even just for

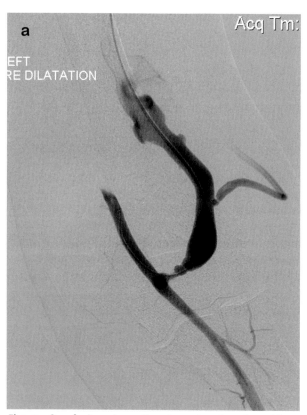
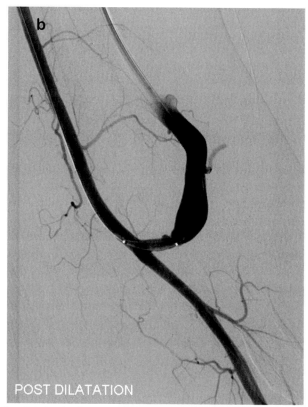

Figure 2. a) Anastomotic stenosis of a brachiocephalic fistula before endovascular treatment. b) After endovascular treatment with a cutting balloon. Larger sheath sizes are required for cutting balloon retrieval, but they do allow imaging with the balloon still *in situ*.

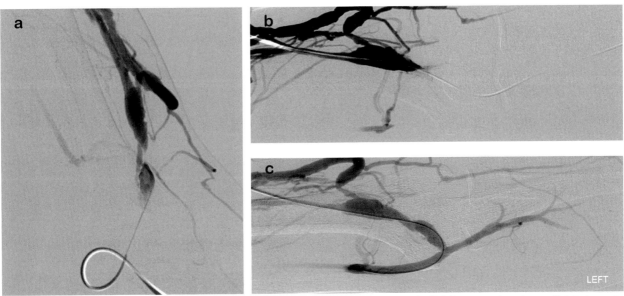

Figure 3. Treatment of a stenosis caused by needle dissection. a) Antegrade fistulogram showing a tight stenosis near the anastomosis. This puncture is too close for endovascular intervention via the same approach. b) Retrograde fistulography does not show the stenosis, but it can still be negotiated. c) This was successfully treated. Multiple collaterals are still present due to a stenosis more centrally in the fistula which was treated later.

needling problems. This should be unnecessary nowadays. Doppler ultrasound is able to examine the whole fistula and identify the position of significant stenoses, if any, in the vast majority of cases. This will allow a decision between endovascular and surgical techniques should intervention be required. It also allows planning of a suitable access site for endovascular treatment, so that imaging and intervention can be performed at the same time.

Fistulography should, therefore, rarely be performed other than as a prelude to intervention. If the anastomosis is normal on duplex, there is no need to image it again, confining percutaneous access to the venous side of the fistula. Conversely, the central veins should be imaged during interventions to any fistula, as this area is not amenable to easy ultrasound examination. Fistulography is, however, required if there is a high suspicion of central venous problems as the cause of fistula problems, or occasionally where large numbers of venous collaterals just make it very difficult on ultrasound examination.

Occasionally, other stenoses are uncovered at fistulography during treatment of a critical peripheral stenosis when poor flow has obscured initial duplex

assessment in the more central parts of the peripheral draining vein. Diagnostic fistulography is also occasionally useful in the non-maturing fistula to assess whether it is simply an anastomotic stenosis causing the problem, or whether there is multifocal disease more centrally.

How to approach the stenosis?

In almost all circumstances, in native fistulas with pre-existing duplex assessment showing significant stenosis, only the venous limb needs to be punctured and only once. It is larger than the brachial or radial artery and less prone to spasm or injury. Patients are used to it! An antegrade or retrograde approach can be planned depending on the position of the stenosis to be treated.

A disadvantage of the retrograde approach is that the stenosis is sometimes not imaged before crossing it (Figure 3) and placement of catheters through such a tight stenosis may itself alter the haemodynamics of the fistula by temporary total occlusion. With prior duplex examination, however, this rarely causes great difficulty. Should it do so, a diagnostic fistulogram via the brachial artery with a 3 French microcatheter will clarify matters. The vein central to a stenosis may be collapsed and cannulation can be facilitated by a temporary tourniquet and ultrasound guidance on occasion.

Series of fistula interventions have been published with good results from antegrade access to the brachial artery [10], but with a significant complication rate. Antegrade 7 French sheaths are comparable in size to some patients' brachial arteries.

A good argument is made for limiting arterial access to small (3 French) catheters for difficult diagnostic problems that do require preliminary diagnostic fistulography, e.g. with multiple collaterals or non-maturing fistulas, and then intervening separately via the venous limb [11]. Wires can even be passed through from an antegrade arterial approach using only a 4 French catheter to facilitate subsequent venous limb access-based intervention. In these circumstances, an axillary artery approach can be useful to keep the operator's hands away from the X-ray beam.

High pressure or standard balloons?

The stenoses are due to neointimal hyperplasia rather than atheroma. This is rubbery material caused by smooth muscle proliferation. Examination of this material makes it surprising that angioplasty works at all. Most operators inflate the balloon for longer periods of time than with atheromatous lesions, but there is no definite evidence for this practice. Many stenoses are resistant to standard balloon dilatation and high pressure balloons are therefore used primarily by many operators. A majority of fistula stenoses are reported to require inflation of the balloon to above 15 ATM [12]. A recent series reported 100% success if aggressive inflation above the manufacturer's conservative recommended inflation pressures were used [13].

Is there a place for cutting balloons?

Cutting balloons have small microtome blades mounted on a balloon. They have been around for 16

years, with usage reported in multiple types of lesion in the coronary and peripheral circulation. The blades incise a few cells' thickness during balloon inflation enabling subsequent dilatation to be performed at lower pressures (4-6 ATM) than standard balloons. The suggestion is that this may decrease barotrauma at this site and hence decrease the rate of redevelopment of neointimal hyperplasia-related stenosis. Although markers of arterial injury are reported as being less with the cutting balloon than with standard balloons, there is no real evidence that this translates into clinical practice. They are significantly more expensive (approximately £500 compared with £60-£120 for standard and high pressure balloons). This, however, could still easily be cost-effective were cutting balloon dilatation to be even a little more durable than standard or high pressure balloons.

A randomised multicentre trial in a large number of patients comparing standard to cutting balloons in the treatment of graft venous stenoses failed to show any difference between the two techniques [14]. Six-month primary patency in both stenosed and thrombosed grafts was comparable to previous series. There were more complications in the cutting balloon group. Against this, only small numbers were performed in each centre and it has been argued that there is a learning curve with any new technology including the cutting balloon. Interestingly, pain scoring was significantly lower with the use of the cutting balloon.

However, these results may not be applicable to native fistulas. A single centre series using the cutting balloon as the primary treatment for native fistula stenoses reports a six-month primary patency rates of 76% [15]. Similar six-month primary patency rates of 81% are reported in a multicentre study [16]. These compare favourably to best reported series for standard angioplasty. A policy of selective use of the cutting balloon in cases where initial dilatation has failed on the same occasion may lead to an increased chance of vessel rupture [17].

A randomised controlled trial between high pressure balloons and cutting balloons as primary treatment for native fistula stenoses would be very worthwhile to answer this question.

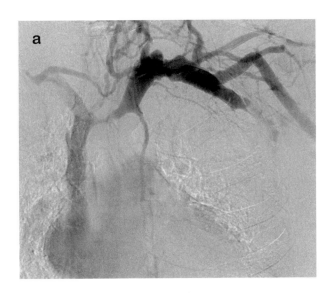

Figure 4. Medium-term successful treatment of a brachiocephalic vein stenosis. a) Antegrade fistulography showing a tight stenosis with collaterals. b) After balloon angioplasty via a femoral venous approach. No problems after one year. Although stents are more durable and effective, they have their own problems and balloon angioplasty can be tried first.

Is there a place for stents?

A policy of selective stent placement for failure of angioplasty or rapid restenosis after angioplasty has been used by several operators. Primary stent placement in large numbers of patients has not been reported. Overall, there is no evidence that primary fistula patency rates are any better than with angioplasty alone in controlled trials [18] and repetitive intervention will still be required. Failed angioplasty should prompt consideration of the pros and cons of surgical revision of the fistula in anything other than an emergency (pre-occlusive or rupture) situation.

What about central vein stenosis?

The treatment of more central venous stenosis (defined as subclavian, brachiocephalic, superior vena cava and iliac veins) is a difficult area. High volume fistula flow is itself a stimulus for stenosis, but additionally, previous central venous access commonly causes venous stenosis. It is well recognised that subclavian venous catheterisation should be avoided in patients likely to require fistula formation.

Once stenosis does occur, it can be treated with balloon angioplasty. Access via the femoral vein can be used to avoid large fistula punctures. The durability of balloon angioplasty is poor with a high incidence of immediate recoil. An overall primary patency rate of 20% at six months is standard, but some patients do well [19] (Figure 4). In general the interval between repetitive angioplasty becomes increasingly short. Stent placement in these circumstances is, therefore, frequently considered and several series report good results. One study [20] reported a six-month primary patency of 80%. The two-year primary patency was 28%, but cumulative patency at the same time was 89%. This is important as the same stent may be required to support a new fistula in the same limb.

The available data would, therefore, support liberal use of stents in this clinical situation. However, good planning and caution should be taken with this approach. There is a small, but not zero, mortality to central venous stenting. Unlike central venous stenting for malignant obstruction, the position of the stent is critical so as not to limit future options for haemodialysis, whether this be future fistula creation or central venous catheter insertion. Venous confluences should not be covered if at all possible. Again it is always possible to defer the procedure after central venography pending full multidisciplinary discussion.

Conclusions

It is important that a multidisciplinary team is involved in the maintenance of good haemodialysis access for this patient group. In the absence of strong evidence for some treatment strategies, local protocols need to be devised and understood by the whole team to achieve reasonable consistency. Due to the complexity of options available, treatment possibilities and timing need to be considered for each individual patient. This is particularly important when the decision is taken to abandon a fistula and create another. Multidisciplinary discussion should involve nephrologists, dialysis nurses and vascular laboratory staff, as well as vascular surgeons and radiologists. Patients also need to be involved in the decision-making process to ensure compliance. Endovascular therapies make a large contribution, but not a total solution for the needs of these patients.

Summary

◆ Native haemodialysis fistulas are the preferred mode of dialysis access and are more durable than grafts.

◆ Veins are a finite resource in each patient and each fistula should be maintained as long as sensibly possible.

◆ Endovascular treatments have a large, but not exclusive part to play in the maintenance of fistula patency.

◆ Duplex assessment allows appropriate interventions to be planned.

◆ Percutaneous access to native fistulas for endovascular intervention is preferable via the venous side.

◆ Treatments are likely to be repetitive.

◆ Stent placement may be effective for central venous stenosis but is not without problems.

◆ Multidisciplinary discussion of treatment options is essential in this patient group.

References

1. Rodriguez JA, Armadans L, Ferrer E, et al. The function of permanent vascular access. Nephrol Dial Transplant 2000; 15(3): 402-8.

2. NKF-DOQI clinical practice guidelines for vascular access. National Kidney Foundation - Dialysis Outcomes Quality Initiative. Am J Kidney Dis 1997; 30(4 suppl 3): S150-S191.

3. Schwab SJ, Raymond JR, Saeed M, et al. Prevention of hemodialysis fistula thrombosis. Early detection of venous stenoses. Kidney Int 1989; 36(4): 707-11.

4. Turmel-Rodrigues L, Pengloan J, Baudin S, et al. Treatment of stenosis and thrombosis in haemodialysis fistulas and grafts by interventional radiology. Nephrol Dial Transplant 2000; 15(12): 2029-36.

5. Turmel-Rodrigues L, Raynaud A, Louail B, et al. Manual catheter-directed aspiration and other thrombectomy techniques for declotting native fistulas for hemodialysis. J Vasc Interv Radiol 2001; 12(12): 1365-71.

6. Tessitore N, Lipari G, Poli A, et al. Can blood flow surveillance and pre-emptive repair of subclinical stenosis prolong the useful life of arteriovenous fistulae? A randomized controlled study. Nephrol Dial Transplant 2004; 19(9): 2325-33.

7. Shahin H, Reddy G, Sharafuddin M, *et al*. Monthly access flow monitoring with increased prophylactic angioplasty did not improve fistula patency. *Kidney Int* 2005; 68(5): 2352-61.
8. Dember LM, Holmberg EF, Kaufman JS. Randomized controlled trial of prophylactic repair of hemodialysis arteriovenous graft stenosis. *Kidney Int* 2004; 66(1): 390-8.
9. Turmel-Rodrigies L, Mouton A, Birmele B, *et al*. Salvage of immature forearm fistulas for haemodialysis by interventional radiology. *Nephrol Dial Transplant* 2001; 16(12): 2365-71.
10. Manninen HI, Kaukanen ET, Ikaheimo R, *et al*. Brachial arterial access: endovascular treatment of failing Brescia-Cimino hemodialysis fistulas - initial success and long-term results. *Radiology* 2001; 218(3): 711-8.
11. Turmel-Rodrigues L, Trerotola S. Off the beaten path: transbrachial approach for native fistula interventions. *Radiology* 2001; 218(3): 617-9.
12. Trerotola SO, Kwak A, Clark TW, *et al*. Prospective study of balloon inflation pressures and other technical aspects of hemodialysis access angioplasty. *J Vasc Interv Radiol* 2005; 16(12): 1613-8.
13. Trerotola SO, Stavropoulos SW, Shlansky-Goldberg R, *et al*. Hemodialysis-related venous stenosis: treatment with ultrahigh-pressure angioplasty balloons. *Radiology* 2004; 231(1): 259-62.
14. Vesely TM, Seigel JB. Use of the peripheral cutting balloon to treat hemodialysis-related stenoses. *J Vasc Interv Radiol* 2005; 16(12): 1593-603.
15. Singer- Jordan J, Papura S. Cutting balloon angioplasty for primary treatment of haemodialysis fistula venous stenoses: preliminary results. *J Vasc Interv Radiol* 2005; 16: 25-9.
16. McBride K, Bhat R, Chakraverty S, *et al*. Peripheral cutting balloon for treating native hemodialysis fistula stenoses: three-year experience. CVIR congress edition, September 2005, 05-A-496-CIRSE. *Cardiovasc Intervent Radiol* 2005; 28(4): 547.
17. Chakraverty S, Meier MA, Aarts JC, *et al*. Cutting-balloon-associated vascular rupture after failed standard balloon angioplasty. *Cardiovasc Intervent Radiol* 2005; 28(5): 661-4.
18. Chalmers N. The role of vascular radiology in hemodialysis access. *Semin Dial* 2002; 15(4): 259-68.
19. Kovalik EC, Neuman GE, Suhocki P, *et al*. Correction of central venous stenoses: use of angioplasty and vascular wallstents. *Kidney Int* 1994; 45(4): 1177-81.
20. Haage P, Vorwerk D, Piroth W, *et al*. Treatment of hemodialysis-related central venous stenosis or occlusion: results of primary Wallstent placement and follow-up in 50 patients. *Radiology* 1999; 212(1): 175-80.

Chapter 29

Endovascular treatment of vascular complications of thoracic outlet syndrome

Nick Woodward MRCP FRCR, Specialist Registrar, Radiology

Andrew Platts FRCS FRCR, Consultant Radiologist

Royal Free Hospital, London, UK

Introduction

Thoracic outlet syndrome (TOS) refers to a range of clinical manifestations caused by the compression of the brachial plexus, subclavian vein and subclavian artery as they exit the thorax and enter the axilla.

Neurogenic TOS results from compression, distortion or abrasion of the brachial plexus. This entity may be difficult to objectively confirm clinically, with relatively limited long-term success from surgery [1]. Vascular TOS, resulting from compression of the subclavian artery or vein, affects 5-10% of patients with thoracic outlet syndromes.

TOS is caused by a range of anatomical anomalies including cervical ribs, first rib abnormalities, scalene muscle segmentation and hypertrophy of the subclavius muscle/tendon [2].

Symptoms of vascular TOS include arm fatigue and paraesthesia with effort (arterial), and cyanosis and engorgement of the affected arm (venous). Arterial complications include post-stenotic dilatation and aneurysm formation of the affected vessel, and distal ischaemia caused by emboli. Venous complications include thrombosis (the Paget-Schroetter syndrome).

Investigation should aim to confirm the site of vascular compromise at the thoracic inlet, and identify the structures responsible. Plain radiography should be performed to identify bony anomalies at the thoracic inlet such as cervical ribs. Other useful modalities include CT and MR angiography (with the arm in both adduction and abduction) [3] and conventional digital subtraction angiography (again in abduction and adduction). CT and MRI have the advantage in that they may also demonstrate the relationship of vascular structures to surrounding structures. Doppler ultrasound is particularly useful in examination of the venous system [4], and has the advantage of being relatively cheap and non-invasive.

The optimal management for vascular TOS is controversial, and ranges from conservative treatment using physiotherapy and anticoagulation, to more aggressive strategies that include surgical thoracic outlet decompression, thrombolysis, angioplasty and endovascular stenting (sometimes in combination).

Venous thoracic outlet syndrome

Primary axillary-subclavian thrombosis (Paget-Schroetter syndrome) occurs in the setting of thoracic outlet compression, and is distinct from secondary thrombosis (such as caused by indwelling subclavian catheters or pacemakers). The vein is compressed or abraded between the clavicle, first rib and subclavius muscle, each of which may be abnormal. Symptoms include pain, cyanosis and venous engorgement, typically in active, young patients and consequently, may lead to disability and inability to work [5]. Presentation may occur after an acute event, or following chronic occupational or recreational trauma (for example in lumberjacks, painters or bodybuilders).

With conservative treatment alone (anticoagulation), many patients are left with some form of chronic disability. Recently, there has been growing consensus that the most effective treatment includes initial catheter-directed thrombolysis followed by surgical decompression of the thoracic outlet [2, 5-9]. The role of percutaneous transluminal angioplasty (PTA) and stent placement is more controversial.

Table 1. Protocols for thrombolysis [2,5,7,10,11].

Authors	Regime	Duration
Coletta et al [5] 2001	Urokinase: • Pulse 250,000 iu • Infusion 120,000 iu/h	24-72 hours
Urschel & Razzuk [2] 2000	Streptokinase: • Bolus 250,000 • Infusion 100,000 U/h Urokinase: • Bolus 4,400 U/kg • Infusion 4,400 U/kg/h	24 to 48 hours (or until lysis of clot) Until clot lysis (mean 26 hours)
Urschel & Patel [11] 2003	Urokinase: • Bolus 4,400 U/kg • Infusion 4,400 U/h tPA: • 2mg/h • 1mg/h	Until clot lysis 8 hours Until lysis (mean time 20 hours)
Angle et al [7] 2001	Urokinase: • 60,000 to 120,000 U/h tPa: • 2 to 3mg/h	 24 to 72 hours
Sharafuddin et al [10] 2002	tPa: • weight-based high dose: 0.025-0.05mg/kg/h • non-weight-based high dose: 3-4mg/h • high volume low-dose: 0.5mg/h (with concomitant heparin)	

Thrombolysis (Figures 1 and 2)

Thrombolysis, recently with alteplase (recombinant tissue plasminogen activator, tPa), previously with urokinase and streptokinase, reduces morbidity compared with anticoagulation [2]. Published protocols have varied over time (Table 1).

Most authors agree that thrombolysis should be followed by early surgery to relieve thoracic outlet obstruction (normally first rib resection) [2,5-7,9,11], with the benefit of both a reduction in recurrent thrombosis and improvement in symptoms. Surgery as early as the day following 24 to 48 hours of thrombolysis appears to be safe [2]. Thrombolysis should be

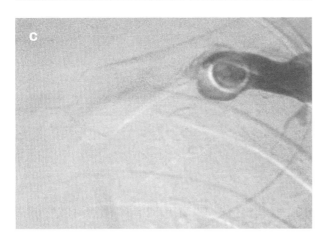

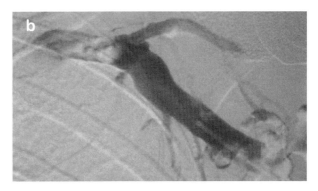

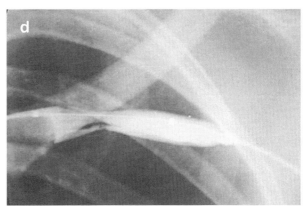

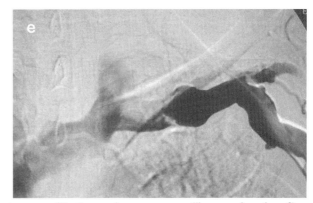

Figure 1. A case of acute venous thoracic outlet syndrome with three days arm swelling and pain after swimming training. a) MRA showing thrombus in the left axillosubclavian vein. b) Catheter venogram showing venous thrombus propagating peripherally from the point of venous compression between the first rib and the clavicle. c) After thrombolysis with rtPa, an underlying tight venous stenosis is revealed. d) Balloon dilatation of the vein. The stenosis is at the point where the vein passes between the clavicle and first rib. e) After dilatation, the thickened and irregular traumatised valve leaflets can be seen. The first rib was resected after two weeks, the patient remaining on anticoagulation in the interval.

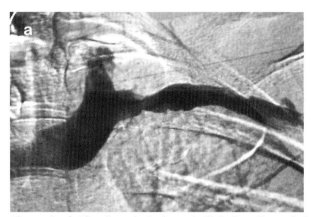 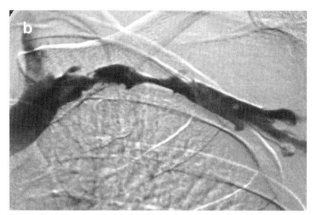

Figure 2. a) After thombolysis and dilatation, the vein is irregular but the patient declined early rib resection. The patient was anticoagulated but rethrombosed at seven weeks. **b)** After repeat thrombolysis and balloon dilatation, this resistant stenosis was revealed. After discussion the patient underwent resection of the first rib and dissection of the vein free from a cuff of dense fibrous tissue.

performed as soon as possible after the acute event, and is usually ineffective six weeks or more after thrombosis, by which time periphlebitis will be well established [2].

Percutaneous transluminal angioplasty (PTA) (Figures 1 and 2)

Residual vein stenosis (due to thickening of the vein wall or valve leaflets) following thrombolysis and thoracic outlet decompression appears to be common [6, 12-14].

Some centres routinely perform early venography following thoracic outlet decompression with a view to angioplasty/stenting, either immediately after surgery [12], or intra-operatively [6].

Schneider et al [6] advocate intra-operative PTA; they identified residual subclavian vein stenosis in 64% of 25 patients, with 92% and 96% of patients having primary and secondary patency respectively, at one year following PTA.

Kreienberg [12] performed PTA in all patients (n=23); 14 patients with residual stenosis of greater than 50% following PTA underwent stent placement. Patients who did not require stent placement following PTA did better, with 100% patency at mean follow-up at four years.

Coletta et al [5] performed venography ten days following decompressive surgery: eight of 18 patients had residual stenosis; two had successful PTA (with

stents being placed in the remaining six). They advocate oral anticoagulation for a period of three months following treatment.

Stenting

There is no evidence to support pre-operative endovascular stent placement. Stent placement prior to thoracic outlet decompression is less effective and makes subsequent surgery more difficult [5,11,12]. Stents are prone to fracture and collapse prior to rib resection [15,16].

Postoperative stent placement, as with PTA, is controversial. Kreienberg et al [12] placed stents in patients with short segment venous strictures following lysis and decompression (14 veins stented; nine patent at mean follow-up of 3.5 years). In the series of Coletta et al [5], six patients (out of 18) received PTA plus stent placement, with follow-up imaging revealing in-stent stenosis in two. Conversely, Urschel does not advocate stent placement: in 384 patients managed with 'optimal therapy' (thrombolysis and prompt transaxillary first rib resection), 380 had a good result (symptoms relieved and returned to work). They contrast this with stent failure in 22 patients who underwent stenting without first rib resection [11].

Patients with symptoms that do not respond to venous thrombolysis may still respond to first rib resection, as this decompresses the venous collaterals. When symptoms persist some respond to the creation of a distal arteriovenous fistula to generate venous collateral formation. The fistula is closed after six weeks with resolution or improvement in symptoms. Patients should be warned that the symptoms will initially be significantly worse, until the fistula is closed.

Table 2. Treatment for venous TOS.

Diagnosis
• Duplex, MRA or CTA

Treatment
• Venography and thrombolysis and PTA of stenosis
• Surgery with resection of first rib and venolysis

Follow-up imaging
• Duplex. If there is evidence of recurrent stenosis, venoplasty may be effective

Resistant cases
• Distal arteriovenous fistula

Summary

In summary, there may be a role for stent placement in a small proportion of patients with residual vein stenosis following thrombolysis and first rib resection. To date, however, the total number of patients is small, with no long-term data on patency. Stents should not be placed prior to first rib resection. There is no level I evidence on which to base treatment decisions. The suggested sequence for treatment of venous thoracic outlet syndrome is outlined in Table 2.

Arterial thoracic outlet syndrome

Arterial TOS (Figure 3) represents approximately 5% of all cases of TOS, usually involving the subclavian artery. Longstanding intermittent compression of the subclavian artery leads to stenosis and post-stenotic

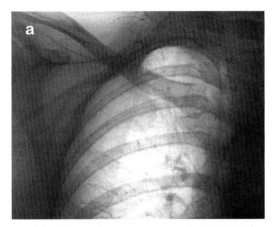
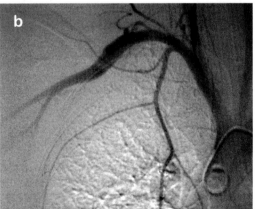
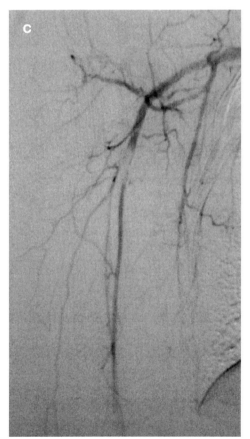

Figure 3. A case of arterial thoracic outlet syndrome with acute arm ischaemia. a) Right cervical rib on unsubstracted angiogram image. b) Subtle stenosis and post-stenotic dilation of distal right subclavian artery. c) Embolus in proximal right brachial artery.

dilatation, with subsequent aneurysm formation. Mural thrombus may form within the aneurysm leading to embolisation and thrombosis. Patients may present with acute embolisation or more chronic symptoms.

Traditional management has been surgical, with resection of the first/cervical ribs and arterial reconstruction as appropriate. Up to 84% of patients have a good response to treatment on long-term follow-up [17]. Coletta et al [5] followed-up ten patients with arterial TOS: nine patients underwent first rib resection and one underwent subclavian artery bypass (in contrast to the multimodality treatment of venous TOS). Nine of ten patients remained asymptomatic on follow-up.

Less evidence exists for an endovascular role in the management of arterial TOS than in venous disease. If distal thrombosis or embolisation is present, catheter-directed thrombolysis can be performed prior to surgery, but should not delay surgery if the viability of the limb is acutely threatened. Urgent surgery may involve embolectomy and surgical vascular reconstruction, but chronic embolisation is not infrequent and the distal vessels may be occluded. The patency rates following angioplasty for subclavian stenosis decrease with time: from 91% initially to 54% at five years in one study [18] and a secondary cumulative patency rate of 72% after 100-month follow-up in another [19]. It seems unlikely that PTA can influence stenosis caused by intermittent extrinsic compression.

Malliet et al [20] reported a small series (three patients) with arterial TOS and subclavian artery aneurysms who underwent first rib resections and stent graft insertion. Two patients had early post-procedure thrombosis of their stent grafts which responded to thrombolysis or thrombectomy.

Summary

Currently, there are no long-term results of angioplasty and/or stenting in arterial TOS. There may be a role in selected cases (for example, stent insertion in subclavian aneurysms, following rib resection), but there is currently no evidence to support routine use, and several anecdotal series caution against widespread adoption of this technique. The suggested sequence for treatment of arterial thoracic outlet syndrome is outlined in Table 3.

Table 3. Treatment for arterial TOS.

Diagnosis
- DSA, MRA / CTA

Treatment
- Acute ischaemia: embolectomy and bypass graft and rib resection
- Acute on chronic
  o Surgery as above
  o Thrombolysis followed by surgical decompression
- Chronic symptoms without ischaemia: surgical decompression
- Most patients will require surgery; angioplasty or stenting may be performed after surgical decompression

Follow-up imaging
- Duplex ultrasound

Summary

◆ There are no level I data relating to the treatment of complications of arterial and venous thoracic outlet syndrome.

◆ Management should be delivered by a multidisciplinary team, based on locally available expertise.

◆ Venous TOS: most patients will require surgical decompression usually after lysis of venous thrombosis.

◆ Arterial TOS: most patients will require surgery.

References

1. Altobelli GG, Kudo T, Haas BT, *et al.* Thoracic outlet syndrome: pattern of clinical success after operative decompression. *J Vasc Surg* 2005; 42(1): 122-8.

2. Urschel Jr HC, Razzuk MA. Paget-Schroetter syndrome: what is the best management? *Ann Thorac Surg* 2000; 69(6): 1663-8.

3. Charon JP, Milne W, Sheppard DG, *et al.* Evaluation of MR angiographic technique in the assessment of thoracic outlet syndrome. *Clinical Radiology* 2004; 59(7): 588-95.

4. Longley DG, Yedlicka JW, Molina EJ, *et al.* Thoracic outlet syndrome: evaluation of the subclavian vessels by color duplex sonography. *Am J Roentgenol* 1992; 158(3): 623-30.

5. Coletta JM, Murray JD, Reeves TR, *et al.* Vascular thoracic outlet syndrome: successful outcomes with multimodal therapy. *Cardiovasc Surg* 2001; 9(1): 11-5.

6. Schneider DB, Dimuzio PJ, Martin ND, *et al.* Combination treatment of venous thoracic outlet syndrome: open surgical decompression and intraoperative angioplasty. *J Vasc Surg* 2004; 40(4): 599-603.

7. Angle N, Gelabert HA, Farooq MM, *et al.* Safety and efficacy of early surgical decompression of the thoracic outlet for Paget-Schroetter syndrome. *Ann Vasc Surg* 2001; 15(1): 37-42.

8. Azakie A, McElhinney DB, Thompson RW, *et al.* Surgical management of subclavian-vein effort thrombosis as a result of thoracic outlet compression. *J Vasc Surg* 1998; 28(5): 777-86.

9. Lee MC, Grassi CJ, Belkin M, *et al.* Early operative intervention after thrombolytic therapy for primary subclavian vein thrombosis: an effective treatment approach. *J Vasc Surg* 1998; 27(6): 1101-7; discussion 1107-8.

10. Sharafuddin MJM, Sun SMA, Hoballah JJM. Endovascular management of venous thrombotic diseases of the upper torso and extremities. *J Vasc Intervent Radiol* 2002; 13(10): 975-90.

11. Urschel J, Patel AN. Paget-Schroetter syndrome therapy: failure of intravenous stents. *Ann Thorac Surg* 2003; 75(6): 1693-6.

12. Kreienberg PB, Chang BB, Darling RC, III, *et al.* Long-term results in patients treated with thrombolysis, thoracic inlet decompression, and subclavian vein stenting for Paget-Schroetter syndrome. *J Vasc Surg* 2001; 33(2 Suppl): S100-5.

13. Machleder HI. Evaluation of a new treatment strategy for Paget-Schroetter syndrome: spontaneous thrombosis of the axillary-subclavian vein. *J Vasc Surg* 1993; 17(2): 305-15.

14. Rutherford RB. Primary subclavian-axillary vein thrombosis: the relative roles of thrombolysis, percutaneous angioplasty, stents, and surgery. *Sem Vasc Surg* 1998; 11(2): 91-5.

15. Bjarnason H, Hunter DW, Crain MR, *et al.* Collapse of a Palmaz stent in the subclavian vein. *Am J Roentgenol* 1993; 160(5): 1123-4.

16. Phipp LH, Scott DJ, Kessel D, *et al.* Subclavian stents and stent-grafts: cause for concern? *J Endovasc Surg* 1999; 6(3): 223-6.

17. Sanders RJ, Haug C. Review of arterial thoracic outlet syndrome with a report of five new instances. *Surg Gynecol Obstet* 1991; 173(5): 415-25.

18. Farina C, Mingoli A, Schultz RD, *et al.* Percutaneous transluminal angioplasty versus surgery for subclavian artery occlusive disease. *Am J Surg* 1989; 158(6): 511-4.

19. Korner M, Baumgartner I, Do DD, *et al.* PTA of the subclavian and innominate arteries: long-term results. *Vasa* 1999; 28(2): 117-22.

20. Malliet C, Fourneau I, Daenens K, *et al.* Endovascular stent-graft and first rib resection for thoracic outlet syndrome complicated by an aneurysm of the subclavian artery. *Acta Chirurgica Belgica* 2005; 105(2): 194-7.

Chapter 30

Virtual reality for endovascular training: current evidence and future predictions

Derek A Gould MB ChB FRCP FRCR, Consultant Interventional Radiologist

Royal Liverpool University Hospital, Liverpool, UK

Introduction

Political and logistical pressures are reducing the time available for trainees to acquire the skills of interventional radiology, while imaging advances have all but eliminated the need for invasive diagnostic imaging, the traditional learning environment for interventional skills. In the wings, exciting new technologies using virtual reality are set to offer training alternatives, although while standards have existed for aviation simulators for over 15 years, none yet exists for medical simulator models. Hence their assimilation into curricula requires thought and planning in relation to their educational methodology, as well as fundamental proof of training efficacy. Simulation will never fully replace the apprenticeship model, but with relevant instructional design and validation methodologies, it heralds a new era in medical education.

The foregoing chapters set the scene for a century in which development of minimally invasive, interventional treatments will, along with advances in pharmacology, oncology and genomics, progressively reduce the existing indications for open operation. This revolution in patient care has been brought about through the use of medical imaging (interventional radiology [IR], cardiology) or light (endoscopy, laparoscopic surgery) to guide therapeutic interventions. This article will focus on the use of simulation, in particular how computers, virtual environments and a human-computer interface might be used to train the vascular elements of IR.

Today the skills of IR are still learnt in an apprenticeship, although this is an historical and defective process requiring expert supervision, placing patients at increased risk, prolonging procedures and ultimately resulting in more expensive patient management [1,2]. Added to this, the traditional training of interventional core skills has used invasive diagnostic studies such as angiography, which have all but been replaced by non-invasive imaging methods such as computed tomography (CT), magnetic resonance (MR) and ultrasound. As a result, trainees in IR in 2006 have fewer cases in which to train. There are also political pressures from Working Time Directives and service reorganisations, which allow less time in which to train [3], with a need to attain competence more rapidly. On top of all this, the shift in workload from other disciplines to IR has raised the interest of other specialties in IR procedures.

The goal of medical training is to raise competence when performing procedures in patients to a recognised, agreed and measurable level.

Assessment of medical skills provides trainees with feedback on their learning needs, evidence for certification and information for appointment committees as to the suitability of an appointee's qualifications to perform the tasks of employment. The certifying authority must also ensure that training and assessment meet the needs and expectations of patients, this pact being the basis of the privilege of medical self-regulation. A curriculum defines the processes for measuring these standards against an agreed level of attainment, with a key set of core competencies indicating the summation of knowledge, rules, attitudes, behaviour and practical skills required for certification. Trainees may, however, attain competence at varying rates, and training and assessment methods need to take this into account, although there is an inherent lack of objectivity in the way in which IR proficiency is currently assessed.

The need for change

The apprenticeship training method has been used for centuries, although information concerning psychomotor skills proficiency is still difficult to obtain, particularly in IR. Traditional methods of skills assessment can introduce bias, and may suffer from a lack of reproducibility and reliability. Objective assessment of skills is becoming important to certification in surgery, where observer-based checklists and global scoring systems have been studied for real world tasks [4-8] and virtual reality tools have been investigated [9-11]. In IR, however, in-training assessment is still used in the UK, although Bakker *et al* have successfully used time path analysis for objective assessment [12]. While standardised patients [13] can evaluate clinical and communication skills, they clearly cannot be used to assess invasive procedural skills.

Objective measurements can be made of the time taken to 'successfully' perform a procedure, or of economy of hand motion [7], although these simple performance objectives (metrics) do not indicate how effectively the procedural steps were performed, nor do they identify errors made. Such indicators are, therefore, surrogate measures and more specific performance metrics are required to ensure measurements are appropriate, fair and reproducible. An objective methodology for assessing competence should apply to a range of test scenarios and must be valid, reliable, blinded, fair, unbiased, accountable, cost-effective and feasible [14]. It should be chosen on the basis of evidence of impact on learning, while providing opportunities for feedback on the trainee's development, progress and learning needs [15]. The assessment process should also follow content which is in keeping with a practice model for the discipline concerned: results of assessment can then provide legitimate evidence for award of a certification ('the attestation of specialised competence in a particular area or subset of clinical practice') by the relevant statutory body[16].

In the training and assessment of IR skills, now and in the future, there is little doubt that the apprenticeship, with its ability to train behaviour and attitudes, will be supplemented, but not entirely replaced, by additional paradigms. These could include models, animals or computer-based simulations. Simple deformable models of anatomy can be punctured by needles under ultrasound guidance, or act as a conduit to train catheter and guidewire skills. Rapid prototyping models can faithfully reproduce CT anatomy, may use pumps to circulate fluid and contrast media, with real fluoroscopy. Such models are, however, expensive, are destroyed by multiple needle punctures and lack a facility to easily alter anatomy and pathology. Training can also use animals, which provide realistic physiology and 'feel'; however, it is difficult to reproduce pathology in animals, as their anatomy is dissimilar to that of humans and maintenance is expensive. There are also political problems, particularly in the UK.

For a number of years, cinema-goers have witnessed, increasingly, the integration of virtual environments into movies, while a generation has come to regard the computer games industry as a rite of passage. Richard Robb (The Mayo Clinic) has described virtual reality (VR) as "a human-computer interface that facilitates highly interactive visualisation and control of computer-generated 3D scenes and related components with sufficient detail and responsiveness so as to evoke sensorial experience similar to that of the real experience". Medical simulator technology is rapidly advancing, has a look and feel to suggest valid content, and possesses assessment methodologies which may address the difficulties of quantifying skills.

The technology

For simulation to convey reality requires replication of the range of perceptions that will, potentially, lead to the observer's suspension of disbelief. It is relatively straightforward to produce realistic visuals, although realistic, near-field depth perception presents some problem to developers. The potential for divergence from realism arises when trying to replicate other senses such as touch. To 'pick up' an object requires an interface device which can convey shape, texture, compliance, mass and weight. This recreation of the physics of the real world (physics-based simulation) aims to emulate real world constraints. The human computer interface should not permit the impossible, e.g. to walk through a wall, or pass a guidewire through the innominate bone.

Could simulation then be of practical value in medical training, such as in IR? Will it be affordable and realistic? Could an expert perform a task as he or she does it in the real world? Will skills learnt by a trainee transfer to procedures on patients?

The technology uses a series of key elements to provide an operator with a facility to interact with a virtual environment (VE) [17]. Central to the visual experience of a medical VR simulation is an anatomical VE, which for medical applications can be derived from medical imaging data, perhaps supplemented by medical illustration. VEs have been developed within medical training simulator models by industry (e.g. Immersion Medical, Simbionix, Mentice, VEST Systems, Medical Simulation Corporation [10, 18-22]) and by a number of academic groups (e.g. CIMIT, Web 3D Consortium, CRaIVE, IRCAD [23-26]).

The operator of the system views the virtual world through a visual display which may use a 2D screen, or a passive 3D screen. Head-mounted systems provide realistic stereoscopic effects, but are uncomfortable to wear for prolonged periods and are not widely used in practice. Active stereo glasses, using synchronised polarising screens to view a 2D screen image, are easier to wear and are almost as effective. Autostereoscopic flat screen systems also show promise for stereo viewing without the need for wearing special glasses [27].

A tracking system and input devices provide a representation of the location and physical presence of the operator within the virtual world, for example in enacting a medical intervention. In tracking motion, optical and magnetic systems can be used to locate reflective fiducials or sensor coils, although neither of these currently allows the transmission of force feedback to the operator. Interface devices provide the haptics, or touch sensation, that are necessary for the 'feel' of medical and IR procedures. Needle puncture of an artery or superficial vein, for example, is normally performed using subtle haptic cues alone. Haptic devices may use tactile gloves, mechanical linkages or gimbal mountings as a direct interface to the operator's hand. Rollers can be used to contact catheters and wires, simulating resistance during catheterisation. A particularly successful haptic device, the PhanTom [28] (Figure 1: Sensable Technologies, Woburn, MA), provides tracking and force feedback and is used in conjunction with a number of 'immersive' visualisation applications (e.g. FakeSpace [29], ReachIn [30], SenseGraphics [31]). In these, the operator's hand moves a baton linked to a series of servo driven junctions. The haptic device is co-located with stereo viewing by using a semi silvered mirror: the hand then appears to lie within the three-dimensional VE of a projected computer screen, and can 'touch' objects where they are 'seen'. To

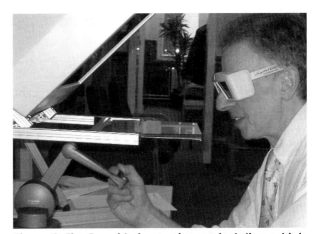

Figure 1. The ReachIn immersive work station, which uses the PhanTom haptic joystick. The operator views the reflected computer screen image as three-dimensional, with his hand 'immersed' in the perceived world.

Arterial needle puncture

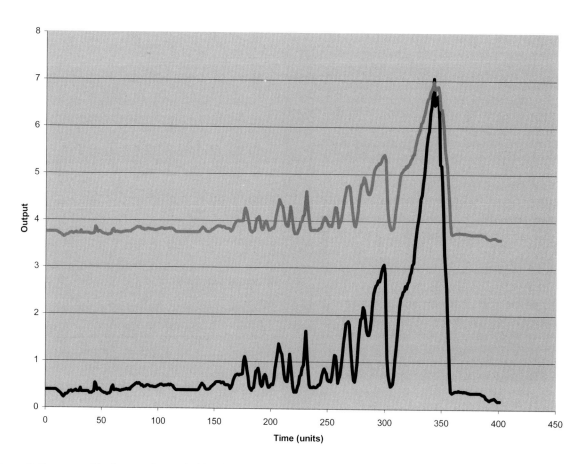

Figure 2. Force profile (grey = force in Newtons; black = output in Volts) during an intra-arterial needle puncture. *Courtesy of Dr. AE Healey, Royal Liverpool University Hospital* [38].

accurately simulate the physics of deformation, cutting and penetration of tissues, anatomical structures in the VE are mathematically rendered. In this way, physics-based modelling provides realistic interactions between instruments and living tissues. While it is not known for certain that highly accurate tactile representation of the real world procedural task is required for training, it is likely that some idea of these forces is necessary for competence.

The physical deformation of tissue is notoriously difficult to model mathematically, as its complex ultra-structure results in both elastic and viscous (visco-elastic) properties, such that tissue deformation is non-linear. Previously, validation of the levels of force feedback in a simulator has been

by the subjective evaluation of experts. In an effort to improve 'feel', workers are now using direct measurement of tissue properties. The component forces of medical instrumentation have been analysed in *in vitro* studies [32-34], although there are differences in the physical properties of living, compared with cadaveric, tissues [35]. Studies have, therefore, been performed to evaluate tissue deformation properties in living animal [35-37] and human [38] tissues, with the aim of attaining more accurate 'feel'. Workers at Liverpool University have used unobtrusive, calibrated sensors (PPS, Los Angeles, California, US) [38,47], worn under surgical gloves, to measure summated forces generated during vascular and visceral needle puncture procedures in patients (Figure 2). Data thus obtained can be incorporated into the underlying mathematical algorithms of simulator models, with the aim of producing accurate output forces during a simulated procedure.

While some geometric simulations (as 'task primitives') can train core skill sets, there remains an arguable need for realism such that boredom is reduced and an operator's emotional responses become those of an actual patient encounter. Using powerful graphics hardware developed by the computer games industry, increasingly realistic simulations can run in (more or less) real time. Realism and complexity should, however, not themselves be objectives of simulation, but should be used to improve assessment, with a more natural task, as presented to the learner, reducing testing artefacts. Improvement in the trainee's assessment would be a requirement before moving to patients and therefore represents a motivating factor.

Simulation does not require patients, who may feel pain and suffer complications, and carries a benefit of throughput and perhaps even of overall cost, particularly if web-based solutions can be introduced. The technology also allows the performance of the unthinkable: the trainee can deliberately make mistakes in safety, to understand the consequences of, and ways of avoiding, error. Simulator models bring the potential to facilitate learning by repetitive practise of tasks of graded difficulty, providing essential feedback to the learner using an assessment methodology referenced to criteria of performance. Simulator-based skills training is thus set to become 'the new apprenticeship', though subsequent progression to procedures on real patients will always require appropriate levels of supervision. In an era where many young graduates have a strong familiarity of interacting with computer graphics from the games industry, the step to using medical simulation as a part of training and assessment will be a natural one.

Validation

A move to using medical simulation to train and certify skills comes with a need to show fitness for purpose. In determining the validity of the training and testing processes, a number of 'validation tests' can

be used [39]. We can examine whether the training scenario resembles the real world task (face validity), and evaluate whether the assessment process measures what it is supposed to measure (content validity). Is the assessment tool actually able to measure the performance indicators (metrics) that reflect the key steps of the target procedure (construct validity)? Does the training process correlate with the outcomes of a gold standard such as apprenticeship (concurrent validity)? Does the performance in a simulator predict future competence when performing procedures in patients (predictive validity)? This latter can be determined by a transfer of training test which shows whether the skills acquired in simulator training can be successfully applied in real procedures. Face and content validity are regarded as of great importance and there is an expectation that, where the training scenario is very like the real world, skills will transfer to procedures in patients. Predictive validation is, however, important to confirm whether this is indeed the case. There is also a need to determine whether skills are maintained over time.

In applying an assessment methodology, whether using standardised patients or a virtual reality simulator, great care must be taken to ensure legitimacy and accuracy of test scores, and the inferences drawn. Defensibility requires thoroughness of selection of the test content, expertise of the test item writers, rigorous standard setting, care of scoring and an appeal mechanism for the examinee. The process of validation is continual and any change in the test, or in the procedure technique, requires repeated or new validation studies. While this may at first sight appear an onerous task, validation could be incorporated within a training and assessment programme, correlating training methods with test outcomes and observer-mediated scores in patient procedures.

Fixed models have been validated in surgery training [40], as well as needle puncture [41] and have been used to train and assess catheter and guidewire skills [42]. Healey *et al* used a vascular, rapid prototyping model to assess experts and novices in vascular catheterisation (Figure 3) [42]. In evaluating consecutive right and left 'renal artery' catheterisation, 36 experts completed the test in an average of 96 seconds (range 225-33). Nineteen trainees with minimal angiographic experience were unable to complete the test within a

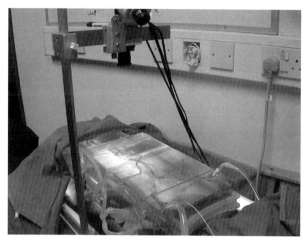

Figure 3. Rapid prototyping model of arterial anatomy for training catheterisation: with video-recording facility. *Courtesy of Dr. AE Healey, Royal Liverpool University Hospital.*

300 second time limit, only two completing the test in an unlimited period. As we have already noted, however, time to completion has limited value as an assessment tool, and more specific measures (metrics) are required for performance assessment.

Applying the technology

A systematic review of 109 studies has looked at whether medical simulation facilitated learning [43]. While the overall quality of the research was considered weak, the best available evidence showed a benefit for simulations when four conditions were met: educational feedback is provided, learners are given the opportunity for repetitive practice, tasks range in difficulty and the exercises based on the simulation are integrated with the curriculum.

The safety record of aviation training attests to the value of standards developed and applied over many years. For example, the Federal Aviation Authority (FAA) will not certify a simulator model for use outside the FAA curriculum. Standards are only just being proposed for medical simulation. The Cardiovascular and Interventional Radiological Society of Europe (CIRSE), the Society of Interventional Radiology (SIR) and the Radiological Society of North America (RSNA) have recently established individual medical simulation task forces, and a joint task force. They

have set out joint recommendations, also supported by the British Society of Interventional Radiology (BSIR), on the development and use of medical simulation to train and assess IR [44]. At the present time, simulation is suitable for use within curricula to acquire familiarity with procedural steps and the instruments used. For use in training and assessment, however, there is a need for simulator development to be more closely associated with the certifying authority or authorities. This would ideally produce a single, comprehensive set of metrics available on open source for incorporation into academic and commercial simulator models. Test validation is recommended to include content, construct, concurrent, and predictive validation with the objective of demonstrating transfer of trained skills to procedures in patients [44].

Metrics relevant to the curriculum can be derived by psychologists or human factors (the interface between man and machine) experts who perform cognitive task analysis [45-47]. Task analysis has recently been performed in IR [47], and while relatively inexpensive to perform, requires involvement of the training and certifying organisations who transparently appoint subject experts to participate in the human factors studies involved [48]. A procedure description is first compiled, encompassing known standards, guidelines and the breadth of practice. This is then decomposed during review of video-recorded procedures, to show the decision-making process, including cues and psychomotor actions. This becomes the task analysis which in turn forms the basis of a further analysis by subject experts to identify the critical performance objectives: these, collectively, are the metrics for assessing performance. Metrics so obtained can be used in checklists or global scoring systems to assess performance, or they can be incorporated into simulators where assessment becomes an automatic and truly objective process. Derived thus, metrics will accurately reflect how a procedure is performed within the curriculum [42,44,47].

Simulation now

A simulator is a computer, with a graphic user interface, and software that includes a simulation engine which can calculate deformation and collision processes involving human tissues. There is a 'mouse' which has been developed as an interface device to accept catheters and guidewires, needles and other instruments. As in all computers, the missing components here are data, which in this case are used to produce patient images, a predetermined level of force feedback ('feel'), and perhaps most importantly, the key measurement points in a procedure (metrics) which are critical to meaningful assessment.

An example of a highly successful training simulator is provided by industry in the MIST-VR laparoscopic simulator (Figure 4: Mentice Corporation, Gothenburg [21]). This simulator trains basic laparoscopic skills using simple geometric representation of procedural tasks. In a predictive validation, there was a 29% reduction in the time to perform a real laparoscopic procedure, with six-fold reduction of errors in patients [9].

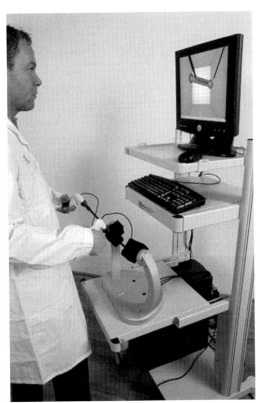

Figure 4. MIST-VR laparoscopic simulator.
Reproduced with permission from Mentice Corporation, Gothenberg, Sweden.

More sophisticated simulator models are becoming available, including endovascular simulators from Simbionix, Immersion, Mentice, and Medical Simulation Corporation [19-22], generally using metrics derived from cardiology programmes. None of these, at the time of writing, has apparently been validated to show a transfer of trained skills to patients, although the outcomes from a number of on-going predictive validation studies of endovascular simulators are awaited with interest. Notwithstanding this, the American FDA has declared that experience on simulators "is (now) an essential pre-requisite to performing carotid artery stenting" [49, 50]. It has been pointed out that the simulator training cited lay within a training package proposed by a stent manufacturer as part of a bid for Food and Drug Administration approval for their carotid artery stent [51].

Despite a lack of successful validation, at the present time the functionality of catheter-based simulators allows a learner to obtain familiarity with procedural steps, and understanding of the use of the various interventional tools and instruments. This has great potential value as many medical errors result from incorrect procedural sequencing. The trainee of tomorrow will also be able to deliberately make such mistakes and errors, exploring their consequences in safety, and the bailout manoeuvres required.

The future

In predicting the impact of technology, short-term progress will often be over-estimated, but what will be accomplished in the longer term is generally under-estimated. As medical practice advances, more interventions will involve visualisation using monitors and computers. Increasingly, therefore, VE-based training systems will approximate real practice and may lead to highly realistic simulation of encounters with patients.

Certifying authorities (e.g. the Royal College of Radiologists in the UK [52]) normally lead development of their curricula (indicating the proficiencies required by the learner), as well as their test items and standards for assessment; the processes with test items in 'VR' simulators should be no different [53]. This, however, creates a problem for the still fledgling simulation industry, in the cost of producing multiple iterations of procedural simulations to fit with different curricula. The solution to this could well lay in the Joint International Task Force recommendations for societies to collaborate in developing uniform sets of metrics.

Medical simulation promises an increased number and availability of training scenarios, with reduced patient risk, improved throughput and perhaps even reduced cost. Current difficulties in validating endovascular simulators are likely to be related to disparity between content (e.g. metrics) and curriculum. With appropriate metrics in place, and the ability to measure them, predictive validation should become more readily achievable.

While medical simulation will indeed provide a robust training alternative, the instructional methodology required must be developed and introduced with objectivity and relevance. There are particular limitations to simulator training if isolated from a curriculum, with its background core skills (imaging, interventional) training. Properly implemented, however, and with successful validation, virtual environments will attain deserved credibility in the critical milieu of medical training. They are poised to introduce a significant move away from traditional apprenticeship training for the first time in over a millennium.

Summary

◆   Virtual environments offer a potential to train and assess core skills in endovascular intervention at a time when apprenticeship training is becoming increasingly compromised.

◆   Despite their outward sophistication, few simulator models have been validated for training. In the absence of validation, simulators may be used for experience of a procedure, for understanding the sequencing of procedural steps and the use of instruments.

◆   Metrics in simulator models should be relevant to the training curriculum. They should, therefore, be derived from a decomposition of the tasks in which the candidate is expected to be competent. Task analysis should be conducted transparently, under the aegis of the certifying authority, by trained psychologists and subject matter experts.

◆   Validation of training and assessment should be carried out in accordance with Joint Task Force recommendations [44].

References

1.   Bridges M, Diamond DL. The financial impact of training surgical residents in the operating room. *Am J Surg* 1999; 177: 28-32.

2.   Crofts TJ, Griffiths JM, Sharma SJ, *et al*. Surgical training: an objective assessment of recent changes for a single health board. *Br Med J* 1997; 314: 814.

3.   Department of Trade and Industry Working Time Regulations. Website. http://www.dti.gov.uk/er/work_time_regs/wtr2.htm# Special. Accessed 28th July 2005.

4.   Martin J, Regehr G, Reznick R, *et al*. Objective structured assessment of technical skill (OSATS) for surgical residents. *Br J Surg* 1997; 84(2): 273-8.

5.   Taffinder N, Smith S, Jansen J, *et al*. Objective measurement of surgical dexterity - validation of the Imperial College Surgical Assessment Device (ICSAD). *Minimally Invasive Therapy and Allied Techniques* 7 (suppl 1) 1998; 11: 2, 13.

6.   European Association of Endoscopic Surgeons: training and assessment of competence. *Surg Endoscopy* 1994; 8: 721-2.

7.   Faulkner H, Regehr G, Martin J. Validation of an objective structured assessment of technical skill for surgical residents. *Acad Med* 1966; 71: 1363-5.

8.   Moorthy K, Munz Y, Sarker SK, *et al*. Objective assessment of technical skills in surgery. *Br Med J* 2003; 327: 1032-7.

9.   Seymour NE, Gallagher AG, Roman SA, *et al*. Virtual reality training improves operating room performance: results of a

randomised, double-blinded study. Yale University & Queen's University, Belfast. *Ann Surg* 2002; 236(4): 58-63; discussion 463-4.

10. Taffinder N, McManus I, Jansen J, *et al.* An objective assessment of surgeons' psychomotor skills: validation of the MIST-VR laparoscopic simulator. *Br J Surg* 1998; 85 (suppl 1): 75.

11. Gallagher AG, Cates CU. Virtual reality training for the operating room and cardiac catheterisation laboratory. *Lancet* 2004: 364: 1538-40.

12. Bakker NH, Tanase D, Reekers JA, *et al.* Evaluation of vascular and interventional procedures with time-action analysis: a pilot study. *J Vasc Interv Radiol* 2002; 13: 483-8.

13. Battles JB, Wilkinson SL, Lee SJ. Using standardised patients in an objective structured clinical examination as a patient safety tool. *Quality & Safety in Health Care* 2004; 13 Suppl 1: 46-50.

14. Skills for the new millennium: report of the societal needs working group. CanMEDS 2000 Project, September 1996.

15. Southgate L, Grant J. Principles for an assessment system for postgraduate medical training. A working paper for the Postgraduate Medical Education Training Board, September 2004.

16. Dauphinee WD. Licensure and certification. In: *International Handbook of Research in Medical Education, Part 2.* Norman GR, Van der Vleuten CPM, Newlble DI, Eds. Kluwer Academic Publishers, 2002: 836.

17. John NW. Basis and principles of virtual reality in medical imaging. In: *Medical Radiology - Diagnostic Imaging, 3D Image Processing. Technique and Clinical Applications.* Caramella D, Bartolozzi C, Eds. Springer-Verlag GmbH & Co. KG, 2002: 35-41.

18. SELECT-IT VEST SYSTEMS AG: Website. http://www.select-it.de. Accessed 7 Apr 2005.

19. SIMBIONIX: Website. www.simbionix.com. Accessed 7 Apr 2005.

20. Immersion Medical: Website. http://www.immersion.com/medical/. Accessed 26 July 2005.

21. Mentice: Website. http://www.mentice.com/. Accessed 26 July 2005.

22. Medical Simulation Corporation: Website. www.medsimulation.com/. Accessed 5 August 2005.

23. Web3D Consortium: Website. http://www.web3d.org/applications/medical/index.html. Accessed 26 July 2005.

24. IRCAD: Website http://www.ircad.fr/virtual_reality/horus.php?lng=en. Accessed 16 January 2006.

25. CRaIVE: Website. www.craive.org.uk. Accessed 26 July 2005.

26. CIMIT: Website. http://www.medicalsim.org/index.htm. Accessed 27 July 2005.

27. Stereographics corporation: Website. http://www.stereographics.com/. Accessed 1st August 2005.

28. Sensable: Website. http://www.sensable.com/. Accessed 27 July 2005.

29. FakeSpace: Website. http://www.fakespace.com/. Accessed 27 July 2005.

30. ReachIn: Website. http://www.reachin.se/. Accessed 27 July 2005.

31. SenseGraphics: Website. http://www.sensegraphics.se/index.html. Accessed 27 July 2005.

32. DiMaio SP, Salcudean SE. Interactive Simulation of Needle Insertion Models. *IEEE Trans Biomed Eng* 2005; 52(7): 1167-79.

33. Alterovitz R, Pouliot J, Taschereau R, *et al.* Simulating needle insertion and radioactive seed implantation for prostate brachytherapy. *Medicine Meets Virtual Reality 11.* Westwood JD, Haluck RS, Hoffman HM, Mogel GT, Phillips R, Robb RA, Eds. IOS press, 2003: 19-25.

34. Kataoka H, Toshikatsu W, Kiyoyuki C, *et al.* Measurement of the tip and friction force acting on a needle during penetration. Medical Image Computing and Computer-Assisted Intervention MICCAI 2002, Tokyo, Japan, September 2002: 216-23.

35. O'Leary MD, Simone C, Washio T, *et al.* Robotic needle insertion: effects of friction and needle geometry. Proceedings of the 2003 IEEE International Conference on Robotics and Automation, Taipei, Taiwan, 2003: 1774-80.

36. Chanthasopeephan T, Desai J, Lau ACW, *et al.* Study of soft tissue cutting forces and cutting speeds. *Medicine Meets Virtual Reality 11.* Westwood JD, Haluck RS, Hoffman HM, Mogel GT, Phillips R, Robb RA, Eds. IOS press, 2004: 56-62.

37. Brouwer I, Ustin J, Bentley L, *et al.* Measuring *in vivo* animal soft tissue properties for haptic modelling in surgical simulation. *Medicine Meets Virtual Reality* 2001. Westwood JD, Haluck RS, Hoffman HM, Mogel GT, Phillips R, Robb RA, Eds. IOS Press, 2001: 69-74.

38. Healey AE, Evans JC, Murphy MG *et al.* In vivo force during arterial interventional radiology needle puncture procedures. *Medicine Meets Virtual Reality 13.* Westwood JD, Haluck RS, Hoffman HM, Mogel GT, Phillips R, Robb RA, Eds. IOS Press, 2005: 178-84.

39. Petrusa ER. Clinical performance assessments. In: *International Handbook of Research in Medical Education, Part 2.* Norman GR, Van der Vleuten CPM, Newlble DI, Eds. Kluwer Academic Publishers, 2002: 688-90.

40. Brehmer M, Tolley DA. Validation of a bench model for endoscopic surgery in the upper urinary tract. *Eur Urol* 2002; 42(2): 175-80.

41. Lathan C, Cleary K, Greco R. Development and evaluation of a spine biopsy simulator. *Studies in Health Technology & Informatics* 1998; 50: 375-6.

42. Gould DA, Johnson SJ, Healey AE, *et al.* Metrics for an interventional radiology curriculum: a case for standardization? MMVR, 14 Long Beach Ca, January 2006.

43. Issenberg SB, McGaghie WC, Petrusa ER, *et al.* Features and uses of high-fidelity medical simulations that lead to effective learning: a BEME systematic review. *Med Teach* 2005; 27(1): 10-28.

44. Gould DA, Reekers JA, Kessel DO, *et al.* Simulation devices in interventional radiology: caveat emptor. *CVIR* 2006: in press.

45. Dick, WO, Carey L, Carey JO. *The Systematic Design of Instruction,* 4th ed. New York: Harper Collins, 1996: chapters 3 and 6.

46. Grunwald T, Clark D, Fisher SS, *et al*. Using cognitive task analysis to facilitate collaboration in development of simulators to accelerate surgical training. In: *Medicine Meets Virtual Reality 12*. Westwood JD, Haluck RS, Hoffman HM, Mogel GT, Phillips R, Robb RA, Eds. IOS Press, 2004: 114-20.

47. Johnson SJ, Healey AE, Evans JC, *et al*. Physical and cognitive task analysis in interventional radiology. *J Clin Radiol* 2005; 61(1): 97-103.

48. Dauphinee WD. Licensure and certification. In: *International Handbook of Research in Medical Education, Part 2*. Norman GR, Van der Vleuten CPM, Newble DI, Eds. Kluwer Academic Publishers, 2002: 859-60.

49. Clinical competence statement on carotid stenting: training and credentialing for carotid stenting - multispeciality consensus recommendations. A report of the SCAI/SVMB/SVS writing committee to develop a clinical competence statement on carotid interventions. *Catheterisation and Cardiovascular Interventions* 2005; 64: 1-11.

50. Gallagher AG, Cates CU. Approval of virtual reality training for carotid stenting; what this means for procedural-based medicine. *JAMA* 2004; 292 (24): 3024-6.

51. Hartman J. Virtual reality training for carotid stenting (letter). *JAMA* 2005; 293(17): 2091.

52. *Structured Training in Clinical Radiology*. 4th Ed. Editorial Board of the Faculty of Clinical Radiology, Royal College of Radiologists, 2004.

53. Dauphinee WD. Licensure and certification. In: *International Handbook of Research in Medical Education, Part 2*. Norman GR, Van der Vleuten CPM, Newble DI, Eds. Kluwer Academic Publishers, 2002: 857.